Echocardiography in Cardiovascular Disease

Echocardiography in Cardiovascular Disease

Guest Editor

Kenya Kusunose

MDPI

Basel • Beijing • Wuhan • Barcelona • Belgrade • Novi Sad • Cluj • Manchester

Guest Editor
Kenya Kusunose
Department of Cardiovascular
Medicine
Tokushima University
Hospital
Tokushima
Japan

Editorial Office
MDPI AG
Grosspeteranlage 5
4052 Basel, Switzerland

This is a reprint of the Special Issue, published open access by the journal *Journal of Cardiovascular Development and Disease* (ISSN 2308-3425), freely accessible at: https://www.mdpi.com/journal/jcdd/special_issues/Echocardiography_Cardiovascular_Disease.

For citation purposes, cite each article independently as indicated on the article page online and as indicated below:

Lastname, A.A.; Lastname, B.B. Article Title. *Journal Name* **Year**, *Volume Number*, Page Range.

ISBN 978-3-7258-7054-7 (Hbk)
ISBN 978-3-7258-7055-4 (PDF)
https://doi.org/10.3390/books978-3-7258-7055-4

Contents

About the Editor

Kenya Kusunose

Kenya Kusunose is affiliated with the University of the Ryukyus in Okinawa, Japan, and works in the field of cardiovascular medicine with a focus on echocardiography. His academic interests include advanced echocardiographic quantification, assessment of cardiac structure and function across a broad spectrum of cardiovascular diseases, and the clinical translation of imaging innovations. He is particularly interested in approaches that improve measurement reproducibility and clinical decision support, including the use of machine learning and other data driven techniques applied to routinely acquired ultrasound data. Through research, collaboration, and education, he aims to advance practical, high-quality echocardiography that can be implemented in everyday clinical care and multicenter studies.

Preface

Echocardiography remains a cornerstone of cardiovascular care because it is widely accessible, repeatable, and directly informs bedside decision making. At the same time, the field is rapidly evolving, with advances in image acquisition, quantitative analysis, and automated interpretation that are changing how we evaluate cardiac structure and function. This Reprint was prepared to provide readers with a curated snapshot of these developments, drawn from the Special Issue Echocardiography and Cardiovascular Disease. The articles assembled here illustrate how rigorous echocardiographic methodology and emerging computational techniques can complement clinical expertise, support consistent reporting, and enhance patient specific risk assessment. We hope this Reprint will be useful to practicing clinicians, imagers, and investigators, and will stimulate further collaboration toward evidence based and data informed cardiovascular imaging.

Kenya Kusunose
Guest Editor

Journal of
Cardiovascular Development and Disease

MDPI

Article

Left Cardiac Remodelling Assessed by Echocardiography Is Associated with Rho-Kinase Activation in Long-Distance Runners

Felipe Contreras-Briceño [1,2,3], Julián Vega [1], Jorge Mandiola [1], María Paz Ocaranza [1,4], Sebastián Herrera [1], Manuel Salinas [1], Rodrigo Fernández [1], Jorge E. Jalil [1,4], Sergio Lavandero [5,6], Mario Chiong [5], Paz Godoy [1], Pablo F. Castro [1], Marta Sitges [7] and Luigi Gabrielli [1,2,*]

1 Advanced Center for Chronic Diseases (ACCDiS), Division of Cardiovascular Diseases, Faculty of Medicine, Pontificia Universidad Católica de Chile, Av. Sergio Livingstone #1007, Santiago 8380492, Chile; fcontrerasb@uc.cl (F.C.-B.); julianvega@gmail.com (J.V.); jmandiola.o@hotmail.com (J.M.); mocaran@uc.cl (M.P.O.); sherrerat@gmail.com (S.H.); kant_76@hotmail.com (M.S.); rodri_fernandezz@hotmail.com (R.F.); jjalil@med.puc.cl (J.E.J.); pazitag.16@gmail.com (P.G.); pcastro@med.puc.cl (P.F.C.)
2 Laboratory of Exercise Physiology, Department of Health Science, Faculty of Medicine, Pontificia Universidad Católica de Chile, Av. Vicuña Mackenna #4860, Santiago 7820436, Chile
3 Physiology Section, Department of Cell Biology, Physiology and Immunology, Faculty of Biology, Universitat de Barcelona, Av. Diagonal #643, 08028 Barcelona, Spain
4 Center of New Drugs for Hypertension (CENDHY), Universidad de Chile & Pontificia Universidad Católica de Chile, Av. Santos Dumont #964, Santiago 8380494, Chile
5 Advanced Center for Chronic Diseases (ACCDiS), Faculty of Chemical & Pharmaceutical Sciences & Faculty of Medicine, Universidad de Chile, Av. Sergio Livingstone #1007, Santiago 8380492, Chile; slavander@uchile.cl (S.L.); mchiong@uchile.cl (M.C.)
6 Department of Internal Medicine, Cardiology Division, University of Texas Southwestern Medical Center, Av. Harry Hines Blvd #5323, Dallas, TX 75390-8573, USA
7 Thorax Institute, IDIBAPS, Hospital Clinic, Av. Carrer del Rosselló #149, 08036 Barcelona, Spain; msitges@clinic.cat
* Correspondence: lgabriel@uc.cl; Tel.: +56-223-543-633

Abstract: This single-blind and cross-sectional study evaluated the role of Rho-kinase (ROCK) as a biomarker of the cardiovascular remodelling process assessed by echocardiography in competitive long-distance runners (LDRs) during the training period before a marathon race. Thirty-six healthy male LDRs (37.0 ± 5.3 years; 174.0 ± 7.0 height; BMI: 23.8 ± 2.8; $\dot{V}O_2$-peak: 56.5 ± 7.3 $mL \cdot kg^{-1} \cdot min^{-1}$) were separated into two groups according to previous training level: high-training (HT, n = 16) ≥ 100 $km \cdot week^{-1}$ and low-training (LT, n = 20) ≥ 70 and < 100 $km \cdot week^{-1}$. Also, twenty-one healthy nonactive subjects were included as a control group (CTR). A transthoracic echocardiography was performed and ROCK activity levels in circulating leukocytes were measured at rest (48 h without exercising) the week before the race. The HT group showed a higher left ventricular mass index (LVMi) and left atrial volume index (LAVi) than other groups ($p < 0.05$, for both); also, higher levels of ROCK activity were found in LDRs (HT = 6.17 ± 1.41 vs. CTR = 1.64 ± 0.66 ($p < 0.01$); vs. LT = 2.74 ± 0.84; ($p < 0.05$)). In LDRs a direct correlation between ROCK activity levels and LVMi (r = 0.83; $p < 0.001$), and LAVi (r = 0.70; $p < 0.001$) were found. In conclusion, in male competitive long-distance runners, the load of exercise implicated in marathon training is associated with ROCK activity levels and the left cardiac remodelling process assessed by echocardiography.

Keywords: athlete's heart; cardiac biomarkers; echocardiography; exercise; functional cardiac capacity

1. Introduction

Physical exercise plays a fundamental role in cardiovascular disease prevention and significantly reduces global mortality [1]. This benefit is associated with different mechanisms linked to structural changes or "adaptation" of the heart [2]. The combination of these adaptations, known as cardiovascular remodelling, involves changes at molecular and cellular levels which translate into structural, electric and functional cardiovascular modifications [3].

The cardiac remodelling process can occur early during the training process [4]. Highly trained runners experience these changes with greater prevalence and intensity, which in most cases are benign and reversible [2]—a condition called "athlete's heart" [5] that includes increased bi-ventricular diameter, left ventricle (LV) parietal thickness, LV mass and bi-atrial volume with systolic and normal diastolic function [6]. The majority of these changes are a physiological adaptation to exercise; however, some patterns may overlap with channelopathies or cardiomyopathies [7]; LV hypertrophy criteria are present in as many as 70% of highly trained athletes [8], and only 12% showed criteria for right ventricular hypertrophy [9].

Advances in image techniques have allowed a better characterization of athlete's heart. It is known that these changes are related with better sports performance [10]; however, some predisposed athletes subjected to high training loads may show a potentially adverse cardiac remodelling ("Phidippides" cardiomyopathy) [6,11]. This adverse cardiac remodelling process is not frequent and is characterized by LV hypertrophy associated with myocardial fibrosis [8], increased coronary atheromatosis, greater right ventricular remodelling and extreme right and left atrial (LA) dilatation [12,13]; there is uncertainty over whether there is a maximum limit of training considered safe, and if it is possible to identify an individual limit for each athlete [13].

The physiological and eventually pathophysiological mechanisms linked to adverse cardiac remodelling in high-performance athletes are not completely clear. In this regard, the dynamics of different biomarkers related to tissue damage, inflammation, oxidative stress and cardiac remodelling have been studied in athletes of different disciplines with no clear significance [6]. A novel pathway related to cell survival and cardiac adaptation to stress is rho-kinase (ROCK) activation [14]. This kinase exerts its role by acting on the cytoskeleton, regulating cell motility (migration), adhesion, and proliferation, assuming a leading role in mediating cardiac remodelling [15,16] in different clinical scenarios [17,18]. The association of ROCK with exercise has been poorly explored. Recently, investigations have reported an increase of ROCK activity induced by aerobic exercise in the skeletal muscle of rats, linked to glucose uptake through insulin receptor substrate 1 (IRS1) phosphorylation [18,19]. In patients with dyslipidemia, moderate aerobic physical exercise (30 min $\times$ 5 days a week) has been related to attenuation of ROCK concentration [20]. The role of insulin pathways during the hypertrophic process and ROCK activation induced by exercise has been recently reported in an interesting review by Anaruma et al. [21]. However, the dynamics of ROCK activation and their association with cardiac remodelling in endurance athletes with highly demanding training protocols, as for a marathon race competition, has not been previously studied. Thus, the primary objective of this study was to evaluate the activity of ROCK and its association with cardiac remodelling assessed by echocardiography in competitive long-distance runners (LDRs) with different training loads before a highly demanding competition (marathon).

2. Materials and Methods

The sample size calculation was done by G*Power® 3.1 software (Heinrich–Heine University, Dusseldorf, Germany) using previous data concerning the association found between echocardiography measurements (negative deformation of the post P wave strain curve, LASa) and $\dot{V}O_2$-max in runners with similar characteristics to the participants in this study (rho = 0.546; p = 0.028) [10]—considering a significance level of 5% and a power of 80%, in a two-tail test, plus 10% of data loss. Thus, thirty-six Caucasian males recreational LDRs were recruited previously to a marathon race (Santiago, 42.2 km). The participants were included 16 weeks before the competition, in the training period called "optimal phase", where the volume of training is increased by running a longer distance each week. Hydric support during preparations follows the recommendation of our sport section group: as a rule, during high intensity or hard physical activity it is recommended to have intakes of 0.6–1 L·h^{-1} with frequent intakes (150–250 mL) every 15–20 min, and always with an isotonic content; also, with frequent body weight checks. The inclusion criteria were: (i) age between 18 and 50 years to minimize possible cardiovascular events linked to the competition, (ii) participation in three or more completed marathons in the last five years, and (iii) recreational status, to obtain a more diverse sample. The exclusion criteria were: (i) presence of any morbidity or disease that alters plasma levels of ROCK (e.g., arterial hypertension, dyslipidemia, insulin resistance, smoking or alcohol consumption habits, renal or liver dysfunction, neoplasia, and chronic respiratory and cardiac diseases) and (ii) use of anti-hypertensive, anorexic, anti-depressant, and/or antibiotics medication. In addition, a control group of healthy and non-active, sedentary subjects (n = 21) was included. The study was approved by the Ethics Committee of Pontificia Universidad Católica de Chile in observance of the Declaration of Helsinki on experimentation in human beings (project n° 16082603). Written informed consent was obtained from the subjects prior to any procedure.

The study was cross-sectional with single blinding in researchers responsible for analyzing the serum samples and performing the echocardiographic reports and statistical analysis; they did not know to which group each subject belonged. After completing an ad hoc questionnaire with open questions concerning sports history, previous injuries, and time availability to training, LDRs were allocated to groups according to feasible weakly exercise volume during the training period before the marathon race. Running 100 km per week as a maximum exercise volume was adopted as a limit to separate the groups; this criterium has been used previously by our research group [10]. Thus, some LDRs were allocated to a high-training group (HT $\geq$ 100 km·week^{-1}, n = 16) and a low-training group (LT $\geq$ 70 and <100 km·week^{-1}, n = 20). Figure 1 shows the study design and assessments performed.

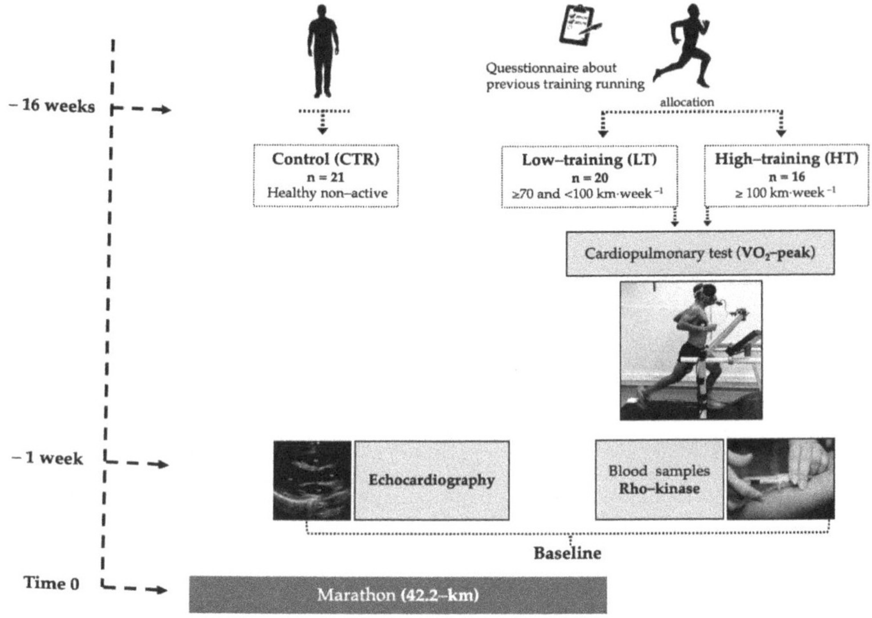

Figure 1. Study design scheme.

Through a venipuncture of the antecubital fossa, peripheral blood mononuclear cells were extracted to determine ROCK activity one week before the marathon competition. ROCK activity was determined in mononuclear cells, using protocols previously described [16]. Briefly, ROCK activation is determined by measuring the phosphorylation of a direct ROCK target, the myosin phosphatase target subunit 1 (MYPT1) of the myosin light chain phosphatase of the light chain of myosin, by Western blot. The antibodies used were anti-myosin phosphatase target subunit 1 (anti-MYPT-1 antibody, rabbit polyclonal, 1/500 cell signaling, Cat 2634) and anti-p-MYPT-1 antibody (phospho-MYPT1-Thr 853 rabbit polyclonal, 1/500, cyclex, Cat CY-P1025). ROCK activity was expressed by the quotient between phosphorylated (p-MYPT1) and total MYPT1 (t-MYPT1). We previously showed in an experimental model that ROCK activity in circulating leukocytes reflects activation of this signaling pathway in the myocardium and aortic wall [22]. Also, troponin-I levels were measured pre- and post-marathon race by a commercially available ELISA kit (CARD-I-KIT ELISA Troponin I, Labmaster, Finland) on an ELISA reader (Tecan-spectra, Austria), and calculated ($ng \cdot mL^{-1}$) as instructed by the manufacturer.

Transthoracic echocardiography (TTE) was performed in all participants using Vivid I echocardiography equipment (General Electric Healthcare, Horten, Norway) with a 2.5/5 MHz sector transducer. Traditional views were acquired from the windows: parasternal, apical, and subcostal for the quantification of the left and right heart chambers according to the American Society of Echocardiography [23]. LV systolic function was assessed by the ejection fraction (EF), calculated by the Simpson's method. LV diastolic function was evaluated using transmitral filling waves and mitral annulus tissue Doppler. LV mass was calculated with the linear method (Devereux's formula) as follows: $0.8 \times 1.04 \times [(IVS + LVID + PWT)^3 - LVID^3] + 0.6$ g [23]. Also, LV longitudinal deformation (longitudinal strain) was carried out using four, three, and two chamber views optimized to achieve >60 frames per second. Images were stored for further analysis by an expert, blinded echocardiographer using the manufacturer's software (EchoPAC, version BT12; GE Healthcare, Horten, Norway).

The physical performance of LDRs was assessed by the cardiopulmonary test (peak aerobic capacity, $\dot{V}O_2$-peak) at the end of the "optimal phase" training period. All LDRs were instructed not to perform physical activity 48 h before the measurement and avoid intakes of alcohol, caffeine, or other stimulants and food for at least three hours before. The $\dot{V}O_2$-peak test was measured on a treadmill ergometer (HP Cosmos, Traunstein, Germany) until voluntary exhaustion, despite oral breathing (respiratory quotient, 1.20 ± 0.05). The exercise protocol consisted of a 3 min rest, a 5 min warm-up (8 $km \cdot h^{-1}$), and a subsequent increase of 2 $km \cdot h^{-1}$ every 150 s, until all criteria for stopping the test were met. Ventilatory data were analysed breath-by-breath using open-circuit spirometry and were expressed under standard temperature, pressure, and dry (STPD) conditions (MasterScreen CPX, Jaeger^{TM}, Würzburg, Germany). Before each test, the gas analyser and the volume transducer were calibrated according to the manufacturer's instructions.

The normality of the data was evaluated using the Shapiro–Wilk test. The ANOVA and Student t-test were used to compare groups. The Pearson correlation test was used for assessing the association between ROCK activity levels and echocardiographic parameters linked to the cardiac remodelling process. The statistical software used was GraphPad Prism 8.0 (GraphPad Software Inc., San Diego, CA, USA). A value of $p <$ 0.05 was considered statistically significant. To evaluate statistical power of the study a post-hoc power analysis was performed [24].

3. Results

Fifty-seven participants were consecutively included (age 37.4 ± 6.1 years). The LDRs achieved values of $\dot{V}O_2$-peak according to their health status (LT: 52.5 ± 8.1 $mL \cdot kg^{-1} \cdot min^{-1}$ vs. HT: 58.5 ± 5.3 $mL \cdot kg^{-1} \cdot min^{-1}$; $p = 0.02$). The HT group completed the marathon race in the least time (231 ± 39 vs. 197 ± 33 min vs. 231 ± 39 LT, p = 0.03). Table 1 shows the participants' characteristics.

The activity of ROCK was different between the groups. HT showed highest ROCK activation (6.17 ± 1.41 vs. 2.74 ± 0.84 LT (p = 0.002), and vs. 1.64 ± 0.66 CTR (p = 0.001); Figure 2). Post-hoc power analysis showed that differences between HT and LT, and HT and CTR groups had 100% power, whereas between LT and CTR group they had 99.6% power.

Table 1. Participant's characteristics.

Variables	Groups			p-Value
	Control (n = 21)	**LT** (n = 20)	**HT** (n = 16)	
Age (years)	35 ± 4	39 ± 5	37 ± 6	0.32
Height (cm)	175 ± 6	174 ± 6	172 ± 7	0.47
Weight (kg)	72 ± 9	73 ± 8	69 ± 8	0.09
Body surface (m^2)	1.89 ± 0.13	1.88 ± 0.12	1.82 ± 0.13	0.08
Creatinine ($mg \cdot dL^{-1}$)	0.99 ± 0.11	0.97 ± 0.10	0.98 ± 0.09	0.63
Hematocrit (%)	42 ± 3	43 ± 3	43 ± 2	0.87
Sodium (mEq/L)	142 ± 2	142 ± 2	142 ± 3	0.44
AST (U/L)	26 ± 7	28 ± 8	29 ± 9	0.67
Uric acid (mg/dL)	5.2 ± 0.8	5.0 ± 0.9	5.6 ± 0.9	0.17
$\dot{V}O_2$-peak ($mL \cdot kg^{-1} \cdot min^{-1}$)	-	52.5 ± 8.1	58.5 ± 5.3	0.02 *
Running experience (years)	-	15 ± 3	17 ± 3	0.81
Time training per week (h)	-	14 ± 2	19 ± 2	0.01 *
Training intensity (%HR máx., 220-age)	-	82 ± 2	81 ± 3	0.78

Data are reported as the mean ± SD; Student's t test, * $p < 0.05$. Abbreviations. CTR: Control; LT: Low training (≥70 and <100 $km \cdot week^{-1}$); HT: High training (≥100 $km \cdot week^{-1}$); AST: Aspartate amino transferase; $\dot{V}O_2$-peak: Peak oxygen consumption.

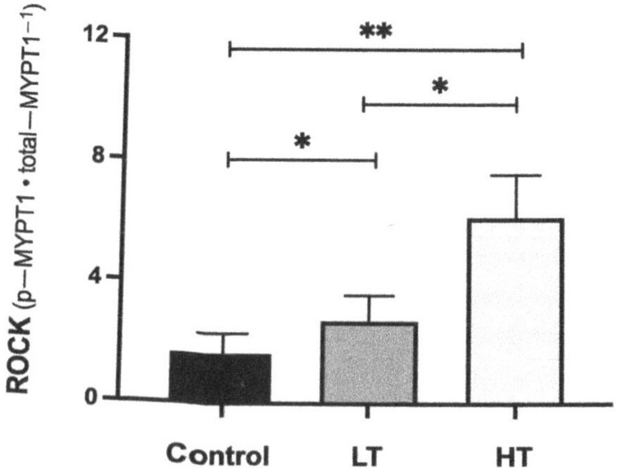

Figure 2. ROCK activity levels by group. Abbreviations: ROCK: Rho kinase activity expressed as p-MYPT1/t-MYPT1 ratio; LT: low training (≥70 and <100 $km \cdot week^{-1}$); HT: high training (≥100 $km \cdot week^{-1}$). * $p < 0.01$. ** $p < 0.001$.

Regarding the quantification of the cardiac chambers by TTE, the results are shown in Table 2.

The HT group showed significantly larger LV linear dimensions than the other groups. Also, they showed a significantly increased LV mass index and LA volume index (Figure 3). LV diastolic function and right ventricle parameters were similar between groups.

Table 2. Heart chambers quantification.

	Groups			
	Control (n = 21)	LT (n = 20)	HT (n = 16)	p-Value
Left Cardiac Cavities				
Interventricular septum (mm)	7.6 ± 0.8; (10.5)	9.0 ± 1.6; (17.7)	10.2 ± 1.2 *; (11.89	<0.001
Posterior wall (mm)	7.6 ± 0.8; (10.5)	8.5 ± 1.2; (14.1)	9.3 ± 2.1 *; (22.6)	0.01
LVEDD (mm)	46 ± 4; (8)	50 ± 5; (10)	58 ± 4 *; (6)	0.04
LVESD (mm)	30 ± 3; (10)	30 ± 4; (13)	33 ± 5; (15)	0.40
Ejection fraction (%)	57 ± 4; (7)	55 ± 6; (10)	54 ± 3; (5)	0.11
LV mas index ($g \cdot m^{-2}$)	58 ± 11; (18)	78 ± 18; (23)	106 ± 27 *; (25)	<0.001
LA diameter (mm)	33 ± 4; (12)	34 ± 3; (8)	36 ± 4; (11)	0.22
LA area (cm^2)	19 ± 5; (26)	22 ± 4; (18)	25 ± 3 *; (12)	<0.001
LA volumen index ($mL \cdot m^{-2}$)	25 ± 9; (36)	30 ± 11; (36)	42 ± 8 *; (19)	<0.001
Global LV longitudinal strain (%)	−21.0 ± −2.0; (9.5)	−19.6 ± −1.6; (8.2)	−19.5 ± −2.4; (12.3)	0.11
E wave ($cm \cdot s^{-1}$)	77 ± 15; (19)	84 ± 12; (14)	78 ± 13; (17)	0.21
A wave ($cm \cdot s^{-1}$)	48 ± 16; (33)	53 ± 10; (19)	50 ± 12; (24)	0.43
Deceleration time (ms)	200 ± 66; (33)	229 ± 65; (28)	233 ± 65; (28)	0.18
e′ lateral ($cm \cdot s^{-1}$)	15.0 ± 1.8; (12.0)	15.0 ± 2.5; (16.7)	15.0 ± 2.3; (15.3)	0.70
e′ medial ($cm \cdot s^{-1}$)	11.0 ± 1.8; (16.4)	10.0 ± 2.0; (20.0)	10.0 ± 2.0; (20.0)	0.75
Right Ventricle				
TAPSE (mm)	25.4 ± 3.3; (12.9)	25.6 ± 4.7; (18.3)	25.8 ± 3.0; (11.6)	0.16
FAC (%)	52.5 ± 3.9; (7.4)	57.3 ± 4.6; (8.0)	56.4 ± 3.7; (6.6)	0.07

Data are reported as the mean ± SD; coefficient of variation (CV). ANOVA test (HT vs. other groups), * $p < 0.05$. Abbreviations: CTR: Control; LT: Low training (≥70 and <100 $km \cdot week^{-1}$); HT: High training (≥100 $km \cdot week^{-1}$); LVEDD: left ventricular-end diastolic diameter; LVESD: left ventricular-end systolic diameter; LV: left ventricle; LA: left atrium; é: mitral annulus tissue Doppler; TAPSE: tricuspid annulus plane systolic excursion; FAC: fractional area change.

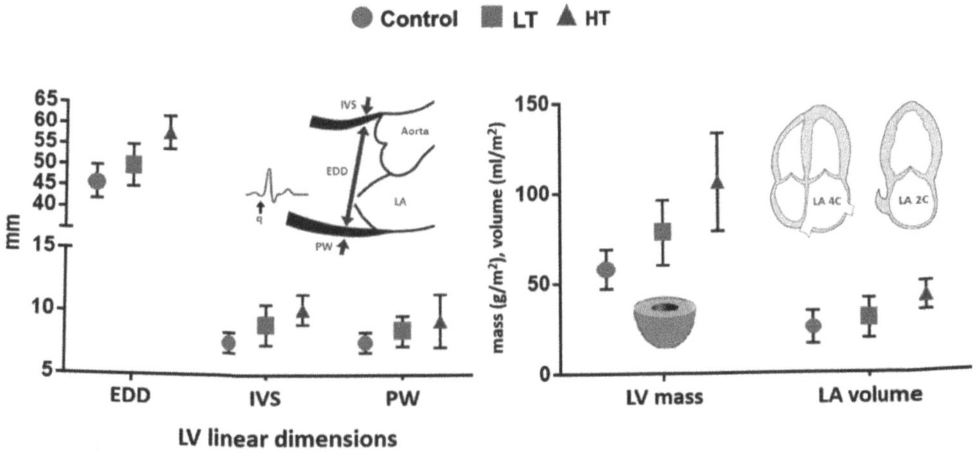

Figure 3. Quantification of left heart chambers. Abbreviations: LT: low training (≥70 and <100 km·week^{-1}); HT: high training (≥100 km·week^{-1}); EDD: end diastolic diameter; IVS: inter ventricular septum; PW: posterior wall; LV: left ventricle; LA: left atrium.

Among LDRs, a direct correlation between ROCK activation in circulating leukocytes, measured by the p-MYPT1/t-MYPT1 ratio, and left cardiac remodelling, evaluated by LV mass index (Figure 4a) and LA volume index, was found (Figure 4b).

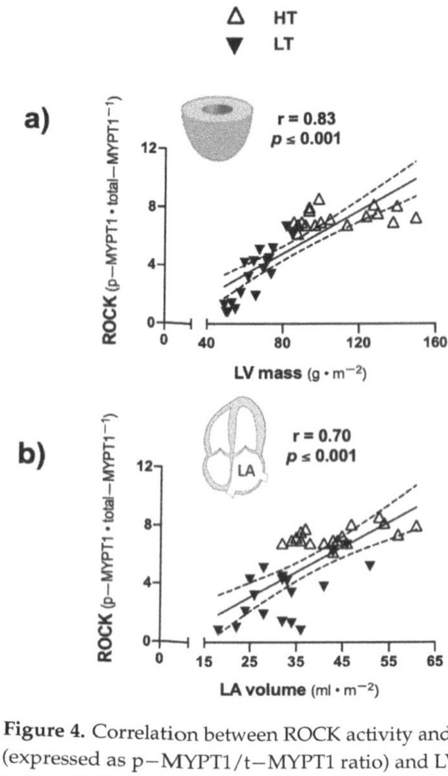

Figure 4. Correlation between ROCK activity and heart remodeling parameters. (**a**) ROCK activity (expressed as p−MYPT1/t−MYPT1 ratio) and LV mass index; (**b**) ROCK activity and LA volume index. Abbreviations: LV: left ventricle; LA: left atrium.

4. Discussion

The main results of this study are that in LDRs, ROCK activation levels in circulation leukocytes were correlated with LV and LA remodelling, as evaluated by indexed LV mass and LA volume. It is expected that with a greater volume of LV cavity the deformation will be less, but we did not find that difference between our groups, probably due to the small differences in the magnitude of left ventricular size between the groups. Also, HT runners showed higher ROCK activity in circulating leukocytes than LT runners and physically healthy, non-active participants. Also, the HT group showed more significant LV diastolic diameter, LV wall thickness, and LV indexed mass, with normal deformation properties and systo-diastolic function; also, in the HT group LA volume was bigger, but with normal filling pressures.

Previous reports revealed that athletes who participate in competitive endurance sports show a heart remodelling process similar to our findings. Athletes showed an increased LA volume and LV mass with normal systolic and diastolic function; these structural changes were more pronounced in those with a more intensive training protocol [6,12,13]. A meta-analysis in athletes with high training regimes showed that acute and prolonged exercise was associated with larger LV volumes and a relative lower LV ejection fraction post-intensive exercise [25]. In this study, the HT group showed a greater left cardiac remodelling process, which potentially gives athletes better performance in highly demanding races [10]; however, these changes could be related to a theoretically excessive and deleterious remodelling process [12], which is in keeping with other reports showing inflammatory and cell remodelling biomarker elevation in athletes, whose complete significance is not fully clarified [22,23].

The ROCK signaling pathway participates in cell survival and cardiac hypertrophy, cardiac fibrosis, and cell apoptosis [15]. Some athletes may develop an extreme cardiac remodelling process, including atrial structure and function changes [12,13,26], worse ventricular performance post-effort [6], and appearance of arrhythmias in long-term follow-up [27,28]. Regarding the physiopathology of previous processes, the ROCK signaling pathway could play an important role in electrical property changes in atrial tissue (connexin expression), as Chen et al. (2018) showed while studying the LA appendage in patients with and without atrial fibrillation [29]. In our study, the HT group showed higher left cardiac cavity remodelling, ROCK activity, and sports performance than other groups; these pathways are probably related to cell survival in stress, and cardiac remodelling allows athletes to better adapt and performance extreme efforts, but there could be an individual point for each subject in which a poor adaptation may be observed. This "point" could lead to an extreme cardiac remodelling process and the risk of future arrhythmias [6] and cardiac dysfunction.

Rho kinase activity is associated with several mechanisms of cardiac injury including ischemic/reperfusion phenomenon [30]. A recent meta-analysis of animal models of myocardial ischemia/reperfusion injury showed that fasudil, a Rho kinase inhibitor, exerts a cardioprotective effect including lowering of troponin-I elevation [31]. Multiple protocols have assessed troponin levels post-different intensities of exercise, but the results have different results and there have been different interpretations on the mechanism of troponin release, which probably depends on multiple individual mechanisms of adaptation to exercise [26,27,32]. In our protocol we did not find troponin-I elevation post-marathon race (troponin-I < 0.156 $ng{\cdot}mL^{-1}$ in all subjects).

Athletes showed a systemic and cellular adaptation to mechanical, inflammatory, and metabolic stress caused by regular and intense exercise training that generated adaptation mechanisms, such as cardiac remodelling and changes in cardiac biomarker expression [33], so that more trained athletes could perform higher workloads, resulting in better performance in highly demanding competitions; however, some subjects could experience extreme and potentially non-adaptive changes [6,13]. Maladaptive changes could be partially explained by experimental models of prolonged intense exercise that showed an increased expression of tumour growth factor-β1 (TGF-β1) in atrial and right ventricular tissue related to myocardial stiffness and myocardial fibrosis [34]. Genetic influences in ROCK activation cannot be ruled out in the formation of cardiac fibrosis associated to a remodelling process induced by intense exercise and regular physical training load. In this regard, normal rodents with genetically higher angiotensin-converting enzyme levels have increased ROCK cascade activation simultaneously in the heart and circulating leukocytes, and they develop higher LV fibrosis levels in response to isoproterenol [35].

Therefore, we suggest that these processes of conditioning and adaptation to continuous effort could result in a "maladaptation" in individual athletes over time, triggering an adverse remodelling process which would be explained by the concept of "hormesis", that is defined as an adaptive cellular response to stressors resulting in a biphasic dose-response—low doses are related to a beneficial adaptation while high doses result in an adverse effect in some specific subjects. Currently, it is unknown precisely what the real meaning of these changes and the behavior of cardiac remodelling biomarkers in apparently non-pathological conditions is and whether they predispose to and partly explain the development of arrhythmias in this subgroup. Moreover, ROCK activity in circulating leukocytes, which reflects activation of this pathway in the myocardium [22], is related to adverse cardiac remodelling in patients with hypertension and cardiac failure [17,18] making the interpretation of our findings more complex.

An aspect that could interfere with our results is the seasonal variations in corporal composition and hydration status during the training period in competitive athletes, affecting plasmatic volume (and cardiac output) and hemodynamic variables that could interfere in the echocardiography measurements obtained in LDRs [36].

One of the main limitations of our study was the reduced number of participants recruited. Therefore, some of the results should be taken cautiously as due to the relatively small sample size, the data may not have the statistical power to expose small effects of training on ROCK activity and cardiac remodelling, possibly resulting in a type II error. However, post-hoc analysis of ROCK activity data showed that the differences had almost 100% power, suggesting that the sample size of this work is sufficient to assess differences in this parameter. Other limitations were the exclusive participation of male athletes, that our conclusions are potentially applicable exclusively to long-distance runners, and that our results are applicable only to the Caucasian ethnic group. Also, the presence of myocardial fibrosis with cardiac resonance was not evaluated. We assumed that athletes had normal systo-diastolic function and normal deformation (global longitudinal strain) of the left ventricle, only with echocardiographic assessment. The applicability of a questionnaire with open questions to assign athletes to runner groups (HT or LT) also is a limitation, mainly because we did not objectively measure the different levels of physical activity completed by runners during the weeks before allocation, for example, reviewing sports activities completed and loaded into training software (e.g., TrainingPeaks™, EnduranceTool™, etc.).

There is no doubt that moderate exercise training leads to good cardiovascular health and longevity [1]. However, there is increasing evidence that more intense exercise can produce potentially excessive cardiac remodelling and arrhythmic events in the long-term follow-up. So, it is essential to have available and accessible clinical tools and biomarkers that help identify those individuals at a greater risk.

5. Conclusions

In male long-distance competitive runners, the load of exercise implicated in marathon training (overload cardiac volume) is associated with ROCK activity levels and a left cardiac remodelling process assessed by echocardiography.

Author Contributions: Conceptualization: L.G., P.F.C., S.L. and M.C.; methodology: L.G., F.C.-B., J.V., S.H., M.S. (Manuel Salinas), J.E.J., J.M., M.P.O., P.G., S.L., M.C. and P.F.C.; software and validation: L.G., F.C.-B., J.V., S.H., R.F. and M.S. (Manuel Salinas); formal analysis: L.G., F.C.-B., P.F.C., S.L., M.P.O. and M.C.; investigation: L.G., F.C.-B., J.V., S.H., J.M., R.F., M.S. (Manuel Salinas),

J.E.J., M.P.O., P.G. and P.F.C.; resources: L.G., P.F.C., S.L. and M.C.; data curation: L.G., F.C.-B., P.F.C., M.P.O. and M.S. (Marta Sitges); writing—original draft preparation: L.G, F.C.-B., M.S. (Manuel Salinas), P.F.C., S.L. and M.C.; writing—review and editing: S.L., M.S. (Marta Sitges), M.C. and P.F.C.; supervision: M.S. (Marta Sitges), M.P.O., S.L, M.C. and P.F.C. All authors have read and agreed to the published version of the manuscript.

Funding: This research was funded by Fondo Nacional de Ciencia y Tecnología (FONDECYT), [grant number 1170963, 2017] and the Fondo de Financiamiento de Centros de Investigación en Áreas Prioritarias (FONDAP) [grant number 15130011, 2014] from the Agencia Nacional de Investigación y Desarrollo (ANID), Chile.

Institutional Review Board Statement: This study was approved by the ethics committee of the Pontificia Universidad Católica de Chile (Institutional Review Board, protocol number 16082603, date of approval: 5 June 2016). The study was carried out according to the Declaration of Helsinki for human experimentation, and we confirm that the study meets the journal's ethical standards.

Informed Consent Statement: All the participants were informed of the purpose, protocol, and procedures before informed consent was obtained from them.

Acknowledgments: The authors would like to thank all participants of this study and Maximiliano Espinosa, Eduardo Moya, and Cynthia Rojas for technical support in measurements done at Laboratory of Exercise Physiology from Pontificia Universidad Católica de Chile.

Conflicts of Interest: The authors declare no conflict of interest.

References

1. Lear, S.; Hu, W.; Rangarajan, S.; Gasevic, D.; Leong, D.; Iqbal, R.; Casanova, A.; Swaminathan, S.; Anjana, R.; Kumar, R.; et al. The effect of physical activity on mortality and cardiovascular disease in 130 000 people from 17 high-income, middle-income, and low-income countries: The PURE study. *Lancet* **2017**, *390*, 2643–2654. [CrossRef]
2. Sharma, S.; Merghani, A.; Mont, L. Exercise and the heart: The good, the bad, and the ugly. *Eur. Heart J.* **2015**, *36*, 1445–1453. [CrossRef]
3. Cohn, J.; Ferrari, R.; Sharpe, N. Cardiac remodeling-concepts and clinical implications: A consensus paper from an International Forum on Cardiac Remodeling. *J. Am. Coll. Cardiol.* **2000**, *35*, 569–582. [CrossRef]
4. Zdravkovic, M.; Perunicic, J.; Krotin, M.; Ristic, M.; Vukomanovic, V.; Soldatovic, I.; Zdravkovic, D. Echocardiographic study of early left ventricular remodeling in highly trained preadolescent footballers. *J. Sci. Med. Sport* **2010**, *13*, 602–606. [CrossRef] [PubMed]
5. Maron, B.; Pelliccia, A. The heart of trained athletes: Cardiac remodeling and the risks of sports, including sudden death. *Circulation* **2006**, *114*, 1633–1644. [CrossRef]
6. Gabrielli, L.; Sitges, M.; Chiong, M.; Jalil, J.; Ocaranza, M.; Llevaneras, S.; Herrera, S.; Fernandez, R.; Saavedra, R.; Yañez, F.; et al. Potential adverse cardiac remodelling in highly trained athletes: Still unknown clinical significance. *Eur. J. Sport Sci.* **2018**, *18*, 1288–1297. [CrossRef] [PubMed]
7. Prakash, K.; Sharma, S. Interpretation of the electrocardiogram in athletes. *Can. J. Cardiol.* **2016**, *32*, 438–451. [CrossRef]
8. Tahir, E.; Starekova, J.; Muellerleile, K.; von Stritzky, A.; Münch, J.; Avanesov, M.; Weinrich, J.; Stehning, C.; Bohnen, S.; Radunski, U.; et al. Myocardial fibrosis in competitive triathletes detected by contrast-enhanced CMR correlates with exercise-induced hypertension and competition history. *J. Am. Cardiovasc. Coll. Cardiovasc. Imaging* **2018**, *11*, 1260–1270. [CrossRef] [PubMed]
9. Zaidi, A.; Ghani, S.; Sheikh, N.; Gati, S.; Bastiaenen, R.; Madden, B.; Papadakis, M.; Raju, H.; Reed, M.; Sharma, R.; et al. Clinical significance of electrocardiographic right ventricular hypertrophy in athletes: Comparison with arrhythmogenic right ventricular cardiomyopathy and pulmonary hypertension. *Eur. Heart J.* **2013**, *34*, 3649–3656. [CrossRef]
10. Gabrielli, L.; Herrera, S.; Contreras-Briceño, F.; Vega, J.; Ocaranza, M.; Yáñez, F.; Fernández, R.; Saavedra, R.; Sitges, M.; García, L.; et al. Increased active phase atrial contraction is related to marathon runner performance. *Eur. J. Appl. Physiol.* **2018**, *118*, 1931–1939. [CrossRef]
11. Gabrielli, L.; Bijnens, B.; Butakoff, C.; Duchateau, N.; Montserrat, S.; Merino, B.; Gutierrez, J.; Paré, C.; Mont, L.; Brugada, J.; et al. Atrial functional and geometrical remodeling in highly trained male athletes: For better or worse? *Eur. J. Appl. Physiol.* **2014**, *114*, 1143–1152. [CrossRef]
12. Gabrielli, L.; Bijnens, B.; Brambila, C.; Duchateau, N.; Marin, J.; Sitges-Serra, I.; Mont, L.; Brugada, J.; Sitges, M. Differential atrial performance at rest and exercise in athletes: Potential trigger for developing atrial dysfunction? *Scand. J. Med. Sci. Sport.* **2016**, *26*, 1444–1454. [CrossRef]
13. Currie, K.; Bailey, K.; Jung, M.; McKelvie, R.; MacDonald, M. Effects of resistance training combined with moderate-intensity endurance or low-volume high-intensity interval exercise on cardiovascular risk factors in patients with coronary artery disease. *J. Sci. Med. Sport* **2015**, *18*, 637–642. [CrossRef] [PubMed]
14. Shimizu, T.; Liao, J. Rho kinases and cardiac remodeling. *Circ. J.* **2016**, *80*, 1491–1498. [CrossRef]

15. Ho, T.; Huang, C.; Huang, C.; Lin, W. Fasudil, a Rho-kinase inhibitor, protects against excessive endurance exercise training-induced cardiac hypertrophy, apoptosis and fibrosis in rats. *Eur. J. Appl. Physiol.* **2012**, *112*, 2943–2955. [CrossRef] [PubMed]
16. Ocaranza, M.; Gabrielli, L.; Mora, I.; Garcia, L.; McNab, P.; Godoy, I.; Braun, S.; Córdova, S.; Castro, P.; Novoa, U.; et al. Markedly increased Rho-kinase activity in circulating leukocytes in patients with chronic heart failure. *Am. Heart J.* **2011**, *161*, 931–937. [CrossRef]
17. Gabrielli, L.; Winter, J.; Godoy, I.; McNab, P.; Padilla, I.; Cordova, S.; Rigotti, P.; Novoa, U.; Mora, I.; García, L.; et al. Increased Rho-kinase activity in hypertensive patients with left ventricular hypertrophy. *Am. J. Hypertens.* **2014**, *27*, 838–845. [CrossRef]
18. Muñoz, V.; Gaspar, R.; Minuzzi, L.; dos Santos Canciglieri, R.; da Silva, A.; de Moura, L.; Cintra, D.; Ropelle, E.; Pauli, J. Rho-kinase activity is upregulated in the skeletal muscle of aged exercised rats. *Exp. Gerontol.* **2019**, *128*. [CrossRef]
19. Muñoz, V.; Gaspar, R.; Esteca, M.; Baptista, I.; Vieira, R.; da Silva, A.; de Moura, L.; Cintra, D.; Ropelle, E.; Pauli, J. Physical exercise increases ROCK activity in the skeletal muscle of middle-aged rats. *Mech. Ageing Dev.* **2020**, *186*. [CrossRef] [PubMed]
20. Bai, H.; Sun, J.; Du, G.; Jiao, F. Association of moderate aerobic exercise & rho-Associated kinase 2 concentration in subjects with dyslipidemia. *Arch. Med. Sci.* **2017**, *13*, 807–812. [CrossRef] [PubMed]
21. Anaruma, C.; Pereira, R.; Cristina da Cruz Rodrigues, K.; Ramos da Silva, A.; Cintra, D.; Ropelle, E.; Pauli, J.; Pereira de Moura, L. Rock protein as cardiac hypertrophy modulator in obesity and physical exercise. *Life Sci.* **2020**, *254*. [CrossRef]
22. Fierro, C.; Novoa, U.; González, V.; Ocaranza, M.; Jalil, J. Simultaneous Rho kinase inhibition in circulating leukocytes and in cardiovascular tissue in rats with high angiotensin converting enzyme levels. *Int. J. Cardiol.* **2016**, *215*, 309–317. [CrossRef]
23. Lang, R.; Badano, L.; Victor, M.; Afilalo, J.; Armstrong, A.; Ernande, L.; Flachskampf, F.; Foster, E.; Goldstein, S.; Kuznetsova, T.; et al. Recommendations for cardiac chamber quantification by echocardiography in adults: An update from the American Society of Echocardiography and the European Association of Cardiovascular Imaging. *J. Am. Soc. Echocardiogr.* **2015**, *28*, 01–39. [CrossRef] [PubMed]
24. Rosner, B. *Fundamental of Biostatistics*, 7th ed.; Brooks/Cole: Boston, MA, USA, 2011.
25. Middleton, N.; Shave, R.; George, K.; Whyte, G.; Hart, E.; Atkinson, G. Left ventricular function immediately following prolonged exercise: A meta-analysis. *Med. Sci. Sports Exerc.* **2006**, *38*, 681–687. [CrossRef]
26. Shave, R.; Baggish, A.; George, K.; Wood, M.; Scharhag, J.; Whyte, G.; Gaze, D.; Thompson, P. Exercise-induced cardiac troponin elevation: Evidence, mechanisms, and implications. *J. Am. Coll. Cardiol.* **2010**, *56*, 169–176. [CrossRef] [PubMed]
27. Nie, J.; Zhang, H.; Kong, Z.; Wang, C.; Liu, Y.; Shi, Q.; George, K. The impact of exercise modality and menstrual cycle phase on circulating cardiac troponin T. *J. Sci. Med. Sport* **2020**, *23*, 309–314. [CrossRef]
28. Calvo, N.; Brugada, J.; Sitges, M.; Mont, L. Atrial fibrillation and atrial flutter in athletes. *Br. J. Sports Med.* **2012**, *46*, 37–43. [CrossRef]
29. Chen, Y.; Su, F.; Han, J.; Jiao, P.; Guo, W. Expression of rho kinase and its mechanism in the left atrial appendage in patients with atrial fibrillation. *Heart Surg. Forum* **2018**, *21*, 44–48. [CrossRef]
30. Kitano, K.; Usui, S.; Ootsuji, H.; Takashima, S.; Kobayashi, D.; Murai, H.; Furusho, H.; Nomura, A.; Kaneko, S.; Takamura, M. Rho-kinase activation in leukocytes plays a pivotal role in myocardial ischemia/reperfusion injury. *PLoS ONE* **2014**, *9*, 01–10. [CrossRef]
31. Huang, Y.; Wu, J.; Su, T.; Zhang, S.; Lin, X. Fasudil, a rho-kinase inhibitor, exerts cardioprotective function in animal models of myocardial ischemia/reperfusion injury: A meta-analysis and review of preclinical evidence and possible mechanisms. *Front. Pharmacol.* **2018**, *9*, 1–14. [CrossRef]
32. Gresslien, T.; Agewall, S. Troponin and exercise. *Int. J. Cardiol.* **2016**, *221*, 609–621. [CrossRef]
33. Schild, M.; Eichner, G.; Beiter, T.; Zügel, M.; Krumholz-Wagner, I.; Hudemann, J.; Pilat, C.; Krüger, K.; Niess, A.; Steinacker, J.; et al. Effects of acute endurance exercise on plasma protein profiles of endurance-trained and untrained individuals over time. *Mediators Inflamm.* **2016**, *2016*, 4851935 . [CrossRef] [PubMed]
34. Benito, B.; Gay-Jordi, G.; Serrano-Mollar, A.; Guasch, E.; Shi, Y.; Tardif, J.; Brugada, J.; Nattel, S.; Mont, L. Cardiac arrhythmogenic remodeling in a rat model of long-term intensive exercise training. *Circulation* **2011**, *123*, 13–22. [CrossRef] [PubMed]
35. Ocaranza, M.; Díaz-Araya, G.; Carreño, J.; Muñoz, D.; Riveros, J.; Jalil, J.; Lavandero, S. Polymorphism in gene coding for ACE determines different development of myocardial fibrosis in rats. *Am. J. Physiol.—Hear. Circ. Physiol.* **2004**, *286*, 498–506. [CrossRef] [PubMed]
36. Meleleo, D.; Bartolomeo, N.; Cassano, L.; Nitti, A.; Susca, G.; Mastrototaro, G.; Armenise, U.; Zito, A.; Devito, F.; Scicchitano, P.; et al. Evaluation of body composition with bioimpedence. A comparison between athletic and non-athletic children. *Eur. J. Sport Sci.* **2017**, *17*, 710–719. [CrossRef] [PubMed]

Journal of Cardiovascular Development and Disease

MDPI

Article

Use of Echocardiography and Heart Failure In-Hospital Mortality from Registry Data in Japan

Kenya Kusunose [1,*,†], Yuichiro Okushi [1,†], Yoshihiro Okayama [2], Robert Zheng [1], Michikazu Nakai [3], Yoko Sumita [3], Takayuki Ise [1], Koji Yamaguchi [1], Shusuke Yagi [1], Daiju Fukuda [1], Hirotsugu Yamada [4], Takeshi Soeki [1], Tetsuzo Wakatsuki [1] and Masataka Sata [1]

1 Department of Cardiovascular Medicine, Tokushima University Hospital, Tokushima 770-8503, Japan; yuuitirou_0110@yahoo.co.jp (Y.O.); pangtong2004@yahoo.ne.jp (R.Z.); isetaka@tokushima-u.ac.jp (T.I.); yamakoji3@tokushima-u.ac.jp (K.Y.); syagi@tokushima-u.ac.jp (S.Y.); daiju.fukuda@tokushima-u.ac.jp (D.F.); soeki@tokushima-u.ac.jp (T.S.); wakatsukitz@tokushima-u.ac.jp (T.W.); masataka.sata@tokushima-u.ac.jp (M.S.)

2 Clinical Research Center for Developmental Therapeutics, Tokushima University Hospital, Tokushima 770-8503, Japan; okayama0317@outlook.com

3 Center for Cerebral and Cardiovascular Disease Information, National Cerebral and Cardiovascular Center, Osaka 564-8565, Japan; nakai.michikazu@ncvc.go.jp (M.N.); ysumi@ncvc.go.jp (Y.S.)

4 Department of Community Medicine for Cardiology, Tokushima University Graduate School of Biomedical Sciences, Tokushima 770-8503, Japan; yamadah@tokushima-u.ac.jp

* Correspondence: kusunosek@tokushima-u.ac.jp; Tel.: +81-88-633-7851; Fax: +81-88-633-7894

† These authors contributed equally to this work.

Abstract: Background: Echocardiography requires a high degree of skill on the part of the examiner, and the skill may be more improved in larger volume centers. This study investigated trends and outcomes associated with the use and volume of echocardiographic exams from a real-world registry database of heart failure (HF) hospitalizations. Methods: This study was based on the Diagnosis Procedure Combination database in the Japanese Registry of All Cardiac and Vascular Datasets (JROAD-DPC). A first analysis was performed to assess the trend of echocardiographic examinations between 2012 and 2016. A secondary analysis was performed to assess whether echocardiographic use was associated with in-hospital mortality in 2015. Results: During this period, the use of echocardiography grew at an average annual rate of 6%. Patients with echocardiography had declining rates of hospital mortality, and these trends were associated with high hospitalization costs. In the 2015 sample, a total of 52,832 echocardiograms were examined, corresponding to 65.6% of all HF hospital admissions for that year. We found that the use and volume of echocardiography exams were associated with significantly lower odds of all-cause hospital mortality in heart failure (adjusted odds ratio (OR): 0.48 for use of echocardiography and 0.78 for the third tertile; both $p < 0.001$). Conclusions: The use of echocardiography was associated with decreased odds of hospital mortality in HF. The volumes of echocardiographic examinations were also associated with hospital mortality.

Keywords: heart failure; echocardiography; mortality; big data

1. Introduction

Heart failure (HF) is a leading cause of cardiovascular death and remains a major socioeconomic issue [1,2]. Despite advances in modern therapy, mortality rates for HF continue to be high. Echocardiography is an easily available, versatile, and cost-effective means of cardiac imaging. This technique does not require intervention, radiation exposure, or radioactive isotopes [3]. It also provides data on cardiac dysfunction, hemodynamic status, valvular heart disease, and myocardial ischemia for treatment of heart failure [4]. There are several recommendations for the use of echocardiography in acute hospitalized HF [5,6]; however, clinical evidence and data on echocardiographic use are limited. Studies on nationwide data in the United States showed that, even if echocardiographic examinations were underused during cardiovascular hospitalizations, the use of echocardiography itself was associated with lower inpatient mortality [7]. On the other hand, echocardiography requires a high degree of skill on the part of the examiner, and skill may be more improved in large volume centers [8]. We hypothesized that higher hospital echocardiographic volumes would be associated with reduced inpatient mortality in patients admitted with acute heart failure. We analyzed trends and outcomes in association with the use and volumes of echocardiography using real-world big data based on HF hospitalizations to check the association between echocardiographic volumes and inpatient mortality.

2. Methods

2.1. Study Population

First, we queried the Japanese Registry of All Cardiac and Vascular Diseases and the Diagnosis Procedure Combination (JROAD-DPC) database to quantify temporal trends in inpatient echocardiographic use between April 2012 and March 2017. Second, we explored the 2015 database to investigate whether the use and volume of echocardiographic exams were associated with all-cause in-hospital mortality in patients with HF. JROAD-DPC is a nationwide registry, a medical database with information on admission and discharge for cardiovascular diseases, clinical examinations and treatment status, patient status and hospital overview. The JROAD-DPC database integrates the information with analysis datasets covering 5.1 million cases between April 2012 and March 2017. The identification of HF (I50.0, I50.1, I50.9) hospitalization was based on the International Classification of Diseases (ICD) diagnosis codes. The diagnosis of HF was defined as the main diagnosis, admission-precipitating diagnosis, or most resource-consuming diagnosis. We defined readmission as an admission after discharge to a DPC hospital due to HF. Data regarding patient age and sex, main diagnosis, comorbidity at admission, length of hospitalization and treatment content were extracted from the database. We identified the numbers of board-certified doctors through the Japanese Circulation Society who were working full time in cardiovascular departments in Japan, and the numbers of transthoracic echocardiographies through the survey of the Japanese Circulation Society. The Institutional Review Board of the Tokushima University Hospital approved the study protocol (no. 3503).

Figure 1 shows the patient selection flowchart. We selected 649,960 patients hospitalized with HF between April 2012 and March 2017. To analyze the associations between echocardiography and all-cause in-hospital mortality in HF, we enrolled 140,768 patients hospitalized for HF at 739 hospitals between April 2015 and March 2016. To reduce the variability of the data collected from this database, we focused on one year of data. We excluded patients from readmission cases (n = 42,660), age < 20 years (n = 284), death in 24 h after admission to exclude counter bias by patients in whom a fatal outcome occurred without sufficient lead time to obtain an echocardiographic examination if clinically indicated (n = 2074), a planned hospitalization to focus on hospital mortality (n = 10,652), and a lack of data (n = 15,042). As a result, a total of 80,496 were selected to assess hospital mortality. We categorized the 739 hospitals into 3 groups according to the number of echocardiographic studies performed annually (first tertile: <2500 cases, second tertile: 2500–4500 cases, third tertile: >4500 cases) and compared the groups of patients admitted to the categorized hospitals.

2.2. Clinical Outcomes

The main outcome was in-hospital mortality (total number of deaths during hospitalization).

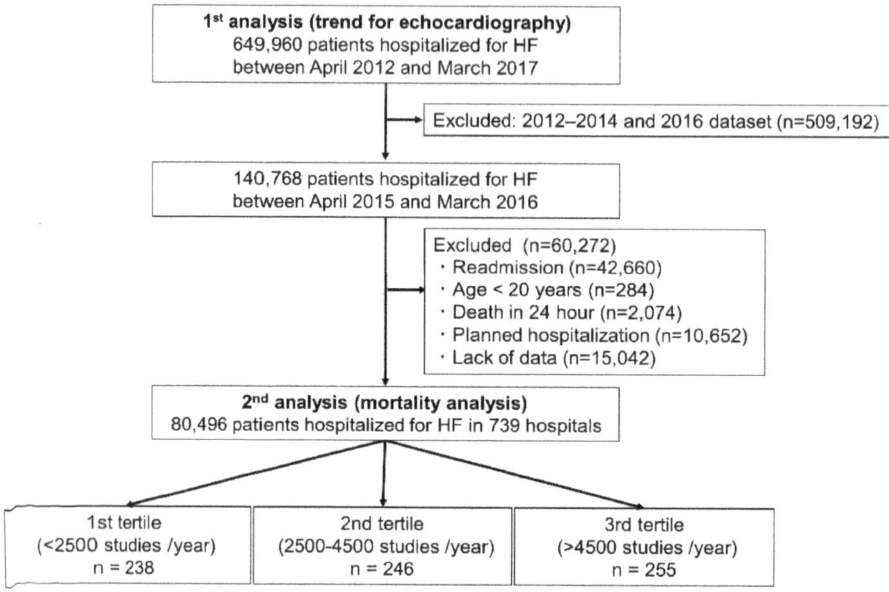

Figure 1. Flowchart of this study. HF, heart failure.

2.3. Statistical Analysis

Temporal trends in the incidence of echocardiographic use between 2012 and 2016 were analyzed. The increase in volume was analyzed by calculating the average annual percentage change from 2012 to 2016. The 2015 sample was dichotomized into three groups based on echocardiographic volumes, and descriptive statistics were generated on frequencies and proportions for categorical variables. Continuous variables are expressed as the mean ± SD for parameters with a normal distribution, as the median (interquartile range; IQR) for parameters with a skewed distribution, and categorical variables as the proportion (%). We estimated the odds ratios (ORs) and their 95% confidence interval (CI) for in-hospital mortality using multivariable models. A forward stepwise multivariable analysis was performed using relevant variables (associated with outcomes), incorporating a p value threshold <0.05 as the entry cutoff. All statistical tests were 2-sided, and p values less than 0.05 were considered statistically significant. Statistical analysis was performed using SAS version 9.4 and JMP 14.0 (SAS Institute Inc., Cary, NC). Odds ratios (ORs) and their 95% confidence interval (CI) for in-hospital mortality were calculated using multivariable models of multinomial logistic regression analysis in 3 groups.

3. Results

3.1. Analysis of Trends

A total of around 90,000 echocardiographic examinations per year were performed at all centers participating in this database from 2012 to 2016. During this period, the use of echocardiography grew at an average annual rate of 6% (Figure 2A). The numbers of in-hospital deaths were 12,206 (mortality: 11.2%), 12,159 (mortality: 10.5%), 13,959 (mortality: 10.6%), 14,895 (mortality: 10.6%), and 16,720 (mortality: 10.9%) in 2012, 2013, 2014, 2015 and 2016, respectively. An evaluation of resource use and patient outcomes found that patients with echocardiographic examinations had relatively lower rates of hospital mortality compared with patients without echocardiographic examinations. There was no trend of mortality among years. On the other hand, patients with echocardiographic examinations were associated with higher hospitalization costs than those without examinations (Figure 2B,C). According to these trends, we undertook a detailed analysis to investigate whether the use of echocardiography may be related to hospital outcomes.

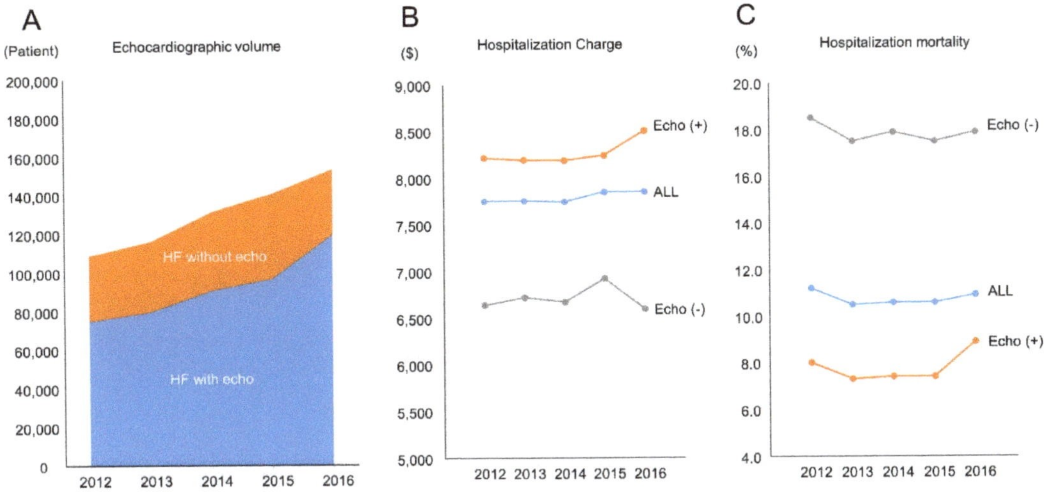

Figure 2. Trends in echocardiography use between 2012 and 2016. (**A**) Echocardiographic volume; (**B**) Hospitalization Charge; (**C**) Hospitalization mortality; HF, heart failure; $, US dollar.

3.2. 2015 Nationwide Inpatient Characteristics

Table 1 and Table S1 display the 2015 sample and the study population stratified by echocardiographic use and categorical variables. A total of 53.6% of patients in this study were male. The mean age was 78 ± 13 years, and half of all patients had hypertension (51.3%). Around 60% of the patients were New York Heart Association (NYHA) class III or IV. A total of 58,921 echocardiograms were examined in 2015, corresponding to 73.2% of all HF hospital admissions for that year. The distributions observed within categorical variables between the echocardiography and non-echocardiography groups of our study population are shown in Table 2. In a comparison of the two sample groups, patients undergoing echocardiography were younger, had a higher BMI, had a higher prevalence of hypertension dyslipidemia atrial fibrillation, and had less chronic kidney disease (all $p < 0.001$) (Table 2). The distribution of other comorbidities was comparable to the echocardiographic status.

Table 1. Baseline hospital characteristics.

Hospital Characteristics	All	1st Tertile	2nd Tertile	3rd Tertile
Number of Institutes	739	238	246	255
BC Doctor	4 (2–6)	2 (1–3)	4 (3–5)	7 (4–10)
TTE	3315 (2070–5361)	1733 (1220–2043)	3294 (2888–3943)	6613 (5293–8543)
Bed	386 (275–536)	279 (198–342)	394 (301–487)	560 (405–701)
CV Bed	35 (28–44)	30 (20–37)	33 (30–42)	41 (33–51)

Data are presented as the median (interquartile range). Abbreviations: BC, board-certified; CV, cardiovascular.

Table 2. Characteristics with and without echocardiography.

	All	Echocardiography (−)	Echocardiography (+)	*p*-Value
N	80,496	21,575	58,921	
Age (year)	78 ± 13	78.4 ± 12.5	77.8 ± 12.7	<0.001
Male (%)	53.6	54.3	53.4	0.0201
BMI (%)	22.8 ± 5.2	22.7 ± 5.4	22.8 ± 5.1	<0.001
NYHA I-II (%)	41.4	43.9	40.5	<0.001
Complication (%)				
HT	51.3	49.3	52.0	<0.001
DM	26.8	26.8	26.8	0.963
DL	17.6	16.5	18.0	<0.001
MI	9.8	9.7	9.8	0.7042
Af	34.3	30.1	35.9	<0.001
PVD	3.9	4.0	3.8	0.1486
Stroke	7.8	8.0	7.7	0.1892
Dementia	5.5	5.6	5.4	0.3819
COPD	7.0	6.9	7.1	0.3131
Liver Disease	0.1	0.2	0.1	0.1098
CKD	14.5	17.0	13.5	<0.001
Cancer	10.8	10.3	11.0	0.0029
Treatment (%)				
HD	5.0	7.1	4.2	<0.001
Artificial Respirator	19.3	22.2	18.2	<0.001
IABP	0.9	0.7	1.0	<0.001
PCPS	0.1	0.2	0.1	0.0271
Inotropes	12.0	11.8	12.0	0.364
PCI	4.7	3.3	5.3	<0.001

Data given as the proportion. See abbreviations in Table 1. Abbreviations: OR, odds ratio.

3.3. Mortality Analysis

In the analysis cohort, in-hospital mortality was 7.7% (n = 6179). Patients with echocardiography had a significantly lower in-hospital mortality (6.0% vs. 12.2%, $p < 0.001$; OR, 0.46, 95% CI: 0.44–0.49). In the univariate logistic regression analysis, many clinical variables were associated with in-hospital mortality. A multivariate logistic regression adjusting for clinical variables (age, body mass index, NYHA class, hypertension, dyslipidemia, atrial fibrillation, stroke, renal failure, liver failure, cancer, artificial respirator, intra-aortic balloon pumping, percutaneous cardiopulmonary support, inotropes, percutaneous coronary intervention, board-certified doctor) using stepwise selection was performed to evaluate for the association between echocardiographic use and the odds of a patient's death. To adjust by the number of doctors, we included board-certified doctors in this analysis. We found that the use of echocardiograms was associated with significantly lower odds of all-cause hospital mortality in heart failure (adjusted OR: 0.48; 95% CI: 0.45 to 0.51; $p < 0.001$) (Table 3).

In the tertile analysis of the number of echocardiographic volumes, the unadjusted OR for in-hospital mortality was significantly lower in the second tertile (OR, 0.72; 95% CI: 0.67–0.77, $p < 0.001$) and third tertile (OR, 0.56; 95% CI: 0.53–0.60, $p < 0.001$) than in the first tertile. In the stepwise analysis, the adjusted OR for in-hospital mortality was 0.86 (95% CI: 0.79–0.98, $p < 0.001$) for the second tertile and 0.78 (95% CI: 0.72–0.85, $p < 0.001$) for the third tertile. Interestingly, the number of echocardiographic examinations and volumes of the institute remained an independent risk factor after adjustment of clinical variables including the numbers of board-certified doctors (Figure 3).

Table 3. Multivariate analysis of covariates for in-hospital mortality in all patients.

	Univariate				Multivariate			
	OR	**Lower**	**Upper**	***p***	**OR**	**Lower**	**Upper**	***p***
Age	1.06	1.06	1.07	<0.001	1.07	1.07	1.07	<0.001
BMI	0.90	0.89	0.91	<0.001	0.95	0.94	0.96	<0.001
Male	1.29	1.23	1.36	<0.001				
NYHA 1–2	1.86	1.76	1.97	<0.001	0.67	0.63	0.71	<0.001
HT	0.35	0.33	0.37	<0.001	0.43	0.40	0.45	<0.001
DM	0.73	0.69	0.78	<0.001				
DL	0.34	0.31	0.38	<0.001	0.56	0.51	0.63	<0.001
MI	1.06	0.97	1.16	0.1743				
Af	0.65	0.61	0.69	<0.001	0.74	0.69	0.79	<0.001
PVD	0.98	0.86	1.13	0.8059				
Stroke	1.77	1.63	1.92	<0.001	1.44	1.32	1.58	<0.001
Dementia	1.87	1.7	2.05	<0.001				
COPD	1.03	0.93	1.14	0.5749				
CKD	1.42	1.33	1.52	<0.001	1.36	1.26	1.47	<0.001
Liver Failure	2.94	1.83	4.75	<0.001	3.14	1.79	5.52	<0.001
Cancer	1.48	1.38	1.60	<0.001	1.52	1.40	1.65	<0.001
HD	1.3	1.17	1.45	<0.001				
Artificial Respirator	3.29	3.12	3.48	<0.001	2.74	2.57	2.93	<0.001
IABP	3.86	3.25	4.58	<0.001	1.46	1.16	1.83	0.0011
PCPS	19.34	13.25	28.23	<0.001	12.19	7.53	19.74	<0.001
Inotropes	6.46	6.11	6.84	<0.001	5.75	5.37	6.14	<0.001
PCI	0.46	0.38	0.54	<0.001	0.24	0.20	0.29	<0.001
TTE	0.46	0.44	0.49	<0.001	0.48	0.45	0.51	<0.001
All Beds	1.00	1.00	1.00	<0.001				
CV Beds	0.99	0.99	0.99	<0.001				
BC Doctor	0.95	0.94	0.95	<0.001	0.97	0.96	0.98	<0.001
Group 1st Tertile vs 2nd	0.72	0.67	0.77	<0.001	0.86	0.79	0.92	<0.001
2nd vs 3rd	0.56	0.53	0.60	<0.001	0.78	0.72	0.85	<0.001
2nd vs 3rd	0.78	0.74	0.83	<0.001	0.92	0.85	0.98	0.0172

Data given as the proportion. See abbreviations in Table 1. Abbreviations: OR, odds ratio.

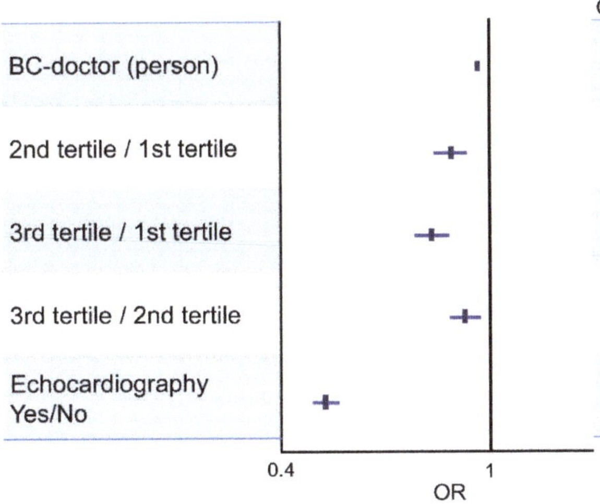

	Death n (%) Comparator	Death n (%) reference	OR	lower	upper	P-value
BC-doctor (person)			0.97	0.96	0.98	<0.001
2nd tertile / 1st tertile	1976 (7.9)	1707 (10.7)	0.86	0.79	0.92	<0.001
3rd tertile / 1st tertile	2496 (6.3)	1707 (10.7)	0.78	0.72	0.85	<0.001
3rd tertile / 2nd tertile	2496 (6.3)	1976 (7.9)	0.92	0.85	0.98	0.0172
Echocardiography Yes/No	3547 (6.0)	2632 (12.2)	0.48	0.45	0.51	<0.001

Figure 3. Odds ratio of in-hospital mortality. BC, board-certified. Dots and lines mean odds ratio (OR) and 95% CI, respectively.

4. Discussion

Echocardiography is common in many clinical aspects of cardiovascular hospitals. However, there are limited data for applications of echocardiography in Japan. Our main findings of this study were: (1) between 2012 and 2016, the use of echocardiography grew at an average annual rate of 6%, (2) patients with echocardiography had declining rates of hospital mortality and these trends were associated with high hospitalization costs, (3) HF patients with echocardiography in the hospitals with larger echocardiographic volumes had significantly lower in-hospital mortality, even after the matching of clinical variables, including the numbers of board-certified doctors.

4.1. *Use of Echocardiogram on HF*

In the United States, the analysis of the largest publicly available all-payer impatient database showed that the incidence of echocardiography per hospitalization gradually increased at annual rates of around 3.0% [7]. However, their analysis suggested that echocardiography may be underused for common and appropriate indications because the incidence of echocardiographic performance per hospitalization was around 2% in 2010. In Japan, 58,921 echocardiograms were examined in 2015, corresponding to 73.2% of all HF hospital admissions for that year, and the incidence of echocardiography is extremely high compared with the United States. This discrepancy reflects differences in study populations because our demographics were specific to the HF inpatient setting and there were high rates of echocardiographic use among cardiovascular hospitals in Japan.

4.2. *Impact of Echocardiograhy on HF Mortality*

In 2015, a total of 58,921 echocardiograms were examined in HF. After adjusting for key variables, we observed that the use of echocardiography was associated with lower odds of hospital mortality in this cohort. Interestingly, the total number of exams performed at institutes was strongly associated with hospital mortality even after the adjustment of the numbers of board-certified doctors. In a previous study for acute coronary syndrome, patients who were admitted to cardiology centers more commonly underwent cardiac catheterization, received evidence-based therapy and had a significantly lower mortality than those admitted to noncardiology centers [9]. Some studies also showed that a large operating volume, number of cardiologists and cardiovascular beds were associated with reduced mortality [10,11]. The similar causal link between examination totals and mortality may be true for echocardiography. Echocardiography is a first-line diagnostic tool that contributes to the initiation of therapy in HF [5,6]. It was well known that echocardiographic decisions improved mortality rates in the clinical setting [12]. In a major academic medical center, 32% of inpatient echocardiographic examinations led to an active change in medical care including cardiovascular managements [13]. The clinical information provided by echocardiography can assist physicians in management decisions and patient risk stratification. Another explanation may show that in large university teaching hospitals with higher resources and advanced procedures in patients with HF, the usage of echocardiography should be higher than in smaller institutions, and the better outcome of patients in the first ones might be explained by easier access to echocardiography and an earlier diagnosis of change in the heart function or of complications, which can lead to a better outcome. In addition, improvement in HF outcomes over time may be attributable to an increasing use of guideline-directed medical therapy, new therapies (such as sacubitril/valsartan), a shift towards more HF with preserved EF and less HF with reduced EF, increasing use of mechanical support, etc. All of these things may be more common in larger centers that do more echoes. These scenarios may support our hypothesis that the use of echocardiography can improve the hospital mortality in HF. According to our results, the quality of care including echocardiography may be associated with outcomes in patients with HF. Because some studies showed that quality of care for patients with HF may be sub-standard and that there is a wide heterogeneity in the quality of care for HF among hospitals in several countries [14,15], the quality of care for patients should be improved in the future. Among patients with HF, in-hospital mortality is reported to vary from around 5.0% to 12.0% [16–19]. Our cohort had a mortality rate of about 10%, which may reflect the current situation in Japan as a hyper-aged society.

4.3. Clinical Implication

Improvement in the prognosis of HF is an essential part of clinical management [5]. According to our data from the large high-risk HF cohort, including around 60% of patients with NYHA III/IV, patients with echocardiography had a lower mortality after the adjustment for clinical variables, including the numbers of board-certified doctors. This study suggests that improving the quality of echocardiographic examinations could be beneficial and that the skill of echocardiography contributes to patients' care and prognosis.

4.4. Limitations

The study based on ICD codes has several limitations. We analyzed only patients with HF hospitalized in facilities contributing to the database, which may lead to selection bias. This database included approximately 50% of Japanese Circulation Society certified hospitals and 29% of all hospitals in Japan [20]. All hospitals were cardiovascular training facilities and their affiliated facilities. We were unable to gather the data from noncardiology wards (e.g., internists or geriatric wards). The database has no information on laboratory data (e.g., NT-proBNP) and specific echocardiographic data (e.g., left ventricular ejection fraction) to assess the prognosis of HF. To overcome this issue, we used treatment devices and isotropic medication as markers of HF severity. All-cause mortality was used as the primary end point in our patient population. The most likely cause of death in our patient population is HF, given the known high-risk nature of our patient population. The patients in this study are mostly Japanese. The results may differ due to racial/cultural differences in other countries. The JROAD-DPC dataset extracts only a record, which contains all types of cardiovascular diseases in any categories of diagnosis based on the DPC dataset in the Ministry of Health, Labor and Welfare in Japan. This J-ROAD dataset has already been validated in past studies [21,22]. Around 40% of acute HF patients had NYHA I–II symptoms in this database. Many patients with even mild symptoms were admitted to hospitals with board-certified doctors, probably due to the insurance system that covers all of its citizens in Japan. In clinical practice, there are a subset of patients less likely to be imaged or to receive aggressive care, in part because it is understood that overall outcomes will be poor. We focused on the 2015 database because the data before 2015 had some missing values including the NYHA functional class. The short period of inclusion was another limitation. Finally, we have excluded almost 40% of the entire cohort for various reasons, and thus there is a selection bias. According to these limitations, this paper should be considered as a hypothesis-generating study.

5. Conclusions

The use of echocardiography was associated with decreased odds of hospital mortality in HF. The number of echocardiographic examinations was also associated with hospital mortality; thus, this study could generate the hypothesis that the skill of echocardiography may be better in the large volume centers and contribute to good outcomes in HF. Our study is based on a highly and retrospectively selected cohort. We believe that larger international studies are warranted to confirm this result.

Supplementary Materials: The following are available online, Table S1: Baseline patient characteristics.

Author Contributions: K.K. conceived the idea for this study. Y.O. (Yuichiro Okushi) and Y.O. (Yoshihiro Okayama) conducted the data analyses. The initial draft of the manuscript was produced by K.K. and Y.O. (Yuichiro Okushi). All authors (K.K., Y.O. (Yuichiro Okushi), Y.O. (Yoshihiro Okayama), R.Z., M.N., Y.S., T.I., K.Y., S.Y., D.F., H.Y., T.S., T.W. and M.S.) were involved in interpreting the results and writing the manuscript. All authors have read and agreed to the published version of the manuscript.

Funding: This work was partially supported by JSPS Kakenhi Grants (20K17084 to Y. Okushi, 19H03654 to M. Sata), and the Takeda Science Foundation (to K. Kusunose).

Institutional Review Board Statement: The study was conducted according to the guidelines of the Declaration of Helsinki, and approved by the Institutional Review Board of Tokushima University (protocol no. 3503).

Informed Consent Statement: Patient consent was waived because the analysis used anonymous clinical data.

Data Availability Statement: Individual anonymized data supporting the analyses contained in the manuscript will be made available upon reasonable written request from researchers whose proposed use of the data for a specific purpose has been approved.

Conflicts of Interest: The authors have no conflict of interest to declare.

Abbreviations

Abbreviations

HF = heart failure, DPC = Diagnosis Procedure Combination, ICD = International Classification of Diseases, NYHA = New York Heart Association.

References

1. Kitai, T.; Miyakoshi, C.; Morimoto, T.; Yaku, H.; Murai, R.; Kaji, S.; Furukawa, Y.; Inuzuka, Y.; Nagao, K.; Tamaki, Y. Mode of death among Japanese adults with heart failure with preserved, midrange, and reduced ejection fraction. *JAMA Netw. Open* **2020**, *3*, e204296. [CrossRef]
2. Vaduganathan, M.; Patel, R.B.; Michel, A.; Shah, S.J.; Senni, M.; Gheorghiade, M.; Butler, J. Mode of Death in Heart Failure With Preserved Ejection Fraction. *J. Am. Coll. Cardiol.* **2017**, *69*, 556–569. [CrossRef]
3. Kirkpatrick, J.N.; Grimm, R.; Johri, A.M.; Kimura, B.J.; Kort, S.; Labovitz, A.J.; Lanspa, M.; Phillip, S.; Raza, S.; Thorson, K.; et al. Recommendations for Echocardiography Laboratories Participating in Cardiac Point of Care Cardiac Ultrasound (POCUS) and Critical Care Echocardiography Training: Report from the American Society of Echocardiography. *J. Am. Soc. Echocardiogr.* **2020**, *33*, 409–422. [CrossRef]
4. Othman, F.; Abushahba, G.; Salustri, A. Adherence to the American Society of Echocardiography and European Association of Cardiovascular Imaging Recommendations for the Evaluation of Left Ventricular Diastolic Function by Echocardiography: A Quality Improvement Project. *J. Am. Soc. Echocardiogr.* **2019**, *32*, 1619–1621. [CrossRef]
5. Tsutsui, H.; Isobe, M.; Ito, H.; Ito, H.; Okumura, K.; Ono, M.; Kitakaze, M.; Kinugawa, K.; Kihara, Y.; Goto, Y.; et al. JCS 2017/JHFS 2017 Guideline on Diagnosis and Treatment of Acute and Chronic Heart Failure- Digest Version. *Circ. J.* **2019**, *83*, 2084–2184. [CrossRef]
6. Writing, C.; Maddox, T.M.; Januzzi, J.L., Jr.; Allen, L.A.; Breathett, K.; Butler, J.; Davis, L.L.; Fonarow, G.C.; Ibrahim, N.E.; Lindenfeld, J.; et al. 2021 Update to the 2017 ACC Expert Consensus Decision Pathway for Optimization of Heart Failure Treatment: Answers to 10 Pivotal Issues About Heart Failure With Reduced Ejection Fraction: A Report of the American College of Cardiology Solution Set Oversight Committee. *J. Am. Coll. Cardiol.* **2021**, *77*, 772–810. [CrossRef]
7. Papolos, A.; Narula, J.; Bavishi, C.; Chaudhry, F.A.; Sengupta, P.P. US hospital use of echocardiography: Insights from the nationwide inpatient sample. *J. Am. Coll. Cardiol.* **2016**, *67*, 502–511. [CrossRef] [PubMed]
8. Mitchell, C.; Rahko, P.S.; Blauwet, L.A.; Canaday, B.; Finstuen, J.A.; Foster, M.C.; Horton, K.; Ogunyankin, K.O.; Palma, R.A.; Velazquez, E.J. Guidelines for Performing a Comprehensive Transthoracic Echocardiographic Examination in Adults: Recommendations from the American Society of Echocardiography. *J. Am. Soc. Echocardiogr.* **2019**, *32*, 1–64. [CrossRef] [PubMed]
9. O'Neill, D.E.; Southern, D.A.; Norris, C.M.; O'Neill, B.J.; Curran, H.J.; Graham, M.M. Acute coronary syndrome patients admitted to a cardiology vs non-cardiology service: Variations in treatment & outcome. *BMC Health Serv. Res.* **2017**, *17*, 354. [CrossRef]
10. Badheka, A.O.; Patel, N.J.; Grover, P.; Singh, V.; Patel, N.; Arora, S.; Chothani, A.; Mehta, K.; Deshmukh, A.; Savani, G.T.; et al. Impact of annual operator and institutional volume on percutaneous coronary intervention outcomes: A 5-year United States experience (2005–2009). *Circulation* **2014**, *130*, 1392–1406. [CrossRef] [PubMed]
11. Kanaoka, K.; Okayama, S.; Yoneyama, K.; Nakai, M.; Nishimura, K.; Kawata, H.; Horii, M.; Kawakami, R.; Okura, H.; Miyamoto, Y.; et al. Number of Board-Certified Cardiologists and Acute Myocardial Infarction Related Mortality in Japan- JROAD and JROAD-DPC Registry Analysis. *Circ. J.* **2018**, *82*, 2845–2851. [CrossRef]

12. Yancy, C.W.; Jessup, M.; Bozkurt, B.; Butler, J.; Casey, D.E., Jr.; Drazner, M.H.; Fonarow, G.C.; Geraci, S.A.; Horwich, T.; Januzzi, J.L.; et al. 2013 ACCF/AHA guideline for the management of heart failure: Executive summary: A report of the American College of Cardiology Foundation/American Heart Association Task Force on practice guidelines. *Circulation* **2013**, *128*, 1810–1852. [CrossRef] [PubMed]
13. Matulevicius, S.A.; Rohatgi, A.; Das, S.R.; Price, A.L.; DeLuna, A.; Reimold, S.C. Appropriate use and clinical impact of transthoracic echocardiography. *JAMA Intern. Med.* **2013**, *173*, 1600–1607. [CrossRef]
14. Gupta, A.; Yu, Y.; Tan, Q.; Liu, S.; Masoudi, F.A.; Du, X.; Zhang, J.; Krumholz, H.M.; Li, J. Quality of care for patients hospitalized for heart failure in China. *JAMA Netw. Open* **2020**, *3*, e1918619. [CrossRef] [PubMed]
15. Emdin, C.A.; Conrad, N.; Kiran, A.; Salimi-Khorshidi, G.; Woodward, M.; Anderson, S.G.; Mohseni, H.; Dargie, H.J.; Hardman, S.M.; McDonagh, T. Variation in hospital performance for heart failure management in the National Heart Failure Audit for England and Wales. *Heart* **2017**, *103*, 55–62. [CrossRef]
16. Honda, S.; Nagai, T.; Sugano, Y.; Okada, A.; Asaumi, Y.; Aiba, T.; Noguchi, T.; Kusano, K.; Ogawa, H.; Yasuda, S. Prevalence, determinants, and prognostic significance of delirium in patients with acute heart failure. *Int. J. Cardiol.* **2016**, *222*, 521–527. [CrossRef]
17. Lee, S.E.; Cho, H.J.; Lee, H.Y.; Yang, H.M.; Choi, J.O.; Jeon, E.S.; Kim, M.S.; Kim, J.J.; Hwang, K.K.; Chae, S.C. A multicentre cohort study of acute heart failure syndromes in Korea: Rationale, design, and interim observations of the Korean Acute Heart Failure (KorAHF) registry. *Eur. J. Heart Fail.* **2014**, *16*, 700–708. [CrossRef]
18. Chioncel, O.; Mebazaa, A.; Harjola, V.P.; Coats, A.J.; Piepoli, M.F.; Crespo-Leiro, M.G.; Laroche, C.; Seferovic, P.M.; Anker, S.D.; Ferrari, R. Clinical phenotypes and outcome of patients hospitalized for acute heart failure: The ESC Heart Failure Long-Term Registry. *Eur. J. Heart Fail.* **2017**, *19*, 1242–1254. [CrossRef] [PubMed]
19. Santos, P.M.; Freire, R.B.; Fernández, A.E.; Sobrino, J.L.B.; Pérez, C.F.; Somoza, F.J.E.; Miguel, C.M.; Vilacosta, I. In-hospital mortality and readmissions for heart failure in Spain. A Study of Index Episodes and 30-Day and 1-year Cardiac Readmissions. *Rev. Española Cardiol.* **2019**, *72*, 998–1004.
20. Yasuda, S.; Nakao, K.; Nishimura, K.; Miyamoto, Y.; Sumita, Y.; Shishido, T.; Anzai, T.; Tsutsui, H.; Ito, H.; Komuro, I.; et al. The Current Status of Cardiovascular Medicine in Japan- Analysis of a Large Number of Health Records From a Nationwide Claim-Based Database, JROAD-DPC. *Circ. J.* **2016**, *80*, 2327–2335. [CrossRef]
21. Nakai, M.; Iwanaga, Y.; Sumita, Y.; Kanaoka, K.; Kawakami, R.; Ishii, M.; Uchida, K.; Nagano, N.; Nakayama, T.; Nishimura, K. Validation of Acute Myocardial Infarction and Heart Failure Diagnoses in Hospitalized Patients with the Nationwide Claim-Based JROAD-DPC Database. *Circ. Rep.* **2021**, *3*, 131–136. [CrossRef] [PubMed]
22. Yamana, H.; Moriwaki, M.; Horiguchi, H.; Kodan, M.; Fushimi, K.; Yasunaga, H. Validity of diagnoses, procedures, and laboratory data in Japanese administrative data. *J. Epidemiol.* **2017**, *27*, 476–482. [CrossRef] [PubMed]

Journal of
Cardiovascular Development and Disease

MDPI

Article

Athlete's Heart in Elite Biathlon, Nordic Cross—Country and Ski-Mountaineering Athletes: Cardiac Adaptions Determined Using Echocardiographic Data

Paul Zimmermann [1,2,3,*], Othmar Moser [3,4], Max L. Eckstein [3], Jan Wüstenfeld [5], Volker Schöffl [2,6,7,8,9], Lukas Zimmermann [2], Martin Braun [1] and Isabelle Schöffl [2,10]

1 Department of Cardiology, Klinikum Bamberg, 96049 Bamberg, Germany; martin.braun@sozialstiftung-bamberg.de
2 Interdisciplinary Center of Sportsmedicine Bamberg, Klinikum Bamberg, 96049 Bamberg, Germany; volker.schoeffl@me.com (V.S.); l.zmann@gmx.de (L.Z.); isabelle.schoeffl@me.com (I.S.)
3 Division of Exercise Physiology and Metabolism, Department of Sport Science, University of Bayreuth, 95440 Bayreuth, Germany; othmar.moser@uni-bayreuth.de (O.M.); Max.Eckstein@unibayreuth.de (M.L.E.)
4 Interdisciplinary Metabolic Medicine Research Group, Division of Endocrinology and Diabetology, Medical University of Graz, 8036 Graz, Austria
5 Insitute for Applied Exercise Science, University Leipzig, 04109 Leipzig, Germany; janwuestenfeld@hotmail.com
6 Department of Traumatology and Orthopaedics, Klinikum Bamberg, 96049 Bamberg, Germany
7 Department of Trauma and Orthopedic Surgery, FAU Erlangen-Nuremberg, 91054 Erlangen, Germany
8 Section Wilderness Medicine, Department of Emergency Medicine, University of Colorado School of Medicine, Denver, CO 80045, USA
9 School of Clinical and Applied Sciences, Leeds Becket University, Leeds LS1 3HE, UK
10 Department of Pediatric Cardiology, University Hospital Erlangen-Nuremberg, 91054 Erlangen, Germany
* Correspondence: paul.zimmermann@arcormail.de; Tel.: +49-951-503-12301

Abstract: Twelve world elite Biathlon (Bia), ten Nordic Cross Country (NCC) and ten ski-mountaineering (Ski-Mo) athletes were evaluated for pronounced echocardiographic physiological cardiac remodeling as a primary aim of our descriptive preliminary report. In this context, sports-related cardiac remodeling was analyzed by performing two-dimensional echocardiography including speckle tracking analysis as left ventricular global longitudinal strain (LV-GLS). A multicenter retrospective analysis of echocardiographic data was performed in 32 elite world winter sports athletes, which were obtained between 2020 and 2021 during the annual medical examination. The matched data of the elite world winter sports athletes (14 women, 18 male athletes, age: 18–35 years) were compared for different echocardiographic parameters. Significant differences could be revealed for left ventricular systolic function (LV-EF, $p = 0.0001$), left ventricular mass index (LV Mass index, $p = 0.0078$), left atrial remodeling by left atrial volume index (LAVI, $p = 0.0052$), and LV-GLS ($p = 0.0003$) between the three professional winter sports disciplines. This report provides new evidence that resting measures of cardiac structure and function in elite winter sport professionals can identify sport specific remodeling of the left heart, against the background of training schedule and training frequency.

Keywords: athlete's heart; Biathlon; Nordic Cross—Country; Ski-mountaineering; cardiac remodeling; echocardiography

1. Introduction

Ski mountaineering (Ski-Mo) is one of the most endurant sports imaginable, as it involves the whole body, mostly performed at altitude involving uphill locomotion, representing a high-energy-demanding elite winter sport [1–6]. Biathlon (Bia) and Nordic Cross Country (NCC) are different to Ski-Mo, yet not less complex and metabolically demanding in their physiological demands, which have been of interest in previous studies [7,8]. The athletic features of these extreme endurance sports should cause pronounced structural and hemodynamical cardiac remodeling of the left heart [9–11]. As the training schedule as well as the conditions during training and competition are comparable between these three winter sports, they represent the athletes in our descriptive preliminary report, in which the most pronounced cardiac adaptations are to be expected.

The term athlete's heart describes different changes and adaptions, namely structural, functional, physiological, and electro-physiological, due to sport-specific cardiac remodeling [12]. Different training stimuli (dynamic vs. static) lead to varying physiological adaptions [13,14]. In this context, especially pronounced changes due to left ventricular (LV) and atrial remodeling can be proven in elite endurance athletes [15]. Inherited and acquired cardiovascular abnormalities such as structural components as hypertrophic cardiomyopathies (HCM), arrhythmogenic ventricular cardiomyopathy (AVCM), or myocarditis—detectable via electrocardiographic (ECG) or echocardiographic evaluation—are sometimes difficult to be distinguished from the physiological adaptations observed in the so-called athlete's heart, especially in athletes performing sports with a high dynamic component [16,17]. Therefore, regular standardized echocardiographic evaluation of athletes is essential, which might contribute to the prevention of undesirable cardiac events in young competitive athletes, because sudden cardiac death in athletes is one of the leading causes of mortality in athletes during sport activities [18–25].

In our preliminary report of elite winter sport athletes, we want to focus on the exercise-induced cardiac remodeling of the athlete's heart by two-dimensional echocardiography including longitudinal peak strain examination [13]. This method, particularly the longitudinal Peak Systolic Strain (LPSS) allows an evaluation of early features of functional and morphological modifications in both ventricles, while conventional morphological echocardiographic parameters fail to distinguish the adaptations in the athlete's heart [13,26–33]. In the last decade, strain analysis by speckle tracking echocardiography has emerged as an effective tool for sports cardiologists to assess the nature of hypertrophy and myocardial contractility especially in athletes [34]. Nevertheless, there is a lack of data about cardiac remodeling in world elite winter sports athletes.

Therefore, the aim of the present descriptive preliminary report is to detect functional and morphological cardiac remodeling in extreme winter sports athlete's heart.

2. Materials and Methods

The local ethics committee of the University of Nurnberg-Erlangen approved the study protocol (17_21 B). The study was conducted in conformity with Good Clinical Practice and the declaration of Helsinki [35]. Before any trial-related activities, our participants were informed about the study protocol and participants gave their written informed consent.

2.1. Study Population

Thirty-two young elite winter sport professionals, all active members of the German National Team, participating in world cups and world championships, were examined during the season 2020/2021. During the severe COVID-19 pandemic situation, no participant was infected or had to be excluded from the analysis due to post-COVID-19 infection syndromes. All participants underwent a sports medicine check-up in their sport medicine performance center—Institute for Applied Exercise Science, University Leipzig and Interdisciplinary Center of Sportsmedicine, Klinikum Bamberg in the preseason preparation summer time. All participants were professional athletes with a total amount of 20–25 training hours per week in high-volume training time and 5–10 training hours in recreation time. Neither arrhythmias nor a known cardiac familiar defect have been detected during their sports career. Figure 1 shows the winter sport professionals selection flowchart.

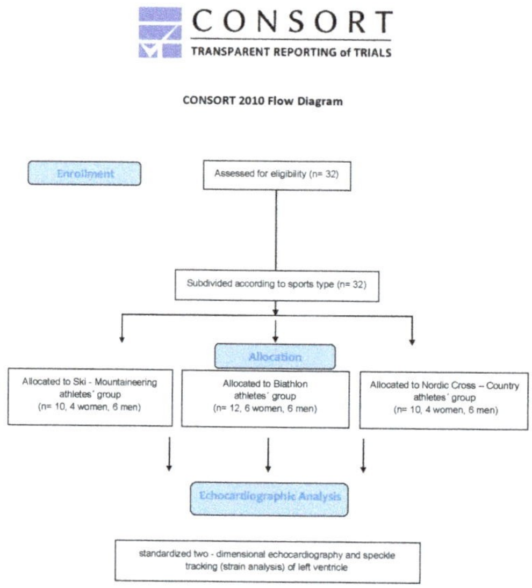

Figure 1. Flowchart of this study.

2.2. Participants Visit

As part of the sports medicine checkup, we performed an echocardiographic functional and morphological assessment using a commercially available echocardiographic system Phillips EPIQ 7 device with an X5-1 aMatrix-array transducer (Phillips Healthcare, Eindhoven, The Netherlands), following a standard protocol [36]. The images were stored and analyzed digitally; for measurements, sequences of at least three heart beats were stored and analyzed. Participants were screened in the preseason preparation summer time and during the echocardiographic examination the heart rate and blood pressure were recorded for the following analysis. Two-dimensional echocardiographic analyses were performed following the general recommendations [36–38]. The systolic LV ejection fraction (LV-EF) was estimated and calculated using biplane Simpson rule, based on the apical four—as well as the apical two-chamber view. Two-dimensional linear dimensions for both ventricles and both atria were performed manually according to the recommendations [36–38]. An estimation of the right ventricular (RV) systolic function using the TAPSE (Tricuspide anular plane systolic excursion) was obtained in the apical four chamber view.

Based on the two-dimensional echocardiographic measurements, the left ventricular mass index (LV Mass index) was calculated with a validated method [39], the relative wall thickness (RWT) of the left ventricle (LV) was calculated as (2× posterior wall thickness)/LVedd [39], and the left atrial volume index (LAVI) was obtained with a validated method for each participant [40].

For assessment of the LV diastolic function, we measured the pulse-wave Doppler in the apical four-chamber view referring to the peak early filling (E wave) and late diastolic filling (A wave) velocities. A tissue Doppler imaging of the lateral mitral anulus in the apical four chamber view was performed (peak early velocity E′) [36,37].

Furthermore, a LV speckle tracking analysis of the athlete's heart was recorded, focusing on the LV-GLS pattern by two-dimensional strain in the apical views. We focused on the analysis of the LV and did not perform RV strain analysis.

Each of the participants was evaluated for the prevalence of right and left heart valve regurgitation as part of the standard echocardiographic assessment.

2.3. Statistical Analyses

Data were analyzed with Graph Pad Prism 8.2.1(279) (Graph Pad Software; San Diego, CA, USA) and Minitap statistic program (Minitab Inc.; State College, PA, USA). Our sample size was not normally distributed; therefore, we evaluated our numerical data group comparisons for ten Ski-Mo athletes, ten NCC athletes, and twelve elite Bia athletes using the analysis of variance testing (ANOVA) and nonparametric testing with post-hoc testing ($p < 0.05$). Afterwards, a gender-specific analysis for the interesting parameters was utilized equally.

3. Results

3.1. Baseline Characterictics and Echocardiographic Assessment

A total of 32 young professional winter sports athletes were examined. The matched data of the three different winter sports were compared for different echocardiographic parameters. In the two-dimensional echocardiographic examination, all participating elite winter sports athletes showed a low–normal to normal LV-EF estimated by the biplane Simpson method and did not show any relevant regurgitation of the left and right heart valves, except mild regurgitation at the mitral and tricuspid valve without any relevant systolic pulmonary artery pressure evaluated by tricuspid peak systolic velocity analysis. The heart rate at baseline as well as the blood pressure were quite low in this elite winter sport population. Anthropometric and echocardiographic data are shown in Tables 1 and 2.

Our measurement values were evaluated referring to the new standards and reference values in standardized transthoracic echocardiography as reported in the 2020 guidelines of the German Society of Cardiology (DGK) for untrained sedentary controls [38].

3.2. Morpholgical and Functional Cardiac Remodeling

All athletes showed a normal systolic LV-EF, but the Bia athletes showed a significantly higher normal systolic LV-EF compared to Ski-Mo and NCC athletes (results shown in Table 2). In this context, analyzing the sex-specific differences of this parameter across the three disciplines, the female Bia-athletes showed a significantly higher LV-EF, compared to Ski-Mo and NCC athletes, whereby in our male participants no significant differences for LV-EF could be revealed (results shown in Table 2). The LV Mass index was calculated as an indexed parameter for all three different winter sports professionals and we could reveal significantly higher values for NCC and Bia athletes in comparison to Ski-Mo athletes (results shown in Table 2 and Figure 2). In this context, Bia and NCC athletes showed a significantly higher RWT in comparison to Ski-Mo athletes (results shown in Table 2).

Table 1. Baseline winter sport professional characteristics. Anthropometric data of the Ski-Mo, NCC and Biathlon athletes.

	Ski–Mo $n = 10$		NCC $n = 10$		Biathletes $n = 12$	
	Male $n = 6$	Female $n = 4$	Male $n = 6$	Female $n = 4$	Male $n = 6$	Female $n = 6$
Age (y)	21.2 ± 1.9	20.8 ± 2.4	26.3 ± 4.1	25.5 ± 0.5	27.3 ± 3.6	29.0 ± 3.2
Height (cm)	178.4 ± 3.7	163.5 ± 8.8	181.3 ± 4.7	171.2 ± 5.8	180.9 ± 5.1	172.8 ± 3.7
Weight (kg)	67.5 ± 0.5	53.2 ± 6.5	72.0 ± 3.0	63.4 ± 5.9	77.1 ± 3.7	62.5 ± 4.1
BMI (kg/m^2)	18.9 ± 1.7	19.8 ± 0.4	22.0 ± 1.1	21.6 ± 1.2	23.6 ± 0.9	20.9 ± 1.0
Resting Blood Pressure	120 ± 5.6	100 ± 8.2	125 ± 8.3	105 ± 7.2	117 ± 7.6	108 ± 6.2
Systolic/Diastolic (mmHg)	82 ± 3.5	72 ± 1.5	78 ± 2.9	71 ± 3.8	77 ± 2.2	70 ± 3.3
Resting Heart Rate (bpm)	40 ± 5.6	44 ± 4.5	42 ± 3.6	46 ± 5.1	41 ± 4.2	45 ± 5.1
BSA (body surface area m^2)	1.75 ± 0.08	1.61 ± 0.12	1.88 ± 0.04	1.81 ±0.07	1.92 ± 0.04	1.77 ± 0.05

Data are presented as a median with standard deviation.

Table 2. Echocardiographic measurements (mean ± SD) of the Ski-mountaineering, Nordic Cross—Country and Biathlon athletes.

	Ski-Mo (I) $n = 10$		NCC (II) $n = 10$		Biathletes (III) $n = 12$		*p*-Value
	Male $n = 6$	Female $n = 4$	Male $n = 6$	Female $n = 4$	Male $n = 6$	Female $n = 6$	
LV edd (mm)	50.83 ± 4.22	45.25 ± 5.96	55.50 ± 3.83	50.75 ± 3.50	55.50 ± 5.24	49.50 ± 1.52	ns
	48.6 ± 5.48		53.6 ± 4.27		52.5 ± 4.83		
LV Mass Index (g/m^2)	97.2 ± 25.2	76.3 ± 26.7	130.7 ± 16.5	106 ± 16.4	133.5 ± 20.6	102.3 ± 14.8	0.0078 *
	88.8 ± 26.6 *		120.8 ± 20.1 *		117.9 ± 23.6 *		
Relative Wall Thickness RWT	0.38 ± 0.03	0.34 ± 0.06	0.40 ± 0.04	0.41 ± 0.04	0.40 ± 0.04	0.42 ± 0.04	Ski-Mo vs. NCC 0.0230 * Ski-Mo vs. Bia 0.0230 *
	0.37 ± 0.05		0.41 ± 0.03		0.41 ± 0.04		
IVSd (mm)	8.67 ± 1.97	8.25 ± 2.50	11.00 ± 0.63	10.50 ± 0.58	10.83 ± 0.98	9.67 ± 1.37	Ski-Mo vs. NCC 0.0266 *, Ski-Mo vs. Bia 0.0337 *
	8.5 ± 2.07		10.4 ± 1.17		10.3 ± 1.29		
LVPWs (mm)	9.97 ± 1.03	7.75 ± 1.50	11.17 ± 0.41	10.50 ± 0.58	12.33 ± 2.07	10.17 ± 1.17	Ski-Mo vs. NCC 0.0161 * Ski-Mo vs. Bia 0.0030 *
	8.9 ± 1.52		10.9 ± 0.57		11.3 ± 1.96		
E/A	2.18 ± 0.58	1.98 ± 0.17	2.48 ± 0.26	2.40 ± 0.77	1.97 ± 0.52	1.75 ± 0.40	NCC vs. Bia 0.0166 *
	2.1 ± 0.45		2.5 ± 0.49		1.9 ± 0.46		
E/E′	6.75 ± 1.71	7 ± 1.79	6.80 ± 0.86	6.13 ± 1.22	7 ± 0.86	6.37 ± 1.04	ns
	6.9 ± 1.66		6.4 ± 1.09		6.7 ± 0.97		
LAVI (mL/m^2)	51.83 ± 12.1	46.25 ± 11.1	150 ± 84.58	89.3 ± 45.7	117.5 ± 37.7	72.8 ± 19.6	0.0052 *
	49.6 ± 11.4		125.7 ± 75.2		95.2 ± 36.9		
RA (cm^2)	19.17 ± 3.87	16.75 ± 2.87	24.83 ± 3.73	18.28 ± 4.72	20.78 ± 3.64	15.50 ± 2.40	ns
	18.2 ± 3.55		22.2 ± 5.16		18.1 ± 4.03		
LV–EF	60,33 ± 4.08	58.00 ± 5.60	61.17 ± 4.96	59.50 ± 4.80	65.83 ± 5.38	73.00 ± 4.34	0.0001 *
	59.4 ± 4.60		60.5 ± 4.70		69.4 ± 5.98		
GLS	−18.26 ± 2.21	−18.83 ± 2.93	−21.21 ± 1.99	−23.25 ± 3.23	−22.62 ± 1.26	−22.34 ± 1.42	0.0003 *
	−18.5 ± 2.38		−22.0 ± 2.61		−22.5±1.29		

Data are presented as mean with standard deviation. *p* value *, statistically significant ($p < 0.05$). Abbreviations: LV edd, left ventricle enddiastolic size; LV, left ventricular; IVSd, interventricular septal wall thickness at diastole; LVPWd, left ventricular posterior wall thickness at diastole; E/A and E/E, parameters for diastolic function of the left ventricle; LAVI, left atrial volume index; RA, right atrium; LV-EF, left ventricular systolic ejection fraction; GLS, global longitudinal strain; ns, non-significant.

Significant differences could be revealed in the echocardiographic analysis referring to LA remodeling of world elite athletes. The LAVI (mL/m^2) was significantly enlarged in our NCC and Bia athletes in comparison to Ski-Mo athletes (results shown in Table 2 and Figure 3). Even sex-related differences between the three subdisciplines could be revealed for male NCC and Bia female athletes, which had significantly larger LAVI than the Ski-Mo athletes (results shown in Table 2).

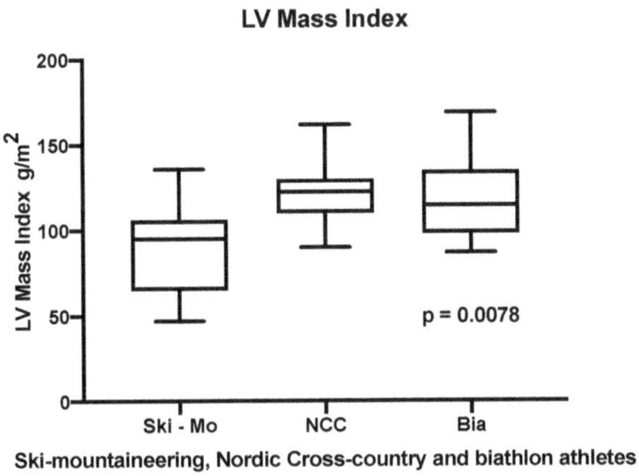

Figure 2. Left ventricular mass index significantly differs in elite winter sports athletes ($p = 0.0078$).

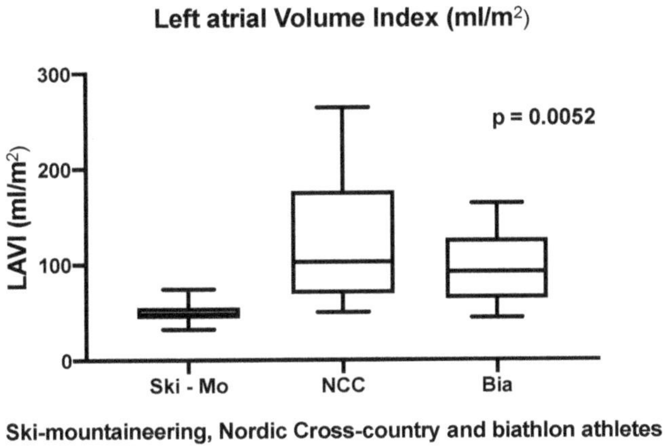

Figure 3. Analysis of the left atrial volume index (LAVI)—significant different results defined by the athletic sporting discipline ($p = 0.0052$).

The athletes differed significantly with regards to the eccentric remodeling of the LV, especially for the interventricular septal wall diameter (IVSd), the left ventricular posterior wall diameter (LVPWd) and RWT. NCC and Bia athletes showed thicker wall diameters than the Ski-Mo athletes, as shown in the Table 2. The gender-specific subanalysis revealed thicker LV wall diameter in the male and female NCC and Bia athletes than in the Ski-Mo athletes (results shown in Table 2).

After proving sport-specific LA cardiac remodeling, the comparison of E/A and E/E′ ratio as criteria for LV diastolic function, revealed significant differences between NCC athletes and Bia athletes with respect to E/A, but not with respect to E/E′. The gender-specific subgroup analysis could not reach significant differences (results shown in Table 2).

No significant results could be revealed for the left ventricle end-diastolic size (LVedd), for the end-diastolic volume (LV EDVedd), the right heart dimensions as right atrial end-systolic diameter (RA endsyst) and right ventricular end-diastolic size (RV edd) as well as the TAPSE of RV in our three different elite winter sport disciplines. The sex-specific analysis across the three cohorts did not reach significant differences for the mentioned five parameters either, i.e., LVedd, LV EDVedd, RA endsyst, RV edd and TAPSE (LVedd and RA endsyst, results shown in Table 2).

Focusing on the speckle tracking analysis with the main emphasis on the LV-GLS, significant differences defined by the athletic sporting discipline could be proven in our small cohort as represented in Figure 4, whereas the LV-GLS significantly differed in men with Ski-Mo athletes having the lowest values ($p = 0.0003$, shown in Table 2).

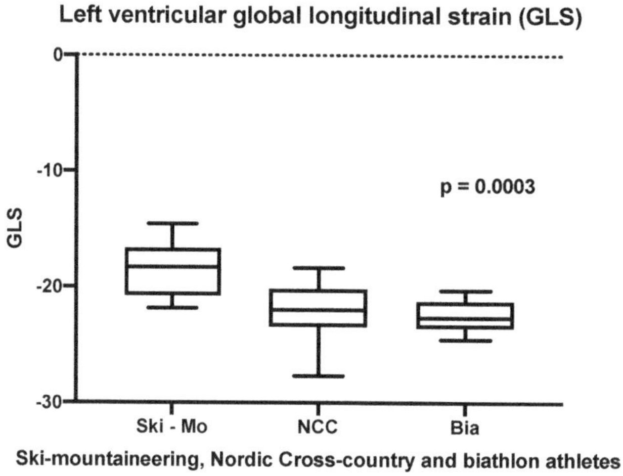

Figure 4. Analysis of the LV-GLS—significant differences defined by the athletic sporting discipline ($p = 0.0003$).

Our measurements of the preliminary descriptive report were compared with the stated data of the German Society of Cardiology (DGK) position statement paper 2020 as generally sedentary control measurements, as presented in Table 3. Therefore, the LVedd diameter in our athletes is estimated to be normal for male participating athletes and in the upper normal range for female participants, and athletes' LV-EF is estimated in the normal range for both. Our LV Mass index measurements, especially in the Bia and NCC athletes, have to be categorized in the upper normal to light extended range in comparison to the DGK sedentary controls. Remodeling of the LV, represented by IVSd and LVPWd, is classified in the upper normal to lightly thickened range in comparison to the DGK recommendations, especially in the Bia and NCC athletes.

Table 3. Comparison of our structural two dimensional echocardiographic data to the stated control data of the position statement paper of DGK (German Society of Cardiology, 2020).

Parameter	OUR Study Data		Reference Value Male	Reference Value Female
	Total Male ($n = 18$)	Total Female ($n = 14$)		
LV edd (mm)	53.9 ± 4.8	48.6 ± 4.1	42–58	38–52
LV-EF (%)	62.4 ± 5.2	64.9 ± 8.6	52–72	54–74
LV Mass Index (g/m^2)	120.4 ± 26.1	95.9 ± 21.9	49–115	43–95
IVSd (mm)	10.2 ± 1.7	9.2 ± 1.7	6–10	6–9
LVPWd (mm)	11.1 ± 1.7	9.6 ± 1.6	6–10	6–9

Data are presented as mean with standard deviation. LV edd, left ventricular enddiastolic size; LV-EF, left ventricular systolic ejection fraction; LV, left ventricular; IVSd, interventricular septal wall thickness at diastole; LVPWd, left ventricular posterior wall thickness at diastole; mm, millimeter; g, grams; m^2, square meters.

4. Discussion

In the present descriptive preliminary report, the morphological and functional cardiac remodeling due to high-performance competition and training volume in elite winter sports athletes was investigated for the first time. The investigated winter sports in this study represent the most endurant competitive sports as they involve the whole body, are often performed at altitude and are associated with high and intense energy demands [1–3,7,8]. They combine ET and ST training components, and include mainly dynamic (isotonic) but also to a lesser degree static (isometric) elements [41].

4.1. Impact of Two Dimensional Echocardiography on Morpholgical and Functional Cardiac Remodeling of the Athlete's Left Heart

The characteristics of the athlete's heart have been investigated mostly in the LV as described by Utomi et al. [15]. The analysis of the systolic LV-EF in our elite winter sport professionals revealed, across the cohorts, significant differences of this weak parameter as seen for higher systolic LV-EF values for our Bia athletes. These results have to be handled carefully due to the fact that all athletes showed a normal systolic LV-EF and that other studies did not reveal significant differences between athletes and non-athletes [42,43]. Our Ski-Mo athletes showed the lowest, but still normal, systolic LV-EF parameters.

Of the three disciplines, Ski-Mo represents the sport with the highest endurance component during training [2]. Most of their training regimen happens at or around ventilatory threshold 1 (VT1). The consequence is an associated bradycardia tendency and a low systolic cardiac function (LV-EF) at rest, when the heart works at a low capacity. In this context, the heart rate and blood pressure at baseline were quite low, as a common known phenomenon in elite athletes [23].

The LVedd and LV EDVedd did not reveal significant differences in our investigated groups of elite athletes, which showed a tendency for bradycardia in general, what has to be taken into consideration by evaluating this parameter. Another morphological remodeling key aspect is the induced LV hypertrophy in older athletes. Therefore, we evaluated in our cohorts the LV mass index, whereby Ski-Mo athletes showed significant lower values compared to NCC and Bia athletes as demonstrated in Table 2.

These results must be handled carefully since the results may be due to inter-group differences in age, height and weight, BMI and BSA. Interindividual differences determined the group of Ski-Mo athletes as the physically smallest and youngest athletes, which might contribute to the obtained differences. Besides the physical status, the differences up to training schedules have to be taken into consideration. All participants in this study were professional athletes with a total amount of 20–25 training hours per week, but the Ski-Mo athletes were the youngest athlete category, with the fewest life time training hours and less years of participation as an elite athlete. The main training focus in Ski-Mo athletes is set on ET sessions, whereas ST sessions represent an essential part in Bia and NCC athletes' training schedule. These circumstances have to be taken into consideration while investigating the progress of exercise-induced cardiac remodeling. Generally, a greater wall thickness of the LV is observed in athletes focusing on ST, i.e., static aspects [44]. In our cohort, these athletes are represented by the NCC and Bia athletes with greater wall thickness than Ski-Mo athletes, while the Ski-Mo athletes show a tendency for eccentric left ventricular wall remodeling due to the higher dynamic aspect of their training. These results—especially proportionately larger LV walls—were firstly proposed and described by Morganroth, but represent a quite common finding, even in our athletes [45]. These variable circumstances have to be taken into consideration once again, while evaluating sport-specific cardiac remodeling, mostly influenced by different aspects due to th the athlete's constitution and different training variables. Nevertheless, our analyzed participants number is small, due to the fact that we only investigated athletes from the German national teams competing at world-class events. Our study has a rather small sample size which is restricted due to the limited spots on a national team. Consequently, drawing a conclusion or reflecting our results for the general population being involved in Ski-Mo,

Bia or NCC would be misleading. Furthermore, as mentioned in the limitations section of our manuscript, an interobserver variability with respect to measurement acquirement must be considered.

Sports-specific remodeling consisted of left heart dimension adaption [46], in a concentric remodeling of the LV. This emerging concentric hypertrophy might be an adaption to sports-specific dynamic efforts in winter sports, but may also be a marker of a beginning heart disease and a regular routine analysis might contribute to prevention of sudden cardiac death in athletes. Our descriptive reporting of significant differences could be proven for LV remodeling, represented as following by RWT and data of LV wall diameters. These trends in data analysis have to be handled carefully due to the mentioned aspects of small size, variable training schedule and physical differences as proven by BMI and BSA inter-athlete differences. Nevertheless, these results show interesting tendencies, which should be confirmed in future studies with a greater number of participants.

In this controversy of training-related cardiac adaption and functional remodeling versus a beginning balanced cardiomyopathy in male endurance athletes, new insights were provided by Utomi et al. [15]. The authors noted morphological features, above all left heart remodeling, with enlarged left heart structures in male athletes in general.

In our study, LA remodeling was observed especially in NCC and Bia athletes. Our evaluated parameter, LAVI, revealed in our small number of participants significantly different results, which implies significantly higher values for the NCC and Bia athletes compared to Ski-Mo athletes. These athletes are represented mainly as a homogenously young and physically small group of male and women athletes. Therefore, our results have to handled with care and can only serve as a description of structural cardiac remodeling of world professional winter sport athletes. Nevertheless, LA remodeling has been described as a typical characteristic in endurance athletes [46]. However, this common finding in highly trained endurance athletes might contribute to the development of an atrial cardiomyopathy, which is characterized by LA enlargement and fibrosis. There is some evidence that an accumulation of lifetime training hours and participation in competitions plays an important role for this development [25,47]. In this context, our results have to handled with care due to the clinical presentation of our athletes, which have even an increased risk for developing an atrial cardiomyopathy during their career and afterwards. These findings might also suggest an atrial remodeling due to firstly structural LAVI as well as secondly to functional remodeling, represented as LA passive and total emptying fraction. Kasikcioglu et al. revealed positive correlations between VO_{2max} and LA passive emptying fraction, which might contribute to improved exercise capacity in athletes and improved cardiac output during exercise [48]. On the other hand, Klasnja et al. found a mild association between measurement of resting left heart cardiac structure and function and peak cardiac output performance, whereas the interpretation of the association should be considered carefully, even in our presented data [49].

The functional remodeling of the LV can be evaluated using the peak early to late diastolic filling ration (E/A ratio) and tissue doppler analysis (E/E′ratio). Higher values are observed in athletes in comparison to non-athletes [50]. We found similar results in our study, which is comparable to previously published data [15]. However, functional remodeling is a controversially discussed topic, as the enhanced maximal cardiac output could be a consequence of enhanced diastolic function on the one hand but is also influenced by putative mechanisms such as volume preload or intrinsic relaxation conditions on the other hand [51]. Our descriptive results emphasize the training-induced adaptations in athletes, which support the thesis of a balanced cardiomyopathy that is supposed to be physiological, but has to be judged with respect to the specific sport and the lifetime training hours. A higher diastolic capacity of the LV might be explained by lower heart rates at rest, improved hemodynamic effects and an increased vagal component in athletes [50].

Nevertheless, discussing the specific cardiac remodeling of the winter sport elite athlete's heart, it has to be stated clearly that the prognostic value of reported echocardiographic assessment is limited and does not provide sensitive results for at least two frequent conditions of sudden cardiac death in athlete's heart. Firstly, coronary artery anomalies and secondly the non-compaction cardiomyopathy of the LV cannot be sensitively detected or ruled out by two-dimensional echocardiographic assessment. Therefore, further cardiac imaging techniques, such as computer tomography or cardiac MRI should be considered [52–54]. In this context, the cardiac MRI screening of Angelini et al. could reveal 1.3% of young people to have high risk cardiovascular conditions, with a surprisingly high value of unknown LV non-compaction cardiomyopathy in this cohort of adolescents. These MRI-based screening protocols might pave the road to accurately identify potential deadly cardiac abnormalities and prevent sudden cardiac death [52].

4.2. Global Longitudinal Strain (GLS) Analysis of the Athlete's Left Ventricle in Winter Sport Professionals

Echocardiographic two-dimensional speckle tracking is a modern method for identifying subtle differences in the adaption of LV strain cardiac pattern or twist mechanism of the LV in athletes [27]. The distinction between physiological adaption and inherited or acquired HCM can be improved by using LV-GLS. In this context, normal LV-GLS is reported between −18% and −25% in healthy individuals, whereas strain imaging in general can reveal early changes and functional abnormalities in cardiac mechanics long before structural damages can be detected [55–57]. In our study limited by the small number of participating athletes, LV-GLS was slightly reduced in Ski-Mo—when compared to NCC and Bia athletes. On the one hand, as mentioned above, Ski-Mo athletes are represented mainly as a homogenously young and physically small group of male and female athletes with less life time training hours compared to the career of the athletes in NCC and Bia. It must be mentioned that our measurements are in the normal range of healthy subjects and were adapted in the preseason preparation summer time. Further sport-season specific echocardiographic follow-ups might be an interesting scientific research topic to evaluate the reversal of echocardiographic strain rate in the context of training intensity and training-related cardiac volume load. An interobserver variability might also finally contribute to our reported slightly existing differences between the different winter sport professionals. Nevertheless, our data confirm previous findings in which highly trained Olympic athletes showed normal GLS and strain rate parameters of the LV with merely mild differences compared with untrained controls [28]. On the other hand, different patterns of LV deformation mechanics were revealed early in young footballers [11,29]. In the end, subtle physiological differences of LV strain pattern analysis have to be interpreted with respect to the performed sport, as reported by Beaumont et al. [27]. In the end, our results emphasize the training-induced adaptions in athlete's heart and although an atrial cardiomyopathy can not be stated clearly, there is evidence for an increased risk for degeneration from a balanced physiological cardiomyopathy to a pathological entity within the lifetime of a sports career. In this context, additional information might be provided by detection of atrial fibrosis in the cardiac MRI.

4.3. Impact of Two Dimensional Echocardiography on Morpholgical and Functional Cardiac Remodeling of the Athlete's Right Heart

The right side of the heart in athletes has also received some interest in the past as well as in the current scientific view. In a systematic review in athletes, Ascenzi et al. [58] detected training-induced RV enlargement. However, RV dilatation is a common phenotypic expression and a differential diagnosis for ARVC. Therefore, the sports-specific background needs to be taken into account in order to discriminate physiological adaption from cardiomyopathies. As a limitation, we did not perform RV strain analysis in our study, nevertheless this topic represents an interesting tool for functional right heart remodeling. In this context, an improved RV apical strain in comparison to a decrease of RV strain in the basal segments is described in athletes in various studies. The specific regional differences within the RV are highlighted, with a broad variability among athletes and in terms of training load [59–61]. Morphological right heart adaption in elite endurance athletes is a common finding in several studies [50], and is reported to show greater right heart remodeling than in ST athletes and untrained controls [62]. Our elite winter sport athletes, which are characterized by ET as a major component as well as speed- and ST units [63], showed comparable results with age- and sex-matched normal data when investigating the right heart echocardiographic parameters (RA and RV size, TAPSE). There was no significant difference between our three elite winter sport professional athlete's groups. However, changes in the right heart are reported to be small and do not prohibit peak performance [50]. Regarding all these different morphological parameters and influencing circumstancing facts, due to the small number of participants, different anatomical athletes' structure and training schedules, our findings can provide guidance for further investigation with a greater number of participating athletes.

4.4. Limitations

Our study has several limitations as mentioned above in the discussion. First of all, the number of professional winter sport athletes is relatively small which is due to the fact that we only investigated high-level athletes from the German national teams competing at world-class events. Secondly, Ski-Mo athletes were the youngest athlete category, implying fewer lifetime training hours and showed a smaller physical constitution than NCC and Bia athletes—these circumstances have to be taken into consideration, while evaluating sport-specific cardiac remodeling and we agree that our paper should be likely regarded as an interesting descriptive preliminary report. Furthermore, the echocardiographic analyses of the participating athletes were performed in a multicenter study design, so that an interobserver variability with respect to measurement acquirement must be considered on the one hand. On the other hand, the mixture of young and experienced athletes especially in the NCC and Bia athlete cohort entails an interindividual variability in relation to anatomical habitus, lifetime training hours and training schedule variability, which might contribute to a certain standard deviation in our measurements. Thirdly, the multicenter measurement was performed in the preseason preparation time in summer. This condition associated with individual training schedules might contribute to individual athlete's heart volume change and result in this difference. Our functional left ventricular analysis has been focused on the LV-GLS and not on the circumferential strain analysis of the LV. No specific strain analysis has been performed in the RV, which is an important limitation of this study and might be performed in further investigations.

5. Conclusions

This is the first study to present data of world class winter sports athletes and morphological and functional remodeling of the left heart.

Our results have to be handled with care due to the mentioned limitations and serve as a preliminary report. Therefore, our results analysis—in general as well as in the gender-specific subgroup—can identify physiological differences in functional and morphological cardiac remodeling, especially due to LV-EF and LV mass index, LA remodeling as measured by LAVI, and differences in the speckle tracking analysis, focusing the LV-GLS. Nevertheless, the individual morphological and secondary functional adaption of the athlete's heart have to be interpreted carefully due to the different types of sports and lifetime training hours. From this aspect, future studies should consider a greater number of participating athletes to verify the impact on sport-specific cardiac remodeling and to further strengthen the evidence base.

Author Contributions: Data curation, P.Z., O.M. and L.Z.; Formal analysis, O.M., M.B. and I.S.; Investigation, P.Z., J.W. and V.S.; Methodology, P.Z. and I.S.; Project administration, P.Z.; Supervision, I.S.; Writing—original draft, P.Z. and I.S.; Writing—review & editing, O.M., J.W., V.S., L.Z., M.L.E. and M.B. All authors have read and agreed to the published version of the manuscript.

Funding: This research received no external funding.

Institutional Review Board Statement: The study was conducted according to the guidelines of the Declaration of Helsinki, and approved by the Ethics Committee of the University of Nurnberg-Erlangen (study protocol 17_21 B).

Informed Consent Statement: Informed consent was obtained from all subjects involved in the study.

Data Availability Statement: Individual anonymized data supporting the analyses of this study contained in this manuscript will be made available upon reasonable written request from researchers whose proposed use of data for a specific purpose has been approved.

Acknowledgments: We want to thank the participants, which were examined in both sport medicine performance center—i.e., Institute for Applied Exercise Science, University Leipzig and Interdisciplinary Center of Sportsmedicine, Klinikum Bamberg. The author thanks Jochen Endrejat for statistical support.

Conflicts of Interest: The authors declare no conflict of interest.

Abbreviations

Bia = Biathletes, NCC = Nordic Cross—Country, Ski-Mo = Ski mountaineering, GLS = global longitudinal strain, HCM = hypertrophic cardiomyopathies, AVCM = arrhythmogenic ventricular cardiomyopathy, LV = left ventricle, LV-EF = left ventricular systolic function, LV edd = left ventricular enddiastolic diameter, BSA = body surface area, LV Mass Index = left ventricular mass index, RA = right atrium, LA = left atrium, LAVI = left atrial volume index, RV = right ventricular, TAPSE = Tricuspide anular plane systolic excursion, RWT = relative wall thickness, ANOVA = analysis of variance testing, BMI = Body mass index, IVSd = interventricular septal wall thickness at diastole, LVPWd = left ventricular posterior wall thickness at diastole, E/A and E/E′= parameters for diastolic function of the left ventricle, DGK = German Society of Cardiology, VT1 = ventilatory threshold 1, ET = endurance training, ST = strength training.

References

1. Buskirk, E.R.; Kollias, J.; Akers, R.F.; Prokop, E.K.; Reategui, E.P. Maximal performance at altitude and on return from altitude in conditioned runners. *J. Appl. Physiol.* **1967**, *23*, 259–266. [CrossRef] [PubMed]
2. Duc, S.; Cassirame, J.; Durand, F. Physiology of Ski Mountaineering Racing. *Int. J. Sports Med.* **2011**, *32*, 856–863. [CrossRef]
3. Menz, V.; Niedermeier, M.; Stehle, R.; Mugele, H.; Faulhaber, M. Assessment of Maximal Aerobic Capacity in Ski Mountaineering: A Laboratory-Based Study. *Int. J. Environ. Res. Public Health* **2021**, *18*, 7002. [CrossRef]
4. Tosi, P.; Leonardi, A.; Schena, L. The energy cost of ski mountaineering: Effects of speed and ankle loading. *J. Sport Med. Phys. Fit.* **2009**, *49*, 25–29.
5. Armstrong, R.B.; Laughlin, M.H.; Rome, L.; Taylor, C.R. Metabolism of rats running up and down an incline. *J. Appl. Physiol.* **1983**, *55*, 518–521. [CrossRef]
6. Balducci, P.; Clémençon, M.; Morel, B.; Quiniou, G.; Saboul, D.; Hautier, C.A. Comparison of Level and Graded Treadmill Tests to Evaluate Endurance Mountain Runners. *J. Sports Sci. Med.* **2016**, *15*, 239–246. [PubMed]
7. Jonsson Kårström, M.; McGawley, K.; Laaksonen, M.S. Physiological Responses to Rifle Carriage during Roller-Skiing in Elite Biathletes. *Front. Physiol.* **2019**, *10*, 1519. [CrossRef]
8. Laaksonen, M.S.; Andersson, E.; Jonsson Kårström, M.; Lindblom, H.; McGawley, K. Laboratory-Based Factors Predicting Skiing Performance in Female and Male Biathletes. *Front. Sports Act. Living* **2020**, *2*, 99. [CrossRef] [PubMed]
9. Karlstedt, E.; Chelvanathan, A.; da Silva, M.; Cleverley, K.; Kumar, K.; Bhullar, N.; Lytwyn, M.; Bohonis, S.; Oomah, S.; Nepomuceno, R.; et al. The impact of repeated marathon running on cardiovascular function in the aging population. *J. Cardiovasc. Magn. Reson.* **2012**, *14*, 58. [CrossRef]
10. Galderisi, M.; Cosyns, B.; Edvardsen, T.; Cardim, N.; Delgado, V.; di Salvo, G.; Donal, E.; Sade, L.E.; Ernande, L.; Garbi, M.; et al. Standardization of adult transthoracic echocardiography reporting in agreement with recent chamber quantification, diastolic function, and heart valve disease recommendations: An expert consensus document of the European Association of Cardiovascular Imaging. *Eur. Heart J.-Cardiovasc. Imaging* **2017**, *18*, 1301–1310. [CrossRef]
11. Stefani, L.; Toncelli, L.; di Tante, V.; Vono, M.C.R.; Cappelli, B.; Pedrizzetti, G.; Galanti, G. Supernormal functional reserve of apical segments in elite soccer players: An ultrasound speckle tracking handgrip stress study. *Cardiovasc. Ultrasound* **2008**, *6*, 14. [CrossRef]
12. Chandra, N.; Bastiaenen, R.; Papadakis, M.; Sharma, S. Sudden Cardiac Death in Young Athletes. *J. Am. Coll. Cardiol.* **2013**, *61*, 1027–1040. [CrossRef] [PubMed]

13. Stefani, L.; Toncelli, L.; Gianassi, M.; Manetti, P.; di Tante, V.; Vono, M.R.C.; Moretti, A.; Cappelli, B.; Pedrizzetti, G.; Galanti, G. Two-dimensional tracking and TDI are consistent methods for evaluating myocardial longitudinal peak strain in left and right ventricle basal segments in athletes. *Cardiovasc. Ultrasound* **2007**, *5*, 7. [CrossRef] [PubMed]
14. Szauder, I.; Kovács, A.; Pavlik, G. Comparison of left ventricular mechanics in runners versus bodybuilders using speckle tracking echocardiography. *Cardiovasc. Ultrasound* **2015**, *13*, 7. [CrossRef] [PubMed]
15. Utomi, V.; Oxborough, D.; Whyte, G.P.; Somauroo, J.; Sharma, S.; Shave, R.; Atkinson, G.; George, K. Systematic review and meta-analysis of training mode, imaging modality and body size influences on the morphology and function of the male athlete's heart. *Heart* **2013**, *99*, 1727–1733. [CrossRef]
16. Pelliccia, A.; Maron, B.J.; Spataro, A.; Proschan, M.A.; Spirito, P. The Upper Limit of Physiologic Cardiac Hypertrophy in Highly Trained Elite Athletes. *N. Engl. J. Med.* **1991**, *324*, 295–301. [CrossRef] [PubMed]
17. Sharma, S.; Merghani, A.; Mont, L. Exercise and the heart: The good, the bad, and the ugly. *Eur. Heart J.* **2015**, *36*, 1445–1453. [CrossRef]
18. Galanti, G.; Toncelli, L.; Tosi, B.; Orlandi, M.; Giannelli, C.; Stefani, L.; Mascherini, G.; Modesti, P.A. Evaluation of left ventricular remodelling in young Afro-Caribbean athletes. *Cardiovasc. Ultrasound* **2019**, *17*, 20. [CrossRef]
19. Maron, B.J. Structural features of the athlete heart as defined by echocardiography. *J. Am. Coll. Cardiol.* **1986**, *7*, 190–203. [CrossRef]
20. Maron, B.J.; Doerer, J.J.; Haas, T.S.; Tierney, D.M.; Mueller, F.O. Sudden Deaths in Young Competitive Athletes. *Circulation.* **2009**, *119*, 1085–1092. [CrossRef]
21. Maron, B.J.; Epstein, S.E.; Roberts, W.C. Causes of sudden death in competitive athletes. *J. Am. Coll. Cardiol.* **1986**, *7*, 204–214. [CrossRef]
22. Maron, B.J.; Haas, T.S.; Ahluwalia, A.; Rutten-Ramos, S.C. Incidence of cardiovascular sudden deaths in Minnesota high school athletes. *Heart Rhythm* **2013**, *10*, 374–377. [CrossRef]
23. Galanti, G.; Stefani, L.; Mascherini, G.; di Tante, V.; Toncelli, L. Left ventricular remodeling and the athlete's heart, irrespective of quality load training. *Cardiovasc. Ultrasound* **2016**, *14*, 46. [CrossRef] [PubMed]
24. Guasch, E.; Benito, B.; Qi, X.; Cifelli, C.; Naud, P.; Shi, Y.; Mighiu, A.; Tardif, J.-C.; Tadevosyan, A.; Chen, Y.; et al. Atrial Fibrillation Promotion by Endurance Exercise. *J. Am. Coll. Cardiol.* **2013**, *62*, 68–77. [CrossRef] [PubMed]
25. Wilhelm, M. Atrial fibrillation in endurance athletes. *Eur. J. Prev. Cardiol.* **2014**, *21*, 1040–1048. [CrossRef] [PubMed]
26. Stefani, L.; Pedrizzetti, G.; de Luca, A.; Mercuri, R.; Innocenti, G.; Galanti, G. Real-time evaluation of longitudinal peak systolic strain (speckle tracking measurement) in left and right ventricles of athletes. *Cardiovasc. Ultrasound* **2009**, *7*, 17. [CrossRef]
27. Beaumont, A.; Grace, F.; Richards, J.; Hough, J.; Oxborough, D.; Sculthorpe, N. Left Ventricular Speckle Tracking-Derived Cardiac Strain and Cardiac Twist Mechanics in Athletes: A Systematic Review and Meta-Analysis of Controlled Studies. *Sports Med.* **2017**, *47*, 1145–1170. [CrossRef]
28. Caselli, S.; Montesanti, D.; Autore, C.; di Paolo, F.M.; Pisicchio, C.; Squeo, M.R.; Musumeci, B.; Spataro, A.; Pandian, N.G.; Pelliccia, A. Patterns of Left Ventricular Longitudinal Strain and Strain Rate in Olympic Athletes. *J. Am. Soc. Echocardiogr.* **2015**, *28*, 245–253. [CrossRef]
29. Charfeddine, S.; Mallek, S.; Triki, F.; Hammami, R.; Abid, D.; Abid, L.; Kammoun, S. Echocardiographic analysis of the left ventricular function in young athletes: A focus on speckle tracking imaging. *Pan Afr. Med. J.* **2016**, *25*, 171. [CrossRef]
30. D'Ascenzi, F.; Caselli, S.; Solari, M.; Pelliccia, A.; Cameli, M.; Focardi, M.; Padeletti, M.; Corrado, D.; Bonifazi, M.; Mondillo, S. Novel echocardiographic techniques for the evaluation of athletes' heart: A focus on speckle-tracking echocardiography. *Eur. J. Prev. Cardiol.* **2016**, *23*, 437–446. [CrossRef]
31. Maufrais, C.; Schuster, I.; Doucende, G.; Vitiello, D.; Rupp, T.; Dauzat, M.; Obert, P.; Nottin, S. Endurance Training Minimizes Age-Related Changes of Left Ventricular Twist-Untwist Mechanics. *J. Am. Soc. Echocardiogr.* **2014**, *27*, 1208–1215. [CrossRef]
32. Santoro, A.; Alvino, F.; Antonelli, G.; Caputo, M.; Padeletti, M.; Lisi, M.; Mondillo, S. Endurance and Strength Athlete's Heart: Analysis of Myocardial Deformation by Speckle Tracking Echocardiography. *J. Cardiovasc. Ultrasound* **2014**, *22*, 196–204. [CrossRef]
33. Tokodi, M.; Lakatos, B.K.; Ruppert, M.; Fábián, A.; Oláh, A.; Sayour, A.A.; Ladányi, Z.; Soós, A.; Merkely, B.; Sengupta, P.P.; et al. Left Ventricular Pressure-Strain-Volume Loops for the Noninvasive Assessment of Volume Overload-Induced Myocardial Dysfunction. *JACC Cardiovasc. Imaging* **2021**, *14*, 1868–1871. [CrossRef]
34. Zacher, J.; Blome, I.; Schenk, A.; Gorr, E. Cardiac adaptations in elite female football- and volleyball-athletes do not impact left ventricular global strain values: A speckle tracking echocardiography study. *Int. J. Cardiovasc. Imaging* **2020**, *36*, 1085–1096. [CrossRef]
35. Harriss, D.J.; MacSween, A.; Atkinson, G. Ethical Standards in Sport and Exercise Science Research: 2020 Update. *Int. J. Sports Med.* **2019**, *40*, 813–817. [CrossRef] [PubMed]
36. Evangelista, A.; Flachskampf, F.; Lancellotti, P.; Badano, L.; Aguilar, R.; Monaghan, M.; Zamorano, J.; Nihoyannopoulos, P. European Association of Echocardiography recommendations for standardization of performance, digital storage and reporting of echocardiographic studies. *Eur. J. Echocardiogr.* **2008**, *9*, 438–448. [CrossRef]
37. Lang, R.; Bierig, M.; Devereux, R.; Flachskampf, F.; Foster, E.; Pellikka, P.; Picard, M.; Roman, M.; Seward, J.; Shanewise, J. Recommendations for chamber quantification. *Eur. J. Echocardiogr.* **2006**, *7*, 1–39. [CrossRef] [PubMed]

38. Hagendorff, A.; Fehske, W.; Flachskampf, F.A.; Helfen, A.; Kreidel, F.; Kruck, S.; la Rosée, K.; Tiemann, K.; Voigt, J.-U.; von Bardeleben, R.S.; et al. Manual zur Indikation und Durchführung der Echokardiographie—Update 2020 der Deutschen Gesellschaft für Kardiologie. *Kardiologe* **2020**, *14*, 396–431. [CrossRef]
39. Hashem, M.-S.; Kalashyan, H.; Choy, J.; Chiew, S.K.; Shawki, A.-H.; Dawood, A.H.; Becher, H. Left Ventricular Relative Wall Thickness Versus Left Ventricular Mass Index in Non-Cardioembolic Stroke Patients. *Medicine* **2015**, *94*, e872. [CrossRef] [PubMed]
40. Lang, R.M.; Badano, L.P.; Mor-Avi, V.; Afilalo, J.; Armstrong, A.; Ernande, L.; Flachskampf, F.A.; Foster, E.; Goldstein, S.A.; Kuznetsova, T.; et al. Recommendations for Cardiac Chamber Quantification by Echocardiography in Adults: An Update from the American Society of Echocardiography and the European Association of Cardiovascular Imaging. *J. Am. Soc. Echocardiogr.* **2015**, *28*, 1–39. [CrossRef]
41. Mitchell, J.H.; Haskell, W.; Snell, P.; van Camp, S.P. Task Force 8: Classification of sports. *J. Am. Coll. Cardiol.* **2005**, *45*, 1364–1367. [CrossRef] [PubMed]
42. Pavlik, G.; Major, Z.; Varga-Pintér, B.; Jeserich, M.; Kneffel, Z. The athlete's heart Part I (Review). *Acta Physiol. Hung.* **2010**, *97*, 337–353. [CrossRef] [PubMed]
43. Pluim, B.M.; Zwinderman, A.H.; van der Laarse, A.; van der Wall, E.E. The Athlete's Heart. *Circulation* **2010**, *101*, 336–344. [CrossRef] [PubMed]
44. Fagard, R. Athlete's heart. *Heart* **2003**, *89*, 1455–1461. [CrossRef] [PubMed]
45. Naylor, L.H.; George, K.; O'Driscoll, G.; Green, D.J. The Athlete's Heart. *Sports Med.* **2008**, *38*, 69–90. [CrossRef]
46. Iskandar, A.; Mujtaba, M.T.; Thompson, P.D. Left Atrium Size in Elite Athletes. *JACC Cardiovasc. Imaging* **2015**, *8*, 753–762. [CrossRef] [PubMed]
47. Zimmermann, P.; Lutter, C. Haemodynamic effects of paroxysmal supraventricular tachycardia in an endurance athlete during exercise testing. *BMJ Case Rep.* **2019**, *12*, e231659. [CrossRef]
48. Kasikcioglu, E.; Oflaz, H.; Akhan, H.; Kayserilioglu, A.; Umman, B.; Bugra, Z.; Erzengin, F. Left Atrial Geometric and Functional Remodeling in Athletes. *Int. J. Sports Med.* **2006**, *27*, 267–271. [CrossRef]
49. Klasnja, A.V.; Jakovljevic, D.G.; Barak, O.F.; Popadic Gacesa, J.Z.; Lukac, D.D.; Grujic, N.G. Cardiac power output and its response to exercise in athletes and non-athletes. *Clin. Physiol. Funct. Imaging* **2013**, *33*, 201–205. [CrossRef]
50. Major, Z.; Csajági, E.; Kneffel, Z.; Kováts, T.; Szauder, I.; Sidó, Z.; Pavlik, G. Comparison of left and right ventricular adaptation in endurance-trained male athletes. *Acta Physiol. Hung.* **2015**, *102*, 23–33. [CrossRef]
51. D'Andrea, A.; Limongelli, G.; Caso, P.; Sarubbi, B.; della Pietra, A.; Brancaccio, P.; Cice, G.; Scherillo, M.; Limongelli, F.; Calabrò, R. Association between left ventricular structure and cardiac performance during effort in two morphological forms of athlete's heart. *Int. J. Cardiol.* **2002**, *86*, 177–184. [CrossRef]
52. Angelini, P.; Cheong, B.Y.; Lenge de Rosen, V.V.; Lopez, J.A.; Uribe, C.; Masso, A.H.; Ali, S.W.; Davis, B.R.; Muthupillai, R.; Willerson, J.T. Magnetic Resonance Imaging–Based Screening Study in a General Population of Adolescents. *J. Am. Coll. Cardiol.* **2018**, *71*, 579–580. [CrossRef]
53. Eckart, R.E.; Scoville, S.L.; Campbell, C.L.; Shry, E.A.; Stajduhar, K.C.; Potter, R.N.; Pearse, L.A.; Virmani, R. Sudden Death in Young Adults: A 25-Year Review of Autopsies in Military Recruits. *Ann. Intern. Med.* **2004**, *141*, 829. [CrossRef]
54. Angelini, P.; Vidovich, M.I.; Lawless, C.E.; Elayda, M.A.; Lopez, J.A.; Wolf, D.; Willerson, J.T. Preventing sudden cardiac death in athletes: In search of evidence-based, cost effective screening. *Tex. Heart Inst. J.* **2013**, *40*, 148–155. [PubMed]
55. Mandraffino, G.; Imbalzano, E.; lo Gullo, A.; Zito, C.; Morace, C.; Cinquegrani, M.; Savarino, F.; Oreto, L.; Giuffrida, C.; Carerj, S.; et al. Abnormal left ventricular global strain during exercise-test in young healthy smokers. *Sci. Rep.* **2020**, *10*, 5700. [CrossRef] [PubMed]
56. Pagourelias, E.D.; Mirea, O.; Duchenne, J.; van Cleemput, J.; Delforge, M.; Bogaert, J.; Kuznetsova, T.; Voigt, J.-U. Echo Parameters for Differential Diagnosis in Cardiac Amyloidosis. *Circ. Cardiovasc. Imaging* **2017**, *10*, e005588. [CrossRef] [PubMed]
57. Yang, C.; Ma, C.S.; Fan, L.; Su, B.; Wang, Y.X.; Jiang, G.D.; Zhou, B.Y. The value of left ventricular longitudinal strain in the diagnosis and differential diagnosis of myocardial amyloidosis. *Zhonghua Yi Xue Za Zhi* **2020**, *100*, 3431–3436.
58. D'Ascenzi, F.; Pelliccia, A.; Solari, M.; Piu, P.; Loiacono, F.; Anselmi, F.; Caselli, S.; Focardi, M.; Bonifazi, M.; Mondillo, S. Normative Reference Values of Right Heart in Competitive Athletes: A Systematic Review and Meta-Analysis. *J. Am. Soc. Echocardiogr.* **2017**, *30*, 845–858. [CrossRef]
59. D'Andrea, A.; Riegler, L.; Golia, E.; Cocchia, R.; Scarafile, R.; Salerno, G.; Pezzullo, E.; Nunziata, L.; Citro, R.; Cuomo, S.; et al. Range of right heart measurements in top-level athletes: The training impact. *Int. J. Cardiol.* **2013**, *164*, 48–57. [CrossRef] [PubMed]
60. D'Ascenzi, F.; Pelliccia, A.; Corrado, D.; Cameli, M.; Curci, V.; Alvino, F.; Natali, B.M.; Focardi, M.; Bonifazi, M.; Mondillo, S. Right ventricular remodelling induced by exercise training in competitive athletes. *Eur. Heart J. Cardiovasc. Imaging* **2016**, *17*, 301–307. [CrossRef] [PubMed]
61. Sitges, M.; Merino, B.; Butakoff, C.; de la Garza, M.S.; Paré, C.; Montserrat, S.; Vidal, B.; Azqueta, M.; Sarquella, G.; Gutierrez, J.A.; et al. Characterizing the spectrum of right ventricular remodelling in response to chronic training. *Int. J. Cardiovasc. Imaging* **2017**, *33*, 331–339. [CrossRef] [PubMed]
62. Pagourelias, E.D.; Kouidi, E.; Efthimiadis, G.K.; Deligiannis, A.; Geleris, P.; Vassilikos, V. Right Atrial and Ventricular Adaptations to Training in Male Caucasian Athletes: An Echocardiographic Study. *J. Am. Soc. Echocardiogr.* **2013**, *26*, 1344–1352. [CrossRef] [PubMed]
63. Sandbakk, Ø.; Hegge, A.M.; Losnegard, T.; Skattebo, Ø.; Tønnessen, E.; Holmberg, H.-C. The Physiological Capacity of the World's Highest Ranked Female Cross-country Skiers. *Med. Sci. Sports Exerc.* **2016**, *48*, 1091–1100. [CrossRef] [PubMed]

Journal of
Cardiovascular Development and Disease

MDPI

Review

Echocardiographic Assessment of Atrial Function: From Basic Mechanics to Specific Cardiac Diseases

Katsuji Inoue [1,*], Hiroshi Kawakami [1], Yusuke Akazawa [1], Haruhiko Higashi [1], Takashi Higaki [2,3] and Osamu Yamaguchi [1]

1 Department of Cardiology, Pulmonology, Hypertension & Nephrology, Ehime University Graduate School of Medicine, Toon 791-0295, Ehime, Japan; kawaka@m.ehime-u.ac.jp (H.K.); z3p1002@gmail.com (Y.A.); hingassy@yahoo.com (H.H.); yamaguti@m.ehime-u.ac.jp (O.Y.)
2 Department of Regional Pediatrics and Perinatology, Ehime University Graduate School of Medicine, Toon 791-029, Ehime, Japan; higaki@m.ehime-u.ac.jp
3 Department of Pediatrics, Ehime University Graduate School of Medicine, Toon 791-0295, Ehime, Japan
* Correspondence: inoue.katsuji.my@ehime-u.ac.jp; Tel.: +81-89-960-5303

Abstract: The left and right atria serve as buffer chambers to control the flow of venous blood for ventricular filling. If an atrium is absent, blood does not flow effectively into the ventricle, leading to venous blood retention and low cardiac output. The importance of atrial function has become increasingly recognized, because left atrial (LA) function contributes to cardiac performance, and loss of LA function is associated with heart failure. LA volume change has been used for LA function assessment in experimental and clinical studies. In conjunction with LA pressure, the LA pressure–volume relationship provides a better understanding of LA mechanics. LA strain measurement by speckle tracking echocardiography was introduced to evaluate three components of LA function as a (booster) pump, reservoir and conduit. Furthermore, increasing evidence supports the theory that LA reservoir strain has prognostic utility in various cardiac diseases. In this review, we summarize LA contribution to maintain cardiac performance by evaluating LA function with echocardiography according to our experiences and previous reports. Furthermore, we discuss LA dysfunction in challenging cardiac diseases of cardiac amyloidosis and adult congenital heart disease.

Keywords: left atrial function; heart failure; pressure–volume loop; left atrial strain; atrial fibrillation; cardiac amyloidosis; adult congenital heart disease

1. Introduction

The atria work as buffer chambers to receive blood from the venous system in a controlled manner and to effectively deliver it to the ventricles. If an atrium is absent, the ventricle carries a considerable hemodynamic burden to maintain cardiac performance. Under such circumstances, preservation of cardiac output depends only on ventricular systolic and diastolic function; otherwise, forward flow is unavoidably produced by an increased pressure in the upper venous system. For example, when the pressure in the pulmonary vein is elevated to force a forward flow into a failing left ventricle, patients complain of heart failure symptoms, such as shortness of breath and dyspnea on exertion. The scenario demonstrates the importance of the left atrial (LA) contribution to overall cardiac function.

The left atrium contributes to cardiac performance through three components, functioning as a (booster) pump, reservoir and conduit. LA pressure and volume change instantaneously during the cardiac cycle. The resultant LA pressure–volume curve shows a figure-eight configuration, which provides important information regarding LA active and passive function.

Echocardiography was first used to assess LA size and function in clinical practice [1]. Two dimensional (2D) echocardiography can be used to quantify LA size, and the LA volume index estimated by 2D echocardiography is a well-known diagnostic and prognostic parameter in patients with heart failure [2,3]. In terms of LA functional assessment, historically, Doppler echocardiography, particularly the pulmonary vein signal, is utilized to understand LA pressure and function. As a screening tool, pulmonary vein flow is relatively underused compared with transmitral flow to evaluate LA function; however, the waveform of pulmonary vein flow enables assessment of the LA pump, reservoir and conduit functions [4,5].

The importance of the atrial contribution to cardiac function has become increasingly recognized in clinical practice. In this review, we summarize LA contribution to prevent heart failure by evaluating LA function with echocardiography according to our experiences and previous reports. Furthermore, we discuss LA dysfunction in challenging cardiac disorders of cardiac amyloidosis and adult congenital heart disease (ACHD).

2. Basic Mechanics of the Left Atrium

The pressure–volume relationship is the gold standard for evaluating myocardial work. Suga presented the concept of the pressure–volume loop area as a novel marker of myocardial work in the left ventricle [6]. Russel, Smiseth, and colleagues developed a noninvasive method to quantify left ventricular (LV) work from the pressure–strain loop area using speckle tracking echocardiography [7].

Regarding the LA pressure–volume relationship, the loop typically has a figure-eight pattern (Figure 1A), with the two loops consisting of the A- and V-loops [8]. The A-loop rotates counterclockwise, which corresponds to LA active contraction and relaxation, while the V-loop rotates clockwise, which corresponds to LA passive dilatation and emptying.

The A-loop area represents LA active function to maintain stroke volume and normal LA pressure despite afterload increase [9]. Although an increase in afterload limits LV work, augmentations of LA pump function (booster function) and LA active relaxation (early reservoir function) immediately react as compensatory mechanisms to prevent 'afterload mismatch' (Figure 1B). However, if atrial fibrillation (AF) is already present, heart failure could develop, because the A-loop is absent due to atrial myopathy (Figure 1C) [8].

The V-loop represents LA passive function. The first half of the upsloping V-loop occurs during the LV ejection period, and the slope begins at the time point of x-trough pressure and ends at that of v-wave pressure. During the LV ejection period, LV myocardial fiber shortens longitudinally, and in turn, the LA wall lengthens as a source of the LA late reservoir function.

The second half of the downsloping V-loop begins at mitral valve opening. After the mitral valve opens, the left atrium behaves as a conduit by producing forward blood flow through LA elastic recoil as well as LV diastolic function. The left atrium reflects LV systolic and diastolic function because of the anatomical continuity between the two chambers [10].

When we focus on LA reservoir function, the left atrium works as a reservoir to maintain cardiac output. An experimental study elegantly revealed that LA reservoir function was determined by LA relaxation, LV longitudinal shortening and LA stiffness [11]. In this phase, the LA pressure rises from the x-trough to v-wave pressure. Importantly, the ratio of the pressure gradient from the x-trough to v-wave pressure to LA volume increase is a surrogate of LA chamber stiffness (Figure 1D). The concept of the LA pressure–volume relationship provides a better understanding of LA intrinsic function as well as LA passive function supported mainly by adjacent LV work.

In this case, the slope connecting the x-trough pressure to the v-wave pressure on the loop becomes steeper than that in other cases with a compliant left atrium (Figure 1A).

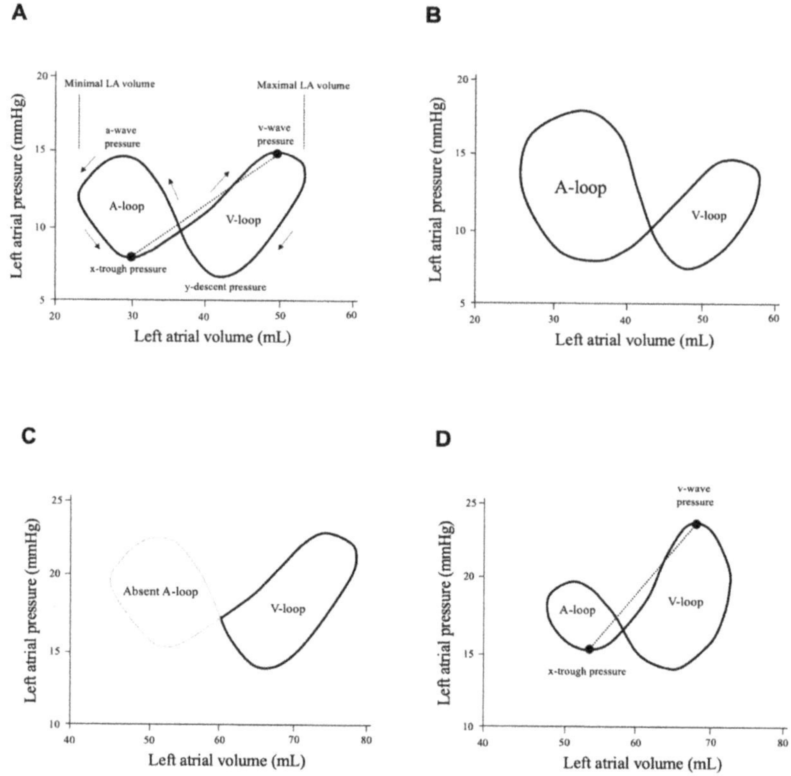

Figure 1. Left atrial pressure–volume loop curve. (**A**) Normal left atrial pressure–volume loop consisting of A- and V-loops. The A-loop is produced by LA contraction (booster pump function) and relaxation (early reservoir function), while the V-loop is produced by LA dilatation (late reservoir function) and emptying (conduit function). LA pressure includes the x-trough and v-wave pressures, and the slope connecting the two pressure points (dotted line) on the loop is defined as the LA stiffness index. (**B**) During afterload increase. When systolic blood pressure increases from 120 to 180 mmHg for instance, left ventricular (LV) systolic and diastolic function worsen due to afterload increase. The A-loop area immediately enlarges to pressure-overloaded LV dysfunction, resulting in the maintenance of stroke volume without a critical elevation in LA pressure. (**C**) Atrial fibrillation occurrence. Atrial fibrillation promotes atrial myopathy, resulting in LA dilatation, functional impairment and perhaps elevated mean LA pressure. The A-loop disappears during atrial fibrillation, and it mainly depends on ventricular function to maintain cardiac performance. (**D**) Left atrial stiffening. The pressure–volume loop in a case of cardiac amyloidosis. Abnormal amyloid proteins deposit into the myocardial wall, including the left atrium. LA, left atrial; LV, left ventricular.

3. Atrial Function in Cardiovascular Diseases

It is recognized that LA function is important to prevent heart failure, particularly if LV function deteriorates. In cases with LV dysfunction, LA dilatation during ventricular systole, which is one of the components of LA 'reservoir function', is limited due to reduced LV longitudinal systolic shortening. Suga reported that LA reservoir function was an important determinant of cardiac output [12]. Thus, heart failure could develop unless a compensatory mechanism operates. Under the circumstances, the left atrium immediately responds by operating its intrinsic 'pump function' to expand a diseased left ventricle and maintain normal cardiac output via the Frank–Starling mechanism [13]. The augmented LA pump function is also linked with enhanced LA relaxation, thus effectively pulling blood from the pulmonary vein to the left atrium [14]. The occurrence of AF is directly associated with an increased incidence of heart failure, especially in patients with LV dysfunction [15,16]. Ablation of the AF is effective to obtain LA reverse remodeling and is expected to reduce the occurrence of heart failure.

LA dilatation is a marker of chronicity of LV diastolic dysfunction. An LA volume index (LAVi) >34 mL/m^2 is an important parameter in estimating LV filling pressure [2]. Meanwhile, AF itself promotes LA dilatation irrespective of LV filling pressure. LA enlargement coexists with LA functional impairment.

LA strain by speckle tracking echocardiography (STE) can be used to evaluate LA function. The EACVI/ASE/Industry Task Force provides standardization of LA strain measurement for clinical and scientific purposes [17]. For the measurement, the Task Force recommends that the zero-strain reference for LA strain curves should be end-diastole, as shown Figure 2. The LA strain curve has two positive peaks corresponding to LA reservoir and pump functions.

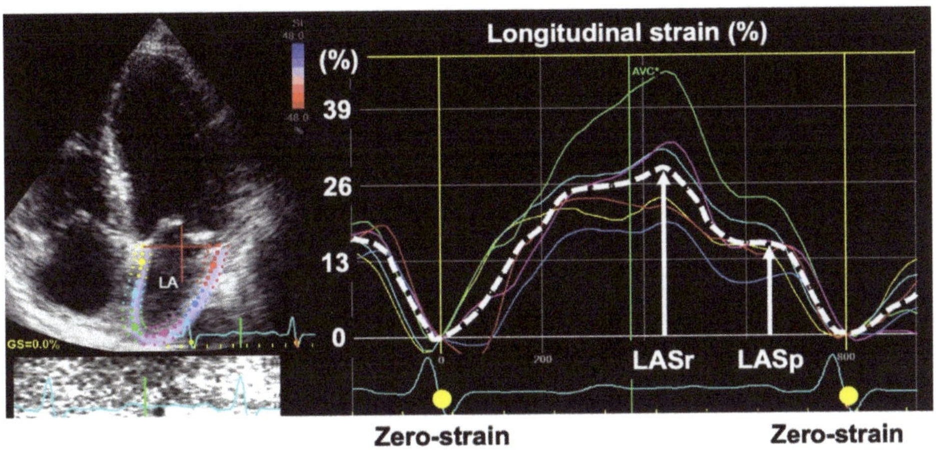

Figure 2. Calculation of left atrial strain. LA strain can be analyzed from a non-foreshortened apical four-chamber view. The zero-strain reference is set at end-diastole according to the recommendation by Badano et al. [17], enabling one to obtain LA strain value even in patients with atrial fibrillation. LA reservoir strain (LASr) is calculated as difference between end-diastole and onset of early LV filling, while LA pump strain (LASp) as difference between onset of atrial contraction and onset of late LV filling. LA, left atrial, LV, left ventricular.

LA functional assessment is emerging to diagnose and predict heart failure in patients with underlying heart diseases. We recently collaborated to conduct a multicenter study of 322 patients with cardiovascular disease of different etiologies [18], resulting that LA reservoir strain < 18% and LA pump strain < 8% predicted elevated LV filling pressure better ($p < 0.05$) than LA volume [18]. Furthermore, LA pump strain > 14% identified normal LV filling pressure with 92% accuracy in patients with preserved LV ejection fraction. These results suggest that LA reservoir strain is an alternative marker to LA volume index for identifying elevated LV filling pressure. In addition, a preservation of LA pump strain indicates LA compensation to maintain normal LV filling pressure in patients with underlying cardiac diseases.

As LA remodeling progresses, LA stiffness increases. The assessment of LA stiffness has been studied from the LA pressure–volume relationship, as mentioned above. Reddy Y et al. reported that LA stiffness progressively increased with LV diastolic dysfunction and AF burden, leading to poor outcomes in patients with heart failure with preserved LV ejection fraction [19]. Cardiac amyloidosis is also a representative cardiac disease with stiff LA syndrome. When we visually focus on LA behavior by echocardiography, LA dilatation is somewhat restricted at the LA reservoir phase in patients with cardiac amyloidosis. This is due to amyloid infiltration in the LA wall leading to progressive loss of atrial function and increased stiffness [20].

In contrast to the left atrium, right atrial (RA) structure and function are not routinely evaluated with echocardiography in clinical practice. In adult congenital heart disease (ACHD), over time, the right-sided heart is often more diseased rather than the left-sided heart. Patients with ACHD suffer from right-sided heart failure presenting as anasarca, ascites and general fatigue. Right ventricular (RV) dilatation is usually observed, and echocardiography enables the estimation of RV size as well as function. The right atrium is also dilated concomitantly with RV remodeling, although the assessment of RA structure and function is less studied in patients with ACHD. Furthermore, the prevalence of AF is rising precipitously with the increase in the aging population, and the right atrium is progressively remodeled. The success rate of AF ablation is unsatisfactory in patients with ACHD with complex cardiac structure and previous surgery.

4. Left Atrial Structure and Function in Atrial Fibrillation

Atrial fibrillation is the most common arrhythmia, and the number of patients with AF has been increasing gradually and steadily worldwide [21,22]. The increasing incidence of AF has contributed to rising health care costs because of the association of AF with stroke, heart failure, and overall mortality [21–23]. Therefore, better preventive and therapeutic steps for the management of this arrhythmia are needed. AF initiates self-perpetuating changes in the structural, functional, and electrophysiological properties of the atrium and promotes atrial remodeling (AF begets AF) [24]. LA structural and functional cardiac abnormalities, including chamber dilatation and systolic/diastolic dysfunction, are all potential risk factors for AF [25–29]. Furthermore, LA structural and electrophysiological remodeling are key markers for risk stratification in patients with AF [1,26–28,30–34].

Considerable evidence exists regarding the usefulness of echocardiographic LA structural and functional parameters for risk stratification (stroke, heart failure, and overall mortality) in patients with AF. In particular, LAVi is a well-established parameter for risk stratification of cardiovascular events and recurrence of catheter ablation (CA) for AF. Osranek et al. reported the results of very long-term follow-up (median 27 years) of 46 patients with well-documented, clinically defined, lone AF [32]. They revealed that patients with large LA volume (LAVi $\geq$ 32 mL/m^2) at baseline had a significantly worse event-free survival after adjustment for age and clinical risk factors (adjusted HR, 4.46). In a systematic review and meta-analysis, Njoku et al. assessed whether LA volume was an independent predictor of AF recurrence following CA, and found that patients with AF recurrence following CA had a higher mean LA volume/LAVi compared with patients with no recurrence [31]. In contrast, many studies have revealed a reduction in LA enlargement after restoration of sinus rhythm by CA (reverse remodeling), and LA reverse remodeling was thought to be a marker for better outcomes (lower recurrence rate) of CA for AF [33,35–39]. In our recent work, we investigated whether the degree of LA volumetric reverse remodeling was associated with long-term outcomes (AF-free survival) after initial CA for AF in 140 patients with LA enlargement (LAVi $\geq$ 34 mL/m^2) at baseline [33]. We found that more than half of the patients (54%) had a normal LA volume (LAVi < 34 mL/m^2) at 1 year follow-up after CA, and those patients had better long-term outcomes (lower recurrence rate) after CA than patients who did not have a normal LA volume. Recent guidelines report the normal ranges and severity partition cutoffs of LA volume abnormality assessed by echocardiography [40]; an LAVi of 34 mL/m^2 can be used as a clear cut-off for risk stratification in a variety of clinical settings in patients with AF.

LA strain assessed by STE can detect early impairment of LA function, such as reduced LA reservoir and (booster) pump function [41,42]. Kuppahally et al. carried out a validation study on the relationship between LA strain and cardiac magnetic resonance and revealed that LA strain was inversely associated with LA fibrosis [43]. Moreover, STE can accurately assess regional myocardial function; thus, LA strain assessed by STE may also be used to evaluate disturbances in the timing of LA contraction (as a LA mechanical dispersion) (Figure 3), which reflect the presence of atrial fibrosis and electrophysiological disorders [44,45]. Watanabe et al. demonstrated that LA mechanical dispersion was increased significantly in patients with low-voltage zones evaluated by electro-anatomical mapping, and the severity of LA dispersion was related to the LA conduction delay in patients undergoing CA for AF [44]. These findings support the conclusion that STE can be a useful tool for evaluation of LA remodeling. Indeed, recent studies demonstrated that LA strain, mainly LA reservoir strain, can be a useful marker for risk stratification of AF in a variety of cardiac conditions [46–55], and can also provide incremental diagnostic and therapeutic value for AF management over LA enlargement [46–48,51]. Furthermore, LA dispersion is greater in patients with AF than in healthy individuals [56–59], and increases in proportion to the duration of AF [56]. LA dispersion predicts progression from paroxysmal to persistent AF [60]. In a community-based study, Kawakami et al. revealed that LA function and dispersion obtained from STE provided incremental information on LA volume and function in the prediction of new-onset AF [61]. LA strain assessed by STE has been also useful in predicting outcomes of AF treatment, including defibrillation and CA. From a functional point of view, LA reservoir strain calculated by STE is considered one of the strongest predictors of AF recurrence [53,55,62]. A recent meta-analysis proved that LA reservoir strain was strongly associated with recurrence of AF after adjusting for age, gender, AF duration, and LA volume, with an excellent predictive value (area under the receiver operating curve of 0.80) [62]. Assessment of LA dispersion using STE may also forecast recurrence after CA for AF. Sarvari et al. evaluated the association of LA dispersion with recurrence after CA for AF in patients with normal LV function and without severe LA enlargement, and demonstrated that LA dispersion was more pronounced in patients with recurrence of AF after CA compared with those without recurrence, and it predicted AF recurrence after adjustment for age, LA volume, e′, and LA function [63]. Although CA is an effective therapy for AF, CA can lead to injury to the atrial myocardium and impairments in neurohormonal functions, leading to "stiff LA syndrome" [64,65]. Therefore, evaluating LA volumetric and functional changes is important after CA for AF, especially in patients with long-standing persistent AF and heart failure. Moreover, reduced LA function and dispersed LA contraction pattern assessed by STE can also contribute to the risk stratification of stroke events in patients with AF [66,67]. Obokata et al. reported that LA strain had an incremental advantage over the CHA_2DS_2-VASc score for predicting the risk of stroke in patients with AF [66]. The greatest advantage of LA strain is the ability to detect early LA function and asynchrony in patients without LA enlargement [51,57,61,63].

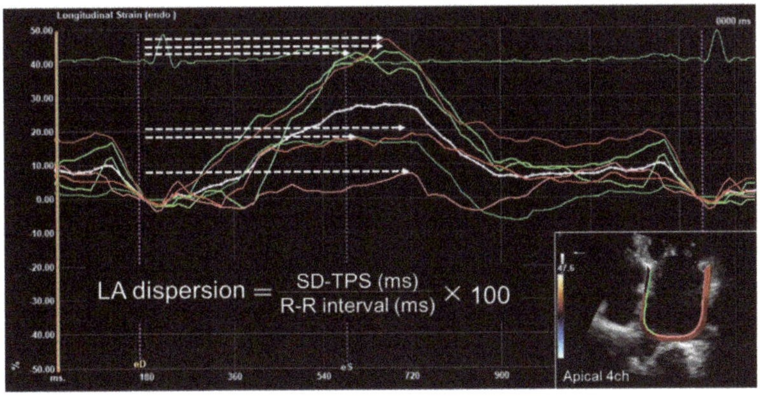

Figure 3. Calculation of left atrial dispersion. LA dispersion is defined as the standard deviation of the time to peak positive strain corrected by the R-R interval (%). White arrows indicate contraction durations defined as the time from the R wave on the electrocardiogram to the maximal time of positive deformation in each LA segment. LA, left atrial.

5. Left Atrial Function in Cardiac Amyloidosis

Cardiac amyloidosis is characterized by extracellular amyloid infiltration in the left ventricle, resulting in a restrictive pathophysiology. Amyloid deposition in the left ventricle causes LV wall thickening and increased ventricular filling pressure, which lead to LV diastolic dysfunction. It has also been reported that amyloid is pathologically deposited not only in the left ventricle, but also in the left atrium. The left atrium in cardiac amyloidosis is hemodynamically impaired similarly to the left ventricle. Amyloid infiltration into the LA wall causes it to thicken and stiffen, increasing its size and impairing its ejection force and strain [68]. By observing and evaluating LA behavior, we can learn much about the pathophysiology of cardiac amyloidosis.

Echocardiography is a key imaging modality in diagnosing cardiac amyloidosis. LA dimension or volume is a simple parameter, which indicates a chronic elevation of LA pressure. However, LA size is insufficient to obtain detailed information about LA function. Several studies with STE demonstrated that LA systolic contraction, reservoir and conduit functions were impaired in cardiac amyloidosis [69,70]. Recently, Bandera and colleagues [20] reported substantial impairment of the three phasic functional atrial components (median reservoir strain 8.9%, conduit strain 6.5%, pump strain 4.0%) evaluated by STE. Furthermore, they demonstrated that patients with amyloidosis with sinus rhythm whose atrial contraction was absent had a poorer prognosis compared with those with sinus rhythm and effective mechanical contraction.

Since the ATTR-ACT study [71], which showed that treatment with tafamidis improved the prognosis of cardiac amyloidosis, early diagnosis and phenotyping of cardiac amyloidosis has become more important. Amyloidosis is a disease characterized by LV hypertrophy, but it is often difficult to differentiate from other diseases presenting with LV hypertrophy, such as hypertrophic cardiomyopathy, hypertensive heart disease, and athlete's heart. In cardiac amyloidosis, the characteristic regional differences in LV longitudinal strain from cardiac base to apex are useful in differentiating the diseases. LV longitudinal strain is preserved at the apex and reduced significantly at the mid and basal segments. This strain pattern with STE is called 'apical sparing' and is specific to cardiac amyloidosis [72–74]. Regarding the left atrium in cardiac amyloidosis, Rausch et al. [75] reported that LA strain parameters at three phases were significantly reduced in the amyloidosis cohort compared to the hypertensive heart disease cohort. A reservoir strain cut-off value of 20% was 86% sensitive and 89% specific for detecting cardiac amyloidosis compared to hypertensive heart disease in their analysis.

Recently, we demonstrated the usefulness of visual assessment of the left atrium to differentiate cardiac amyloidosis from hypertrophic cardiomyopathy [76]. As shown in Figure 4, we classified the LA dilatation motion into three grades (preserved: grade 1, abnormal: grade 2, and restricted: grade 3) based on the apical four-chamber view and defined it as the LA dilatation grade (Inoue grade). Among 127 subjects, all 57 (45%) who presented with Inoue grade 1 had hypertrophic cardiomyopathy. In contrast, 28 patients (22%) were classified as Inoue grade 3, 20 of whom had cardiac amyloidosis. Thus, patients with cardiac amyloidosis had a higher Inoue grade than those with hypertrophic cardiomyopathy ($p < 0.01$). This diagnostic parameter is not only an indicator for the diagnosis of cardiac amyloidosis, but also a predictor of prognosis.

Impaired LA function in cardiac amyloidosis leads to decreased cardiac output and the development of heart failure. Another problem related to the clinical course of cardiac amyloidosis is the high incidence of arrhythmias. In particular, AF is commonly encountered and is the most troublesome arrhythmia in this condition. Donnellan et al. reported that AF occurred in 265 (69%) of 383 patients with amyloidosis in a retrospective cohort study [77]. They also identified risk factors associated with the development of AF, including older age, advanced cardiac amyloidosis stage, and higher LA volume index. AF can also cause cardiogenic stroke due to thrombus formation in the left atrium (mainly in the LA appendage). In general, a thrombus is unlikely to form in the left atrium when sinus rhythm is maintained, but in cardiac amyloidosis, thrombus formation can occur even in sinus rhythm. Martinez-Naharro et al. [78] reported that the prevalence of intracardiac thrombi was 6.2% in 324 patients with cardiac amyloidosis (256 males, 79%; 71 ± 11 years of age). Of the 20 patients with intracardiac thrombi, 13 had AF, and seven had sinus rhythm. All patients with AF and intracardiac thrombi were receiving long-term anticoagulation therapy. Therefore, cardiac amyloidosis is a disease that requires careful attention to thromboembolic events, even in patients with normal sinus rhythm or receiving anticoagulation therapy.

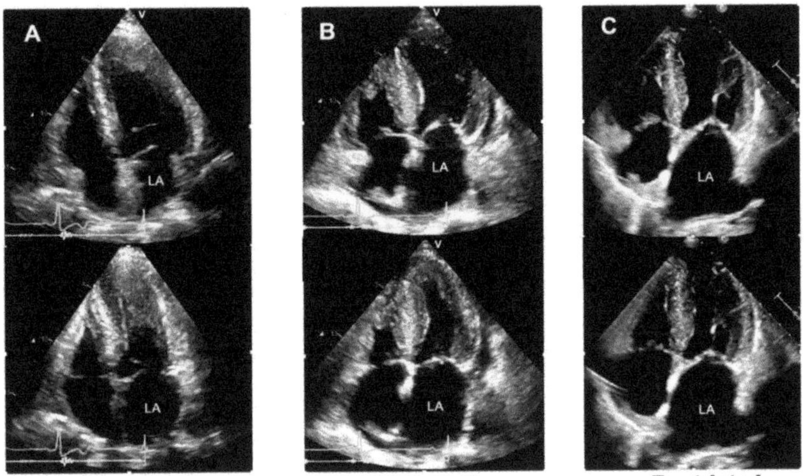

Figure 4. Visual assessment (grading) of left atrial reservoir function. (**A**) A case of hypertrophic cardiomyopathy. (**B**,**C**) Two cases of cardiac amyloidosis. The upper panel in each case is a frame when the LA size is minimized, while the lower panel is a frame when the LA size is maximized. In a patient with hypertrophic cardiomyopathy, the LA dilatation grade (Inoue grade) was preserved (**A**). In contrast, two patients with cardiac amyloidosis showed abnormal (**B**) and restricted (**C**) LA dilatation, indicating LA stiffening. LA, left atrial.

Echocardiography has the potential to enable early diagnosis of cardiac amyloidosis. By focusing not only on the left ventricle, but also on the left atrium, we can better understand the cardiac pathology and provide appropriate treatment for patients with cardiac amyloidosis.

6. Atrial Structure and Function in Adult Congenital Heart Disease

The diagnosis and management of congenital heart disease (CHD) has been a major success story of modern medicine. More than 90% of children with CHD survive into adulthood, and the number of adults with congenital heart disease (i.e., ACHD) is increasing [79]. It is recognized that CHD is associated with lifelong comorbidity that impacts health services utilization and costs. In particular, heart failure (HF) is a serious problem affecting 20–50% of the ACHD population [80]. Diastolic dysfunction correlates with poor prognosis in various forms of ACHD [81]. In adult acquired heart disease, the assessment of LA function has recently emerged as a powerful parameter of diastolic dysfunction [82]. Although the application of these LA functional assessments to patients with ACHD remains questionable, this knowledge should be actively pursued. The application of these LA functional assessments to patients with ACHD remains questionable. We will focus on "Atrial septal defect" and "Fontan Palliation", two common forms of ACHD, and review the current understanding of the assessment of atrial structure and function in ACHD.

6.1. Atrial Septal Defect

Traditionally, an atrial septal defect (ASD) has been repaired surgically. Recently, however, percutaneous transcatheter device occlusion has been used. A previous report showed that there was more significant intra-atrial systolic dyssynchrony with device closure than with surgical closure in strain imaging, suggesting that the bulky device impairs synchronous contraction [83]. In addition, at long-term follow-up, LA reservoir, conduit, and contraction functions were reduced in the device closure group compared with the healthy control group, but there was no difference in these functions in the surgical closure group. These data after ASD treatment suggest that device closure negatively affects LA function [84]. Although it has been reported that the annual incidence of new-onset AF in patients with ASD after device closure was 4.1% [85], the prognostic impact of the reduced LA function remains unknown, and further evidence must be accumulated. On the other hand, a study investigating pre-procedural risk factors for paroxysmal AF occurring after ASD device closure found that the combination of the standard deviations of RA time to peak strain, a marker of RA dyssynchrony, and the RA expansion index, a marker of RA reservoir function, provided a stronger estimate of paroxysmal AF independently of LA dysfunction [86]. These findings highlight the importance of understanding both LA and RA function in predicting the prognosis of patients with ASD.

Although rare, RA dysfunction due to impaired RV dilatation can lead to a right-to-left shunt via ASD. A case report described a patient who underwent pulmonary valvuloplasty for pulmonary stenosis with RV hypertrophy and developed a right-to-left shunt via ASD [87]. STE indicated an impaired reservoir function of the RA with a slight increase in booster function. However, STE analysis is not always possible due to difficulty in visualizing the free wall of the RA. In a case with a residual leak after ASD device implantation, RA dysfunction caused a right-to-left shunt (Figure 5A). In this case, STE analysis was difficult, but the enlarged RA area and decreased RA fractional area change suggested RA dysfunction (Figure 5B) [88].

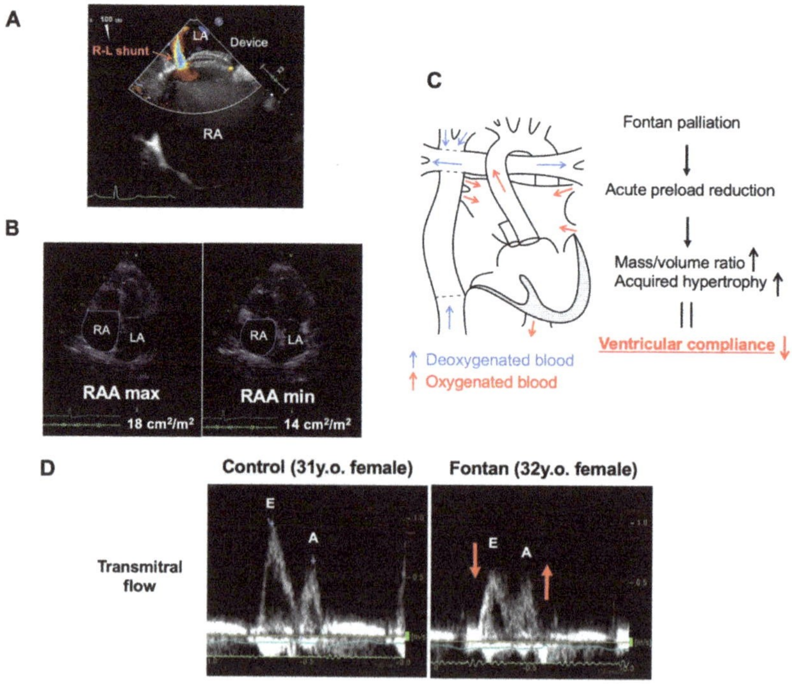

Figure 5. *Cont.*

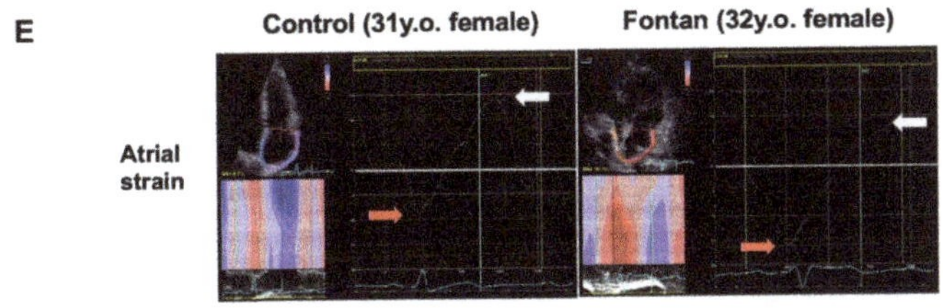

Figure 5. Atrial function in atrial septal defect and Fontan palliation. (**A**) TEE showing a right-to-left (R-L) shunt from a residual leak after ASD device closure with RA dysfunction. (**B**) Four-chamber views of end-systole (RAA max) and end-diastole (RAA min). The decreased RA fractional area change (FAC) suggests RA dysfunction. (**C**) Illustration of the Fontan circulation and the process of impairment of systemic ventricular relaxation after Fontan palliation. (**D**) Transmitral Doppler early diastolic (E-wave) and late diastolic (A-wave) velocities in a control subject, and the SV peak E-wave and A-wave inflow velocities in a patient with Fontan palliation (EC-TCPC). (**E**) Representative atrial strain curves in a patient with Fontan palliation (EC-TCPC) and a control subject. Peak negative (red arrow) and positive (white arrow) atrial strain are noted. TEE, transesophageal echocardiography; ASD, atrial septal defect; RA, right atrial; RAA, right atrial area; EC-TCPC, extracardiac total cavopulmonary connection.

6.2. Fontan Palliation

Fontan [89] reported successful performance of a right-sided cardiac bypass in patients with a functional single ventricle (SV) for the first time in 1971. Since then, with modifications in operative techniques and postoperative management, early survival has improved [90–92]. However, little has been investigated regarding atrial function late after the Fontan palliation.

By separating the pulmonary and systemic circulations, the Fontan palliation imposes an acute preload reduction on a previously volume-loaded ventricle. After the Fontan palliation [93,94], an increased mass/volume ratio and acquired hypertrophy of the ventricles occur, with concomitant impairment of systemic ventricular relaxation (Figure 5C). A persistent late impairment of isovolumic relaxation time and diminishing SV peak early diastolic velocity compared to controls have also been reported [95], suggesting a trend towards reduced ventricular compliance. In a previous study, the SV peak early diastolic (E-wave) was decreased, and the late diastole (A-wave) inflow velocity was increased compared with that in healthy subjects [96] (Figure 5D). This reliance on increased atrial contractility may be a response to the elevated ventricular end-diastolic pressures after the Fontan palliation. These findings were demonstrated in STE-based studies [96,97]. The SV atrial deformation parameters were significantly altered compared with healthy subjects, with markedly impaired conduit strain, reduced reservoir strain, and increased reliance on active strain for ventricular filling (Figure 5E). These differences may have important implications for their long-term outcomes; further studies are needed to clarify the role of atrial function in SV cardiac performance.

7. Conclusions

According to recent developments in diagnostic, therapeutic and preventive medicine, the survival rate has improved in patients with heart failure. However, the number of individuals with heart failure is increasing, because cardiac structural and functional remodeling still exists despite medical and interventional therapies. Atrial enlargement and dysfunction indicate a history of hemodynamic burden and disease severity. The assessment of atrial structure and function by echocardiography enables an understanding of the underlying risk of heart failure, thus promoting early preventive and therapeutic interventions to decrease heart failure occurrence.

Author Contributions: Conceptualization, K.I. and writing—original draft preparation, K.I., H.K., Y.A., H.H. and review and editing, T.H. and supervision, O.Y. All authors have read and agreed to the published version of the manuscript.

Funding: This research received no external funding.

Institutional Review Board Statement: This article was conducted according to the Declaration of Helsinki and approved by the ethics committee of Ehime University Graduate School of Medicine (IRB: 1905015).

Informed Consent Statement: Patient consent was waived because it was performed by the opt-out method of our hospital websites.

Data Availability Statement: No datasets were analyzed in this review article.

Acknowledgments: The authors would like to thank Maki Miyazaki, Namiko Sakuoka, and Yukari Shikano for excellent technical assistance on echocardiography.

Conflicts of Interest: The authors declare no conflict of interest regarding to this review article.

References

1. Hoit, B.D. Left atrial size and function: Role in prognosis. *J. Am. Coll. Cardiol.* **2014**, *63*, 493–505. [CrossRef] [PubMed]
2. Nagueh, S.F.; Smiseth, O.A.; Appleton, C.P.; Byrd, B.F., 3rd; Dokainish, H.; Edvardsen, T.; Flachskampf, F.A.; Gillebert, T.C.; Klein, A.L.; Lancellotti, P.; et al. Recommendations for the Evaluation of Left Ventricular Diastolic Function by Echocardiography: An Update from the American Society of Echocardiography and the European Association of Cardiovascular Imaging. *J. Am. Soc. Echocardiogr.* **2016**, *29*, 277–314. [CrossRef] [PubMed]
3. Paulus, W.J.; Tschope, C.; Sanderson, J.E.; Rusconi, C.; Flachskampf, F.A.; Rademakers, F.E.; Marino, P.; Smiseth, O.A.; De Keulenaer, G.; Leite-Moreira, A.F.; et al. How to diagnose diastolic heart failure: A consensus statement on the diagnosis of heart failure with normal left ventricular ejection fraction by the Heart Failure and Echocardiography Associations of the European Society of Cardiology. *Eur. Heart J.* **2007**, *28*, 2539–2550. [CrossRef]
4. Tabata, T.; Thomas, J.D.; Klein, A.L. Pulmonary venous flow by doppler echocardiography: Revisited 12 years later. *J. Am. Coll. Cardiol.* **2003**, *41*, 1243–1250. [CrossRef]
5. Fukuda, N.; Oki, T.; Iuchi, A.; Tabata, T.; Yamada, H.; Ito, S.; Takeichi, N.; Shinohara, H.; Socki, T.; Shinomiya, H.; et al. Tricuspid inflow and regurgitant flow dynamics after mitral valve replacement: Differences relating to surgical repair of the tricuspid valve. *J. Heart Valve Dis.* **1997**, *6*, 184–188.
6. Suga, H. Total mechanical energy of a ventricle model and cardiac oxygen consumption. *Am. J. Physiol.* **1979**, *236*, H498–H505. [CrossRef]
7. Russell, K.; Eriksen, M.; Aaberge, L.; Wilhelmsen, N.; Skulstad, H.; Remme, E.W.; Haugaa, K.H.; Opdahl, A.; Fjeld, J.G.; Gjesdal, O.; et al. A novel clinical method for quantification of regional left ventricular pressure-strain loop area: A non-invasive index of myocardial work. *Eur. Heart J.* **2012**, *33*, 724–733. [CrossRef]
8. Weimar, T.; Watanabe, Y.; Kazui, T.; Lee, U.S.; Moon, M.R.; Schuessler, R.B.; Damiano, R.J., Jr. Differential impact of short periods of rapid atrial pacing on left and right atrial mechanical function. *Am. J. Physiol. Heart Circ. Physiol.* **2012**, *302*, H2583–H2591. [CrossRef]
9. Inoue, K.; Asanuma, T.; Masuda, K.; Sakurai, D.; Higaki, J.; Nakatani, S. Compensatory increase of left atrial external work to left ventricular dysfunction caused by afterload increase. *Am. J. Physiol. Heart Circ. Physiol.* **2015**, *308*, H904–H912. [CrossRef]
10. Smiseth, O.A.; Inoue, K. The left atrium: A mirror of ventricular systolic and diastolic function. *Eur. Heart J. Cardiovasc. Imaging* **2020**, *21*, 270–272. [CrossRef]
11. Barbier, P.; Solomon, S.B.; Schiller, N.B.; Glantz, S.A. Left atrial relaxation and left ventricular systolic function determine left atrial reservoir function. *Circulation* **1999**, *100*, 427–436. [CrossRef] [PubMed]
12. Suga, H. Importance of atrial compliance in cardiac performance. *Circ. Res.* **1974**, *35*, 39–43. [CrossRef] [PubMed]
13. Braunwald, E.; Frahm, C.J.; Ross, J., Jr. Studies on Starling's law of the heart. V. Left ventricular function in man. *J. Clin. Investig.* **1961**, *40*, 1882–1890. [CrossRef] [PubMed]
14. Toma, Y.; Matsuda, Y.; Moritani, K.; Ogawa, H.; Matsuzaki, M.; Kusukawa, R. Left atrial filling in normal human subjects: Relation between left atrial contraction and left atrial early filling. *Cardiovasc. Res.* **1987**, *21*, 255–259. [CrossRef]
15. Hoit, B.D.; Shao, Y.; Gabel, M. Left atrial systolic and diastolic function accompanying chronic rapid pacing-induced atrial failure. *Am. J. Physiol.* **1998**, *275*, H183–H189. [CrossRef]
16. Benjamin, E.J.; Levy, D.; Vaziri, S.M.; D'Agostino, R.B.; Belanger, A.J.; Wolf, P.A. Independent risk factors for atrial fibrillation in a population-based cohort. The Framingham Heart Study. *JAMA* **1994**, *271*, 840–844. [CrossRef]
17. Badano, L.P.; Kolias, T.J.; Muraru, D.; Abraham, T.P.; Aurigemma, G.; Edvardsen, T.; D'Hooge, J.; Donal, E.; Fraser, A.G.; Marwick, T.; et al. Standardization of left atrial, right ventricular, and right atrial deformation imaging using two-dimensional speckle tracking echocardiography: A consensus document of the EACVI/ASE/Industry Task Force to standardize deformation imaging. *Eur. Heart J. Cardiovasc. Imaging* **2018**, *19*, 591–600. [CrossRef]

18. Inoue, K.; Khan, F.H.; Remme, E.W.; Ohte, N.; Garcia-Izquierdo, E.; Chetrit, M.; Monivas-Palomero, V.; Mingo-Santos, S.; Andersen, O.S.; Gude, E.; et al. Determinants of left atrial reservoir and pump strain and use of atrial strain for evaluation of left ventricular filling pressure. *Eur. Heart J. Cardiovasc. Imaging* **2021**, *18*, 61–70. [CrossRef]
19. Reddy, Y.N.V.; Obokata, M.; Verbrugge, F.H.; Lin, G.; Borlaug, B.A. Atrial Dysfunction in Patients With Heart Failure With Preserved Ejection Fraction and Atrial Fibrillation. *J. Am. Coll. Cardiol.* **2020**, *76*, 1051–1064. [CrossRef]
20. Bandera, F.; Martone, R.; Chacko, L.; Ganesananthan, S.; Gilbertson, J.A.; Ponticos, M.; Lane, T.; Martinez-Naharro, A.; Whelan, C.; Quarta, C.; et al. Clinical Importance of Left Atrial Infiltration in Cardiac Transthyretin Amyloidosis. *JACC Cardiovasc. Imaging* **2022**, *15*, 17–29. [CrossRef]
21. Lloyd-Jones, D.M.; Wang, T.J.; Leip, E.P.; Larson, M.G.; Levy, D.; Vasan, R.S.; D'Agostino, R.B.; Massaro, J.M.; Beiser, A.; Wolf, P.A.; et al. Lifetime risk for development of atrial fibrillation: The Framingham Heart Study. *Circulation* **2004**, *110*, 1042–1046. [CrossRef]
22. Lip, G.Y.H.; Brechin, C.M.; Lane, D.A. The global burden of atrial fibrillation and stroke: A systematic review of the epidemiology of atrial fibrillation in regions outside North America and Europe. *Chest* **2012**, *142*, 1489–1498. [CrossRef] [PubMed]
23. Mozaffarian, D.; Benjamin, E.J.; Go, A.S.; Arnett, D.K.; Blaha, M.J.; Cushman, M.; Das, S.R.; de Ferranti, S.; Despres, J.P.; Fullerton, H.J.; et al. Executive Summary: Heart Disease and Stroke Statistics-2016 Update: A Report From the American Heart Association. *Circulation* **2016**, *133*, 447–454. [CrossRef] [PubMed]
24. Wijffels, M.C.; Kirchhof, C.J.; Dorland, R.; Allessie, M.A. Atrial fibrillation begets atrial fibrillation. A study in awake chronically instrumented goats. *Circulation* **1995**, *92*, 1954–1968. [CrossRef]
25. Cha, Y.M.; Redfield, M.M.; Shen, W.K.; Gersh, B.J. Atrial fibrillation and ventricular dysfunction: A vicious electromechanical cycle. *Circulation* **2004**, *109*, 2839–2843. [CrossRef]
26. Tsang, T.S.; Barnes, M.E.; Bailey, K.R.; Leibson, C.L.; Montgomery, S.C.; Takemoto, Y.; Diamond, P.M.; Marra, M.A.; Gersh, B.J.; Wiebers, D.O.; et al. Left atrial volume: Important risk marker of incident atrial fibrillation in 1655 older men and women. *Mayo Clin. Proc.* **2001**, *76*, 467–475. [CrossRef] [PubMed]
27. Tsang, T.S.; Gersh, B.J.; Appleton, C.P.; Tajik, A.J.; Barnes, M.E.; Bailey, K.R.; Oh, J.K.; Leibson, C.; Montgomery, S.C.; Seward, J.B. Left ventricular diastolic dysfunction as a predictor of the first diagnosed nonvalvular atrial fibrillation in 840 elderly men and women. *J. Am. Coll. Cardiol.* **2002**, *40*, 1636–1644. [CrossRef]
28. Fatema, K.; Barnes, M.E.; Bailey, K.R.; Abhayaratna, W.P.; Cha, S.; Seward, J.B.; Tsang, T.S. Minimum vs. maximum left atrial volume for prediction of first atrial fibrillation or flutter in an elderly cohort: A prospective study. *Eur. J. Echocardiogr. J. Work. Group Echocardiogr. Eur. Soc. Cardiol.* **2009**, *10*, 282–286. [CrossRef]
29. Vlachos, K.; Letsas, K.P.; Korantzopoulos, P.; Liu, T.; Georgopoulos, S.; Bakalakos, A.; Karamichalakis, N.; Xydonas, S.; Efremidis, M.; Sideris, A. Prediction of atrial fibrillation development and progression: Current perspectives. *World J. Cardiol.* **2016**, *8*, 267–276. [CrossRef]
30. Zhuang, J.; Wang, Y.; Tang, K.; Li, X.; Peng, W.; Liang, C.; Xu, Y. Association between left atrial size and atrial fibrillation recurrence after single circumferential pulmonary vein isolation: A systematic review and meta-analysis of observational studies. *Europace* **2012**, *14*, 638–645. [CrossRef]
31. Njoku, A.; Kannabhiran, M.; Arora, R.; Reddy, P.; Gopinathannair, R.; Lakkireddy, D.; Dominic, P. Left atrial volume predicts atrial fibrillation recurrence after radiofrequency ablation: A meta-analysis. *Europace* **2018**, *20*, 33–42. [CrossRef] [PubMed]
32. Osranek, M.; Bursi, F.; Bailey, K.R.; Grossardt, B.R.; Brown, R.D., Jr.; Kopecky, S.L.; Tsang, T.S.; Seward, J.B. Left atrial volume predicts cardiovascular events in patients originally diagnosed with lone atrial fibrillation: Three-decade follow-up. *Eur. Heart J.* **2005**, *26*, 2556–2561. [CrossRef]
33. Kawakami, H.; Inoue, K.; Nagai, T.; Fujii, A.; Sasaki, Y.; Shikano, Y.; Sakuoka, N.; Miyazaki, M.; Takasuka, Y.; Ikeda, S.; et al. Persistence of left atrial abnormalities despite left atrial volume normalization after successful ablation of atrial fibrillation. *J. Arrhythmia* **2021**, *37*, 1318–1329. [CrossRef] [PubMed]
34. Tsang, T.S.; Abhayaratna, W.P.; Barnes, M.E.; Miyasaka, Y.; Gersh, B.J.; Bailey, K.R.; Cha, S.S.; Seward, J.B. Prediction of cardiovascular outcomes with left atrial size: Is volume superior to area or diameter? *J. Am. Coll. Cardiol.* **2006**, *47*, 1018–1023. [CrossRef] [PubMed]
35. Machino-Ohtsuka, T.; Seo, Y.; Ishizu, T.; Yanaka, S.; Nakajima, H.; Atsumi, A.; Yamamoto, M.; Kawamura, R.; Koshino, Y.; Machino, T.; et al. Significant improvement of left atrial and left atrial appendage function after catheter ablation for persistent atrial fibrillation. *Circ. J. Off. J. Jpn. Circ. Soc.* **2013**, *77*, 1695–1704. [CrossRef]
36. Sotomi, Y.; Inoue, K.; Tanaka, K.; Toyoshima, Y.; Oka, T.; Tanaka, N.; Nozato, Y.; Orihara, Y.; Koyama, Y.; Iwakura, K.; et al. Persistent left atrial remodeling after catheter ablation for non-paroxysmal atrial fibrillation is associated with very late recurrence. *J. Cardiol.* **2015**, *66*, 370–376. [CrossRef]
37. Walters, T.E.; Nisbet, A.; Morris, G.M.; Tan, G.; Mearns, M.; Teo, E.; Lewis, N.; Ng, A.; Gould, P.; Lee, G.; et al. Progression of atrial remodeling in patients with high-burden atrial fibrillation: Implications for early ablative intervention. *Heart Rhythm* **2016**, *13*, 331–339. [CrossRef]
38. Oka, T.; Inoue, K.; Tanaka, K.; Ninomiya, Y.; Hirao, Y.; Tanaka, N.; Okada, M.; Inoue, H.; Nakamaru, R.; Koyama, Y.; et al. Left Atrial Reverse Remodeling After Catheter Ablation of Nonparoxysmal Atrial Fibrillation in Patients With Heart Failure with Reduced Ejection Fraction. *Am. J. Cardiol.* **2018**, *122*, 89–96. [CrossRef]

39. Kuppahally, S.S.; Akoum, N.; Badger, T.J.; Burgon, N.S.; Haslam, T.; Kholmovski, E.; Macleod, R.; McGann, C.; Marrouche, N.F. Echocardiographic left atrial reverse remodeling after catheter ablation of atrial fibrillation is predicted by preablation delayed enhancement of left atrium by magnetic resonance imaging. *Am. Heart J.* **2010**, *160*, 877–884. [CrossRef]
40. Lang, R.M.; Badano, L.P.; Mor-Avi, V.; Afilalo, J.; Armstrong, A.; Ernande, L.; Flachskampf, F.A.; Foster, E.; Goldstein, S.A.; Kuznetsova, T.; et al. Recommendations for cardiac chamber quantification by echocardiography in adults: An update from the American Society of Echocardiography and the European Association of Cardiovascular Imaging. *J. Am. Soc. Echocardiogr.* **2015**, *28*, 1–39.e14. [CrossRef]
41. Nesbitt, G.C.; Mankad, S.; Oh, J.K. Strain imaging in echocardiography: Methods and clinical applications. *Int. J. Cardiovasc. Imaging* **2009**, *25*, 9–22. [CrossRef] [PubMed]
42. Marwick, T.H. Methods used for the assessment of LV systolic function: Common currency or tower of Babel? *Heart* **2013**, *99*, 1078–1086. [CrossRef] [PubMed]
43. Kuppahally, S.S.; Akoum, N.; Burgon, N.S.; Badger, T.J.; Kholmovski, E.G.; Vijayakumar, S.; Rao, S.N.; Blauer, J.; Fish, E.N.; Dibella, E.V.; et al. Left atrial strain and strain rate in patients with paroxysmal and persistent atrial fibrillation: Relationship to left atrial structural remodeling detected by delayed-enhancement MRI. *Circ. Cardiovasc. Imaging* **2010**, *3*, 231–239. [CrossRef] [PubMed]
44. Watanabe, Y.; Nakano, Y.; Hidaka, T.; Oda, N.; Kajihara, K.; Tokuyama, T.; Uchimura, Y.; Sairaku, A.; Motoda, C.; Fujiwara, M.; et al. Mechanical and substrate abnormalities of the left atrium assessed by 3-dimensional speckle-tracking echocardiography and electroanatomic mapping system in patients with paroxysmal atrial fibrillation. *Heart Rhythm* **2015**, *12*, 490–497. [CrossRef]
45. Ciuffo, L.; Tao, S.; Gucuk Ipek, E.; Zghaib, T.; Balouch, M.; Lima, J.A.C.; Nazarian, S.; Spragg, D.D.; Marine, J.E.; Berger, R.D.; et al. Intra-Atrial Dyssynchrony During Sinus Rhythm Predicts Recurrence After the First Catheter Ablation for Atrial Fibrillation. *JACC Cardiovasc. Imaging* **2018**, *12*, 310–319. [CrossRef]
46. Pathan, F.; Sivaraj, E.; Negishi, K.; Rafiudeen, R.; Pathan, S.; D'Elia, N.; Galligan, J.; Neilson, S.; Fonseca, R.; Marwick, T.H. Use of Atrial Strain to Predict Atrial Fibrillation After Cerebral Ischemia. *JACC Cardiovasc. Imaging* **2018**, *11*, 1557–1565. [CrossRef]
47. Hirose, T.; Kawasaki, M.; Tanaka, R.; Ono, K.; Watanabe, T.; Iwama, M.; Noda, T.; Watanabe, S.; Takemura, G.; Minatoguchi, S. Left atrial function assessed by speckle tracking echocardiography as a predictor of new-onset non-valvular atrial fibrillation: Results from a prospective study in 580 adults. *Eur. Heart J.—Cardiovasc. Imaging* **2012**, *13*, 243–250. [CrossRef]
48. Abhayaratna, W.P.; Fatema, K.; Barnes, M.E.; Seward, J.B.; Gersh, B.J.; Bailey, K.R.; Casaclang-Verzosa, G.; Tsang, T.S. Left atrial reservoir function as a potent marker for first atrial fibrillation or flutter in persons > or = 65 years of age. *Am. J. Cardiol.* **2008**, *101*, 1626–1629. [CrossRef]
49. Her, A.Y.; Kim, J.Y.; Kim, Y.H.; Choi, E.Y.; Min, P.K.; Yoon, Y.W.; Lee, B.K.; Hong, B.K.; Rim, S.J.; Kwon, H.M. Left atrial strain assessed by speckle tracking imaging is related to new-onset atrial fibrillation after coronary artery bypass grafting. *Can. J. Cardiol.* **2013**, *29*, 377–383. [CrossRef]
50. Imanishi, J.; Tanaka, H.; Sawa, T.; Motoji, Y.; Miyoshi, T.; Mochizuki, Y.; Fukuda, Y.; Tatsumi, K.; Matsumoto, K.; Okita, Y.; et al. Left atrial booster-pump function as a predictive parameter for new-onset postoperative atrial fibrillation in patients with severe aortic stenosis. *Int. J. Cardiovasc. Imaging* **2014**, *30*, 295–304. [CrossRef]
51. Hubert, A.; Galand, V.; Donal, E.; Pavin, D.; Galli, E.; Martins, R.P.; Leclercq, C.; Carré, F.; Schnell, F. Atrial function is altered in lone paroxysmal atrial fibrillation in male endurance veteran athletes. *Eur. Heart J.—Cardiovasc. Imaging* **2018**, *19*, 145–153. [CrossRef] [PubMed]
52. Moreno-Ruiz, L.A.; Madrid-Miller, A.; Martinez-Flores, J.E.; Gonzalez-Hermosillo, J.A.; Arenas-Fonseca, J.; Zamorano-Velazquez, N.; Mendoza-Perez, B. Left atrial longitudinal strain by speckle tracking as independent predictor of recurrence after electrical cardioversion in persistent and long standing persistent non-valvular atrial fibrillation. *Int. J. Cardiovasc. Imaging* **2019**, *35*, 1587–1596. [CrossRef] [PubMed]
53. Motoki, H.; Negishi, K.; Kusunose, K.; Popovic, Z.B.; Bhargava, M.; Wazni, O.M.; Saliba, W.I.; Chung, M.K.; Marwick, T.H.; Klein, A.L. Global left atrial strain in the prediction of sinus rhythm maintenance after catheter ablation for atrial fibrillation. *J. Am. Soc. Echocardiogr.* **2014**, *27*, 1184–1192. [CrossRef]
54. Yoon, Y.E.; Oh, I.Y.; Kim, S.A.; Park, K.H.; Kim, S.H.; Park, J.H.; Kim, J.E.; Lee, S.P.; Kim, H.K.; Kim, Y.J.; et al. Echocardiographic Predictors of Progression to Persistent or Permanent Atrial Fibrillation in Patients with Paroxysmal Atrial Fibrillation (E6P Study). *J. Am. Soc. Echocardiogr.* **2015**, *28*, 709–717. [CrossRef] [PubMed]
55. Yasuda, R.; Murata, M.; Roberts, R.; Tokuda, H.; Minakata, Y.; Suzuki, K.; Tsuruta, H.; Kimura, T.; Nishiyama, N.; Fukumoto, K.; et al. Left atrial strain is a powerful predictor of atrial fibrillation recurrence after catheter ablation: Study of a heterogeneous population with sinus rhythm or atrial fibrillation. *Eur. Heart J. Cardiovasc. Imaging* **2015**, *16*, 1008–1014. [CrossRef] [PubMed]
56. Mochizuki, A.; Yuda, S.; Oi, Y.; Kawamukai, M.; Nishida, J.; Kouzu, H.; Muranaka, A.; Kokubu, N.; Shimoshige, S.; Hashimoto, A.; et al. Assessment of left atrial deformation and synchrony by three-dimensional speckle-tracking echocardiography: Comparative studies in healthy subjects and patients with atrial fibrillation. *J. Am. Soc. Echocardiogr.* **2013**, *26*, 165–174. [CrossRef] [PubMed]
57. Kobayashi, Y.; Okura, H.; Kobayashi, Y.; Okawa, K.; Banba, K.; Hirohata, A.; Tamada, T.; Obase, K.; Hayashida, A.; Yoshida, K. Assessment of atrial synchrony in paroxysmal atrial fibrillation and impact of pulmonary vein isolation for atrial dyssynchrony and global strain by three-dimensional strain echocardiography. *J. Am. Soc. Echocardiogr.* **2014**, *27*, 1193–1199. [CrossRef]

58. Furukawa, A.; Ishii, K.; Hyodo, E.; Shibamoto, M.; Komasa, A.; Nagai, T.; Tada, E.; Seino, Y.; Yoshikawa, J. Three-Dimensional Speckle Tracking Imaging for Assessing Left Atrial Function in Hypertensive Patients With Paroxysmal Atrial Fibrillation. *Int. Heart J.* **2016**, *57*, 705–711. [CrossRef]
59. Shang, Z.; Su, D.; Cong, T.; Sun, Y.; Liu, Y.; Chen, N.; Yang, J. Assessment of left atrial mechanical function and synchrony in paroxysmal atrial fibrillation with two-dimensional speckle tracking echocardiography. *Echocardiography* **2017**, *34*, 176–183. [CrossRef]
60. Sakabe, K.; Fukuda, N.; Fukuda, Y.; Morishita, S.; Shinohara, H.; Tamura, Y. Interatrial dyssynchrony on tissue Doppler imaging predicts progression to chronic atrial fibrillation in patients with non-valvular paroxysmal atrial fibrillation. *Heart* **2009**, *95*, 988–993. [CrossRef]
61. Kawakami, H.; Ramkumar, S.; Nolan, M.; Wright, L.; Yang, H.; Negishi, K.; Marwick, T.H. Left Atrial Mechanical Dispersion Assessed by Strain Echocardiography as an Independent Predictor of New-Onset Atrial Fibrillation: A Case-Control Study. *J. Am. Soc. Echocardiogr.* **2019**, *32*, 1268–1276.e3. [CrossRef] [PubMed]
62. Ma, X.X.; Boldt, L.H.; Zhang, Y.L.; Zhu, M.R.; Hu, B.; Parwani, A.; Belyavskiy, E.; Radha Krishnan, A.K.; Krisper, M.; Kohncke, C.; et al. Clinical Relevance of Left Atrial Strain to Predict Recurrence of Atrial Fibrillation after Catheter Ablation: A Meta-Analysis. *Echocardiography* **2016**, *33*, 724–733. [CrossRef] [PubMed]
63. Sarvari, S.I.; Haugaa, K.H.; Stokke, T.M.; Ansari, H.Z.; Leren, I.S.; Hegbom, F.; Smiseth, O.A.; Edvardsen, T. Strain echocardiographic assessment of left atrial function predicts recurrence of atrial fibrillation. *Eur. Heart J. Cardiovasc. Imaging* **2016**, *17*, 660–667. [CrossRef] [PubMed]
64. Packer, M. Effect of catheter ablation on pre-existing abnormalities of left atrial systolic, diastolic, and neurohormonal functions in patients with chronic heart failure and atrial fibrillation. *Eur. Heart J.* **2019**, *40*, 1873–1879. [CrossRef] [PubMed]
65. Gibson, D.N.; Di Biase, L.; Mohanty, P.; Patel, J.D.; Bai, R.; Sanchez, J.; Burkhardt, J.D.; Heywood, J.T.; Johnson, A.D.; Rubenson, D.S.; et al. Stiff left atrial syndrome after catheter ablation for atrial fibrillation: Clinical characterization, prevalence, and predictors. *Heart Rhythm* **2011**, *8*, 1364–1371. [CrossRef]
66. Obokata, M.; Negishi, K.; Kurosawa, K.; Tateno, R.; Tange, S.; Arai, M.; Amano, M.; Kurabayashi, M. Left atrial strain provides incremental value for embolism risk stratification over CHA(2)DS(2)-VASc score and indicates prognostic impact in patients with atrial fibrillation. *J. Am. Soc. Echocardiogr.* **2014**, *27*, 709–716.e4. [CrossRef] [PubMed]
67. Kupczynska, K.; Michalski, B.W.; Miskowiec, D.; Kasprzak, J.D.; Szymczyk, E.; Wejner Mik, P.; Lipiec, P. Incremental value of left atrial mechanical dispersion over CHA2 DS2 -VASc score in predicting risk of thrombus formation. *Echocardiography* **2018**, *35*, 651–660. [CrossRef] [PubMed]
68. Modesto, K.M.; Dispenzieri, A.; Cauduro, S.A.; Lacy, M.; Khandheria, B.K.; Pellikka, P.A.; Belohlavek, M.; Seward, J.B.; Kyle, R.; Tajik, A.J.; et al. Left atrial myopathy in cardiac amyloidosis: Implications of novel echocardiographic techniques. *Eur. Heart J.* **2005**, *26*, 173–179. [CrossRef]
69. Nochioka, K.; Quarta, C.C.; Claggett, B.; Roca, G.Q.; Rapezzi, C.; Falk, R.H.; Solomon, S.D. Left atrial structure and function in cardiac amyloidosis. *Eur. Heart. J. Cardiovasc. Imaging* **2017**, *18*, 1128–1137. [CrossRef]
70. Aquaro, G.D.; Morini, S.; Grigoratos, C.; Taborchi, G.; Di Bella, G.; Martone, R.; Vignini, E.; Emdin, M.; Olivotto, I.; Perfetto, F.; et al. Electromechanical dissociation of left atrium in patients with Cardiac Amyloidosis by Magnetic Resonance: Prognostic and clinical correlates. *Int. J. Cardiol. Heart Vasc.* **2020**, *31*, 100633. [CrossRef]
71. Maurer, M.S.; Schwartz, J.H.; Gundapaneni, B.; Elliott, P.M.; Merlini, G.; Waddington-Cruz, M.; Kristen, A.V.; Grogan, M.; Witteles, R.; Damy, T.; et al. Tafamidis Treatment for Patients with Transthyretin Amyloid Cardiomyopathy. *N. Engl. J. Med.* **2018**, *379*, 1007–1016. [CrossRef] [PubMed]
72. Phelan, D.; Collier, P.; Thavendiranathan, P.; Popovic, Z.B.; Hanna, M.; Plana, J.C.; Marwick, T.H.; Thomas, J.D. Relative apical sparing of longitudinal strain using two-dimensional speckle-tracking echocardiography is both sensitive and specific for the diagnosis of cardiac amyloidosis. *Heart* **2012**, *98*, 1442–1448. [CrossRef] [PubMed]
73. Saito, M.; Imai, M.; Wake, D.; Higaki, R.; Nakao, Y.; Sumimoto, T.; Yokomoto, Y.; Ogimoto, A.; Suzuki, M.; Kawakami, H.; et al. Semiquantitative assessment of the relative apical sparing pattern of longitudinal strain for cardiac amyloidosis identification. *Echocardiography* **2020**, *37*, 1422–1429. [CrossRef] [PubMed]
74. Liu, D.; Hu, K.; Niemann, M.; Herrmann, S.; Cikes, M.; Stork, S.; Gaudron, P.D.; Knop, S.; Ertl, G.; Bijnens, B.; et al. Effect of combined systolic and diastolic functional parameter assessment for differentiation of cardiac amyloidosis from other causes of concentric left ventricular hypertrophy. *Circ. Cardiovasc. Imaging* **2013**, *6*, 1066–1072. [CrossRef] [PubMed]
75. Rausch, K.; Scalia, G.M.; Sato, K.; Edwards, N.; Lam, A.K.; Platts, D.G.; Chan, J. Left atrial strain imaging differentiates cardiac amyloidosis and hypertensive heart disease. *Int. J. Cardiovasc. Imaging* **2021**, *37*, 81–90. [CrossRef]
76. Higashi, H.; Inoue, K.; Inaba, S.; Nakao, Y.; Kinoshita, M.; Miyazaki, S.; Miyoshi, T.; Akazawa, Y.; Kawakami, H.; Uetani, T.; et al. Restricted left atrial dilatation can visually differentiate cardiac amyloidosis from hypertrophic cardiomyopathy. *ESC Heart Fail.* **2021**, *8*, 3198–3205. [CrossRef]
77. Donnellan, E.; Wazni, O.M.; Hanna, M.; Elshazly, M.B.; Puri, R.; Saliba, W.; Kanj, M.; Vakamudi, S.; Patel, D.R.; Baranowski, B.; et al. Atrial Fibrillation in Transthyretin Cardiac Amyloidosis: Predictors, Prevalence, and Efficacy of Rhythm Control Strategies. *JACC Clin. Electrophysiol.* **2020**, *6*, 1118–1127. [CrossRef]

78. Martinez-Naharro, A.; Gonzalez-Lopez, E.; Corovic, A.; Mirelis, J.G.; Baksi, A.J.; Moon, J.C.; Garcia-Pavia, P.; Gillmore, J.D Hawkins, P.N.; Fontana, M. High Prevalence of Intracardiac Thrombi in Cardiac Amyloidosis. *J. Am. Coll. Cardiol.* **2019**, *73* 1733–1734. [CrossRef]
79. Baumgartner, H. Geriatric congenital heart disease: A new challenge in the care of adults with congenital heart disease? *Eur Heart J.* **2014**, *35*, 683–685. [CrossRef]
80. Diller, G.P.; Kempny, A.; Alonso-Gonzalez, R.; Swan, L.; Uebing, A.; Li, W.; Babu-Narayan, S.; Wort, S.J.; Dimopoulos, K. Gatzoulis, M.A. Survival Prospects and Circumstances of Death in Contemporary Adult Congenital Heart Disease Patients Under Follow-Up at a Large Tertiary Centre. *Circulation* **2015**, *132*, 2118–2125. [CrossRef]
81. Panesar, D.K.; Burch, M. Assessment of Diastolic Function in Congenital Heart Disease. *Front. Cardiovasc. Med.* **2017**, *4*, 5 [CrossRef] [PubMed]
82. Thomas, L.; Marwick, T.H.; Popescu, B.A.; Donal, E.; Badano, L.P. Left Atrial Structure and Function, and Left Ventricular Diastolic Dysfunction: JACC State-of-the-Art Review. *J. Am. Coll. Cardiol.* **2019**, *73*, 1961–1977. [CrossRef] [PubMed]
83. Ma, X.J.; Huang, G.Y.; Liu, F.; Wu, L.; Sheng, F.; Tao, Z.Y. The impacts of transcatheter occlusion for congenital atrial septal defect on atrial volume, function, and synchronicity in children: A three-dimensional echocardiography study. *Echocardiography* **2008** *25*, 1101–1111. [CrossRef] [PubMed]
84. Seo, J.S.; Park, Y.A.; Wi, J.H.; Jin, H.Y.; Han, I.Y.; Jang, J.S.; Yang, T.H.; Kim, D.K.; Kim, D.S. Long-Term Left Atrial Function after Device Closure and Surgical Closure in Adult Patients with Atrial Septal Defect. *J. Cardiovasc. Imaging* **2021**, *29*, 123–132 [CrossRef]
85. Spies, C.; Khandelwal, A.; Timmermanns, I.; Schrader, R. Incidence of atrial fibrillation following transcatheter closure of atrial septal defects in adults. *Am. J. Cardiol.* **2008**, *102*, 902–906. [CrossRef]
86. Vitarelli, A.; Mangieri, E.; Gaudio, C.; Tanzilli, G.; Miraldi, F.; Capotosto, L. Right atrial function by speckle tracking echocardiography in atrial septal defect: Prediction of atrial fibrillation. *Clin. Cardiol.* **2018**, *41*, 1341–1347. [CrossRef]
87. Iio, C.; Inoue, K.; Tashiro, R.; Higaki, T.; Higaki, J. Secundum atrial septal defect resulting in hypoxaemia. *Eur. Heart J. Cardiovasc. Imaging* **2014**, *15*, 103. [CrossRef]
88. Fukuda, Y.; Tanaka, H.; Motoji, Y.; Ryo, K.; Sawa, T.; Imanishi, J.; Miyoshi, T.; Mochizuki, Y.; Tatsumi, K.; Matsumoto, K.; et al. Utility of combining assessment of right ventricular function and right atrial remodeling as a prognostic factor for patients with pulmonary hypertension. *Int. J. Cardiovasc. Imaging* **2014**, *30*, 1269–1277. [CrossRef]
89. Fontan, F.; Baudet, E. Surgical repair of tricuspid atresia. *Thorax* **1971**, *26*, 240–248. [CrossRef]
90. Gentles, T.L.; Mayer, J.E., Jr.; Gauvreau, K.; Newburger, J.W.; Lock, J.E.; Kupferschmid, J.P.; Burnett, J.; Jonas, R.A.; Castaneda, A.R.; Wernovsky, G. Fontan operation in five hundred consecutive patients: Factors influencing early and late outcome. *J. Thorac. Cardiovasc. Surg.* **1997**, *114*, 376–391. [CrossRef]
91. Amodeo, A.; Galletti, L.; Marianeschi, S.; Picardo, S.; Giannico, S.; Di Renzi, P.; Marcelletti, C. Extracardiac Fontan operation for complex cardiac anomalies: Seven years' experience. *J. Thorac. Cardiovasc. Surg.* **1997**, *114*, 1020–1030, discussion 1030-1021. [CrossRef]
92. Veldtman, G.R.; Nishimoto, A.; Siu, S.; Freeman, M.; Fredriksen, P.M.; Gatzoulis, M.A.; Williams, W.G.; Webb, G.D. The Fontan procedure in adults. *Heart* **2001**, *86*, 330–335. [CrossRef] [PubMed]
93. Penny, D.J.; Rigby, M.L.; Redington, A.N. Abnormal patterns of intraventricular flow and diastolic filling after the Fontan operation: Evidence for incoordinate ventricular wall motion. *Br Heart J* **1991**, *66*, 375–378. [CrossRef] [PubMed]
94. Frommelt, P.C.; Snider, A.R.; Meliones, J.N.; Vermilion, R.P. Doppler assessment of pulmonary artery flow patterns and ventricular function after the Fontan operation. *Am. J. Cardiol.* **1991**, *68*, 1211–1215. [CrossRef]
95. Akagi, T.; Benson, L.N.; Gilday, D.L.; Ash, J.; Green, M.; Williams, W.G.; Freedom, R.M. Influence of ventricular morphology on diastolic filling performance in double-inlet ventricle after the Fontan procedure. *J. Am. Coll. Cardiol.* **1993**, *22*, 1948–1952. [CrossRef]
96. Khoo, N.S.; Smallhorn, J.F.; Kaneko, S.; Kutty, S.; Altamirano, L.; Tham, E.B. The assessment of atrial function in single ventricle hearts from birth to Fontan: A speckle-tracking study by using strain and strain rate. *J. Am. Soc. Echocardiogr.* **2013**, *26*, 756–764. [CrossRef]
97. Li, S.J.; Wong, S.J.; Cheung, Y.F. Atrial and ventricular mechanics in patients after Fontan-type procedures: Atriopulmonary connection versus extracardiac conduit. *J. Am. Soc. Echocardiogr.* **2014**, *27*, 666–674. [CrossRef]

Journal of
Cardiovascular
Development and Disease

MDPI

Review

Exercise Stress Echocardiography in the Diagnostic Evaluation of Heart Failure with Preserved Ejection Fraction

Tomonari Harada [1], Kazuki Kagami [1,2], Toshimitsu Kato [1], Hideki Ishii [1] and Masaru Obokata [1,*]

1 Department of Cardiovascular Medicine, Gunma University Graduate School of Medicine, Maebashi 371-8511, Gunma, Japan; tharada@gunma-u.ac.jp (T.H.); mirror.1028k@gmail.com (K.K.); t-kato@gunma-u.ac.jp (T.K.); hkishii@med.nagoya-u.ac.jp (H.I.)
2 Division of Cardiovascular Medicine, National Defense Medical College, Tokorozawa 359-8513, Saitama, Japan
* Correspondence: obokata.masaru@gunma-u.ac.jp; Tel.: +81-27-220-8145

Abstract: More than half of patients with heart failure have a preserved ejection fraction (HFpEF). The prevalence of HFpEF has been increasing worldwide and is expected to increase further, making it an important health-care problem. The diagnosis of HFpEF is straightforward in the presence of obvious objective signs of congestion; however, it is challenging in patients presenting with a low degree of congestion because abnormal elevation in intracardiac pressures may occur only during physiological stress conditions, such as during exercise. On the basis of this hemodynamic background, current consensus guidelines have emphasized the importance of exercise stress testing to reveal abnormalities during exercise, and exercise stress echocardiography (i.e., diastolic stress echocardiography) may be used as an initial diagnostic approach to HFpEF owing to its noninvasive nature and wide availability. However, evidence supporting the use of this method remains limited and many knowledge gaps exist with respect to diastolic stress echocardiography. This review summarizes the current understanding of the use of diastolic stress echocardiography in the diagnostic evaluation of HFpEF and discusses its strengths and limitations to encourage future studies on this subject.

Keywords: diagnosis; expired gas analysis; heart failure with preserved ejection fraction

1. Introduction

The burden of heart failure (HF) is increasing worldwide, and more than half of patients with HF have a preserved left ventricular (LV) ejection fraction (HFpEF) [1]. Owing to aging populations and the increasing prevalence of metabolic comorbidities, such as obesity, metabolic syndrome, and diabetes mellitus, the prevalence and incidence of HFpEF relative to HF with reduced ejection fraction (HFrEF) is expected to increase further [2]. The limited treatment options for HFpEF and the increasing burden of this disease result in a substantial unmet clinical need in the modern era.

In contrast to HFrEF, the diagnosis of HFpEF is challenging because patients have a normal ejection fraction. In addition, many patients have normal hemodynamics at rest and show abnormal hemodynamic responses only during exercise [1,3]. Accumulating evidence has demonstrated the utility of exercise stress testing (exercise stress echocardiography or invasive hemodynamic exercise testing) in revealing diastolic reserve limitation and, subsequently, elevation in LV filling pressures during exercise. As a result, exercise stress testing has been increasingly recommended for the diagnostic evaluation of HFpEF [4–9]. For this purpose, exercise stress echocardiography (i.e., diastolic stress echocardiography) plays a central role in clinical practice owing to its noninvasive nature and wide availability [4]. However, evidence supporting the use of this method remains limited and many knowledge gaps remain. In this review, we will summarize the current understanding of the use of diastolic stress echocardiography for the diagnosis of HFpEF, highlighting its strengths and limitations.

2. Pathophysiological Background Supporting the Importance of Exercise Stress Echocardiography for the Diagnosis of HFpEF

The diagnosis of HFrEF is straightforward and requires the detection of a decreased ejection fraction on echocardiography in patients with symptoms of HF (e.g., dyspnea, peripheral edema, and jugular venous distention). In contrast, HFpEF is more difficult to evaluate because the patients' LV ejection fraction is preserved, making it difficult to distinguish HFpEF from other disorders presenting with HF-like symptoms (e.g., pulmonary diseases) [3,10,11]. In such cases, the diagnosis relies on objective evidence of congestion or elevated LV filling pressures [10], including the detection of pulmonary congestion on chest radiography or computed tomography, high natriuretic peptide levels, echocardiographic signs of LV diastolic dysfunction, or abnormal central hemodynamics directly measured through cardiac catheterization. Nevertheless, the diagnosis of HFpEF is not simple because many patients, especially those with no or a low degree of congestion, have normal LV filling pressures at rest [4,12]. Thus, the methods for identifying HFpEF among euvolemic patients have poor sensitivity (~60%), even during right heart catheterization, when performed at rest [4]. In patients with HFpEF, intracardiac pressures dramatically increase during the stress of exercise [4,13–17]. On the basis of this hemodynamic background, the ability of exercise stress echocardiography to reveal abnormalities that develop only during stress has been receiving increasing attention [4,8,18,19].

3. Exercise Echocardiography Methods

3.1. Clinical Indications

Diastolic stress echocardiography is indicated in patients who are suspected of having HFpEF based on clinical history, symptoms, or physical findings but had no clear evidence of elevated filling pressures from assessments performed at rest, such as echocardiography or measurement of natriuretic peptide levels [3,4,10,20]. Patients with apparent congestion or abnormal findings indicative of elevated LV filling pressures (e.g., high left atrial pressure according to the European Association of Cardiovascular Imaging [EACVI]/American Society of Echocardiography [ASE] algorithm) do not need to be referred for exercise testing because of a sufficiently high pretest probability. Meanwhile, diastolic stress echocardiography should not be performed in patients with no features of HFpEF because even a positive exercise test does not increase the post-test probability of definitively diagnosing HFpEF (as, theoretically, the positive predictive value depends on disease prevalence) [21]. Therefore, diastolic stress echocardiography is most useful in patients with an intermediate pretest probability for HFpEF.

Two scoring systems are available for estimating the pretest probability of HFpEF: the H_2FPEF and HFA-PEFF scores [8,22]. The H_2FPEF score is a weighted composite score of four clinical factors (obesity, two or more antihypertensive medications, atrial fibrillation, and age > 60 years) and two echocardiographic parameters (ratio of early diastolic mitral inflow velocity to mitral annular tissue velocity [E/e' ratio] > 9 and estimated pulmonary artery systolic pressure > 35 mmHg), ranging from 0 to 9 points [22]. The HFA-PEFF score is a consensus-based algorithm proposed by the Heart Failure Association (HFA) of the European Society of Cardiology (ESC) that is composed of three domains (functional, morphological, and natriuretic peptide domains) and ranges from 0 to 6 points [8]. Patients with an intermediate pretest probability based on these metrics (H_2FPEF score of 2–5 points or HFA-PEFF score of 2–4 points) are indicated for diastolic stress echocardiography to refine the diagnosis of HFpEF [23]. Studies have also demonstrated that both scores predict reduced exercise capacity and clinical outcomes in patients with HFpEF [19,24–27].

3.2. Exercise Stress Methods

Exercise requires integrated physiologic responses in the cardiovascular system, including biventricular contractility, lusitropic effect, chronotropic response, systemic and pulmonary vasodilation, and venous return, involving the central and peripheral nervous systems, lungs, coronary circulation, and skeletal muscle [16,28–30]. Patients with HFpEF may develop abnormalities in several of these components, leading to symptoms of dyspnea and exercise intolerance [15–17,31]. When a patient is able to exercise, dynamic exercise (e.g., treadmill or bicycle ergometer testing) should be selected because it can cause physiologic stress to the cardiovascular system [7]. Isometric exercise (sustained isometric handgrip exercise) can be performed in some patients to produce afterload-mediated stress [32–34]. A preload stress test through passive leg raises or the leg-positive pressure maneuver might also represent a non-exercise test to reveal LV diastolic dysfunction [35,36]. However, multiple abnormalities contribute to LV diastolic dysfunction and elevated LV filling pressures in HFpEF [15–17,31]. Therefore, the use of handgrip exercises or a preload stress test is less likely to be an alternative to dynamic exercise because it only partially stresses the cardiovascular system (i.e., handgrip exercise does not considerably affect the heart rate, preload, or venous return) [5,37].

Supine bicycle stress echocardiography is the recommended modality for diastolic stress echocardiography, as it has important advantages over treadmill exercise, as follows [7,8,38]: it allows continuous image acquisition throughout the test rather than only immediately post-exercise; it uses the semi-left lateral decubitus position, which facilitates the acquisition of images during exercise; and it has a much lower risk of falling down than treadmill exercise. However, as most physical activities in daily living are performed in an upright position, upright bicycle ergometer exercise is likely to produce more physiological stress than supine bicycle exercise if diagnostic-quality images can be obtained during exercise [39,40]. Notably, because the exercise position can affect central hemodynamics, the results must be interpreted with caution [41]. An increase in LV filling pressures may be more prominent owing to greater preload augmentation in the supine position than in the upright position [4,39,40,42].

3.3. Stress Protocols, Image Acquisition, and Targeted Parameters

No universally adopted protocols exist for diastolic stress echocardiography. The EACVI/ASE guidelines recommend a multistage protocol, starting at 25 watts (W) at a 60 rpm cadence with the load increasing by 25 W every 3 min until peak exercise [7,20]. Other researchers have proposed a ramp stress protocol, starting at 15 W with 5 W increments every minute to a submaximal target heart rate of 100–110 bpm. During supine bicycle exercise echocardiography, echocardiographic images should be obtained at baseline, at each stage of exercise, and during the early recovery phase [7]. The advantage of image acquisition is the chance to determine the E/e' ratio before the fusion of the mitral E and A velocities (Figure 1).

The EACVI/ASE guidelines recommend measuring the transmitral flow velocities, mitral annular tissue velocities, and tricuspid regurgitant velocity (TRV) to detect abnormal LV diastolic function reserve and the resulting increase in LV filling pressures [7,20]. The E/e' ratio plays a key role in estimating LV filling pressures during exercise stress echocardiography [7,20]. A simultaneous catheterization–echocardiography study demonstrated a moderate correlation between the E/e' ratio and invasively measured pulmonary capillary wedge pressure (PCWP) during exercise (r = 0.54–0.58) [4], although some studies raised questions about the ability of the E/e' ratio to indicate changes in LV filling pressures [43–45]. The most common diagnostic limitation is the inability to evaluate the E/e' ratio when the diastolic velocities are fused during high heart rates [4]. The EACVI/ASE guidelines recommend the acquisition of images during the submaximal phase before the fusion of the mitral E and A velocities (heart rate, 100–110 bpm) or during the early recovery period [7]. Previous studies using exercise right heart catheterization have consistently shown that an abnormal increase in left-side filling pressure occurs early during submaximal (20-W) exercise in patients with HFpEF [4,5,16,46,47]. This observation may support the utility of E/e' ratio measurement during submaximal supine exercise in diagnosing HFpEF [4]; however, further studies are required to determine the diagnostic value of the E/e' ratio during submaximal exercise, ideally using simultaneous invasive exercise hemodynamic testing. Conversely, PCWP may rapidly return to baseline levels early in the recovery phase even in patients with HFpEF (1 min post-exercise) [5]. Thus, PCWP may be normal when the E and A waves are no longer fused (Figure 1). It is also important to remember that E/e′ ratio cannot be applied to patients with specific diseases, such as mitral stenosis, severe mitral regurgitation, mitral annular calcification, mitral valve repair, or a prosthetic mitral valve, or in the presence of regional wall motion abnormalities [48].

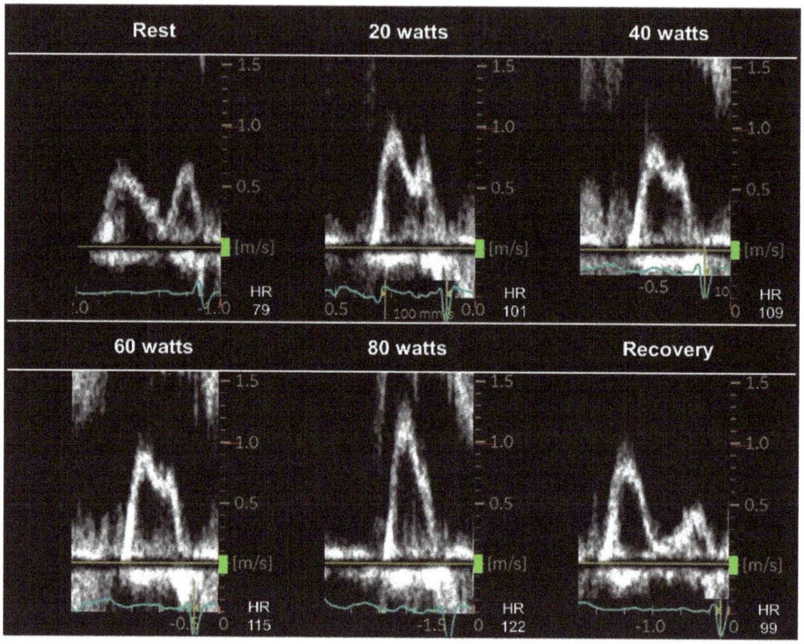

Figure 1. Changes in the transmitral inflow profile at rest and throughout exercise in a patient with heart failure and preserved ejection fraction. During peak exercise (80 watts), the transmitral E and A waves were indistinguishable owing to fusion. Continuous image acquisition allowed for the identification of an E wave of 100 cm/s at 60–watt exercise, and the E/e′ ratio at this stage was elevated (E/e′ ratio, 15.5). Invasive exercise right heart catheterization revealed that the pulmonary capillary wedge pressure (PCWP) was normal at rest (9 mmHg); however, it increased to 26 mmHg during peak exercise (80 watts). Although the E and A waves were no longer fused in the early recovery phase, the E/e′ ratio was 12.9. The invasively measured PCWP decreased to 19 mmHg (<25 mmHg) at 1 min post–exercise. HR, heart rate.

Pulmonary hypertension (PH) in HF is primarily caused by a passive elevation in downstream LV filling pressures [49]. Thus, the assessment of PH during diastolic stress echocardiography is important to evaluate the severity of increases in LV filling pressures during the stress of exercise, and this can be achieved by measuring the TRV [7,8,20]. An isolated increase in the TRV during exercise is insufficient to diagnose HFpEF because it may be secondary to pulmonary vascular disease (pre-capillary component) or high cardiac output (CO). The presence of a concomitant increase in the TRV and E/e′ ratio can increase the probability of elevated LV filling pressures [8,50,51]. Importantly, exercise-induced PH predicts poor clinical outcomes in patients with HFpEF [52,53]. The current practice in assessing PH during exercise relies on TRV alone rather than the combination of TRV and right atrial pressure (RAP) [7,8,20,54]. This may be related to the technical difficulty in imaging the inferior vena cava during exercise; however, the exclusion of RAP leads to a serious underestimation of the severity of PH during exercise in some patients in whom RAP may increase dramatically (~40 mmHg) [14,15,17,55]. Prior studies reported a close relationship between RAP and peripheral venous pressure at rest [56,57]. Our group recently demonstrated that the measurement of peripheral venous pressure may be a reliable alternative to RAP measurement during diastolic stress echocardiography [58].

Accumulating evidence has shown that lung ultrasound can reliably demonstrate pulmonary congestion as multiple B-lines in patients with HF [59]. Echocardiographic B-lines (lung comets) can be visualized as vertical, laser-like, hyperechoic artifacts that arise from the pleural line and extend to the bottom of the screen without fading [60,61]. B-lines may develop or quickly worsen in response to exercise in patients with HF, and "wet spots" may appear in the third intercostal space in two regions along the anterior axillary and mid-axillary lines, where B-lines most prominently develop during supine exercise [62]. An increased number of B-lines during exercise is correlated with hemodynamic congestion (Figure 2) (higher PCWP and pulmonary arterial pressures), as well as with reduced exercise capacity and worse clinical outcomes in HFpEF [63–67].

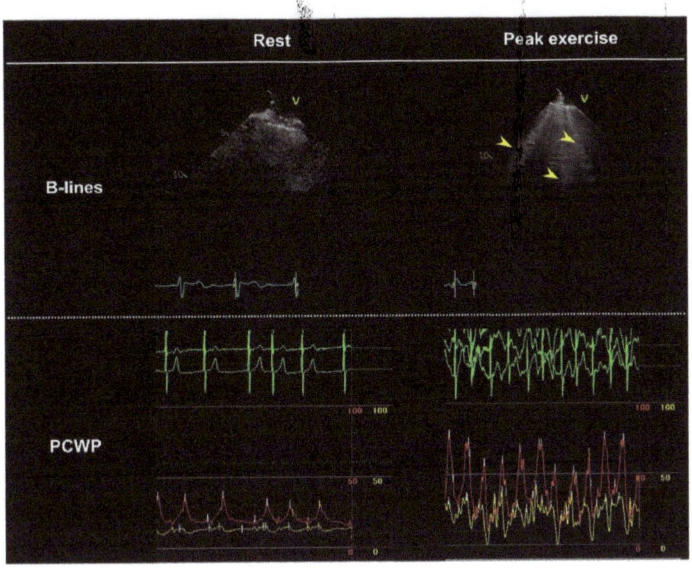

Figure 2. Exercise-induced ultrasound B-lines with simultaneously measured pulmonary capillary wedge pressure (PCWP) in a patient with heart failure and preserved ejection fraction. The patient demonstrated mildly elevated PCWP (19 mmHg, red line) without ultrasound B-lines at rest. During peak exercise (40 watts), the PCWP increased to 33 mmHg with marked V waves (71 mmHg), and multiple B-lines developed (yellow arrowheads).

Notably, the assessment of ultrasound B-lines may be less influenced by the movement of the heart during exercise, contributing to a high data acquisition rate. However, the limitations in assessing B-lines in diastolic stress echocardiography also need to be considered. The presence of B-lines is not specific to pulmonary congestion but rather indicates interstitial syndrome [60,68]. Thus, its diagnostic value is limited in patients with concomitant interstitial lung diseases. B-lines can be evaluated in 28 chest regions [7]; however, scanning all 28 regions may reduce the time for imaging other parameters [63]. The most important limitation is the lack of consensus on the interpretation of results. Further studies are required to establish the cutoff value of the number of B-lines to define elevated LV filling pressures during exercise in patients with HFpEF.

Depending on the assumed differential diseases, additional echocardiographic parameters can be evaluated, including the following: regional wall motion; mitral regurgitation; pulmonary venous flow velocities; right ventricular systolic function (tricuspid annular plane systolic excursion, tricuspid lateral annular systolic velocity, or right ventricular longitudinal strain); tricuspid regurgitation; and inferior vena cava measurements. For example, regional wall motion abnormalities can be additionally evaluated in patients suspected of having HFpEF with multiple coronary risk factors. This approach might allow for a better pathophysiological characterization that may lead to a specific treatment strategy (Figure 3) [11].

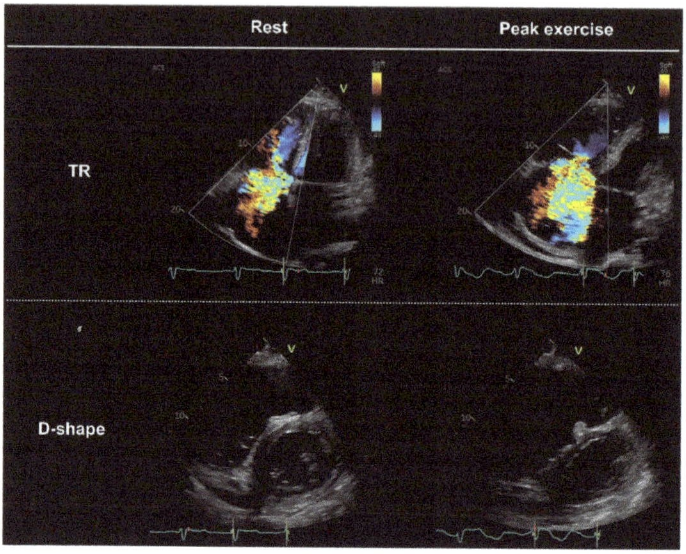

Figure 3. Heightened ventricular interdependence due to worsening tricuspid regurgitation (TR) during exercise in a patient with heart failure and preserved ejection fraction. The patient had persistent atrial fibrillation and moderate-to-severe TR at rest. The TR velocity was 2.5 m/s, and the estimated right atrial pressure based on inferior vena cava measurements was 15 mmHg. During peak exercise (20 watts), the TR dramatically worsened with incomplete coaptation of the tricuspid valves, resulting in paradoxical reduction in TR velocity (1.9 m/s). A significant increase in TR during exercise caused greater ventricular interdependence, contributing to reduced exercise capacity (peak oxygen consumption [VO_2], 7.1 mL/min/kg).

3.4. Interpretation of Test Results and Diagnosis of HFpEF

The EACVI/ASE proposed a consensus-based scheme to define abnormal diastolic function based on the E/e′ ratio, TRV, and e′ velocity (Figures 4 and 5) [7,20].

Although this algorithm is pathophysiologically sound, its requirement of satisfying all three criteria may reduce the feasibility and sensitivity of diagnosing HFpEF. A study reported that during peak exercise, the E/e′ ratio was not measurable in approximately 20% and TRV was measurable in only approximately 50% of patients [4]. The HFA of the ESC suggested an algorithm that emphasizes the exercise E/e′ ratio, adding 2 points for isolated E/e′ elevation and 3 points for a concomitant increase in the E/e′ ratio and TRV to the resting HFA-PEFF score (Figure 5) [8]. This may be more probabilistically reasonable than the EACVI/ASE guidelines (i.e., patients with elevated E/e′ and TRV are more likely to have HFpEF). Thereby, the development or increasing number of B-lines may indicate an increased probability of HFpEF [3,63].

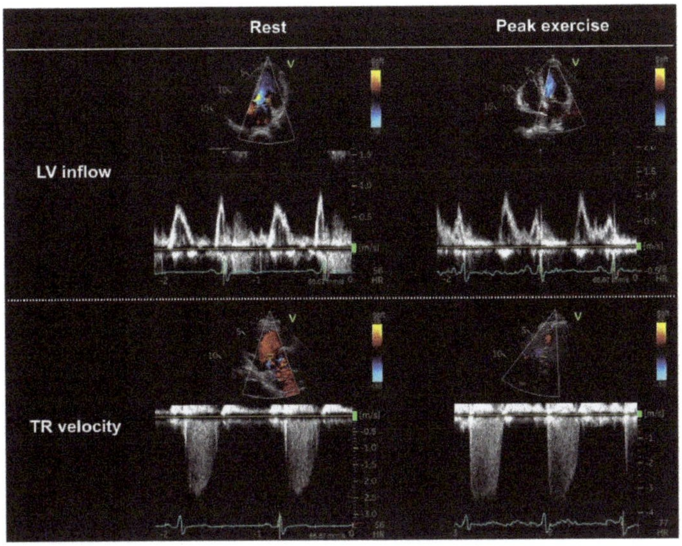

Figure 4. Key parameters in diastolic stress echocardiography. A 72-year-old woman who presented with exertional dyspnea was referred for diastolic stress echocardiography. She had a normal ejection fraction (61%), slightly elevated B-type natriuretic peptide (NP) levels (48.2 pg/mL), borderline E/e′ ratio (10.9), and a normal tricuspid regurgitation (TR) velocity (2.4 m/s). During peak exercise, the E wave and E/e′ ratio increased (16.9), with a concomitant elevation in TR velocity (3.8 m/s). LV, left ventricular.

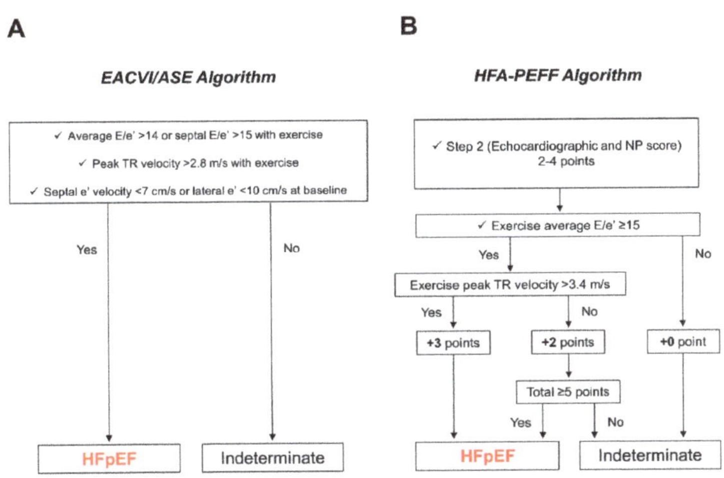

Figure 5. EACVI/ASE recommendations and HFA-PEFF algorithm for the diagnosis of HFpEF using exercise stress echocardiography. (**A**) In the EACVI/ASE recommendations, the test is considered abnormal (i.e., HFpEF) when all three criteria are met. (**B**) In the HFA-PEFF algorithm, the E/e′ ratio and TR velocity during exercise are used to add points to the resting HFA-PEFF score calculated in step 2. If the total score is ≥5 points, the diagnosis of HFpEF is confirmed. ASE, American Society of Echocardiography; EACVI, European Association of Cardiovascular Imaging; HFA-PEFF algorithm, a consensus-based algorithm proposed by the Heart Failure Association of the European Society of Cardiology; HFpEF, heart failure with preserved ejection fraction; TR, tricuspid regurgitation; NP, natriuretic peptide.

The most important limitation of exercise stress echocardiography is imaging quality. Acquiring diagnostic-quality images is more challenging during exercise in patients with obesity, which is very common in HFpEF. When echocardiographic imaging has poor quality or equivocal findings, invasive exercise hemodynamic testing is recommended to confirm the diagnosis [8].

4. Potential Value of Simultaneous Expired Gas Analysis

Cardiopulmonary exercise testing (CPET) is a gold standard test for evaluating exercise capacity and provides valuable information on exercise physiology involving the pulmonary, cardiovascular, and peripheral oxidative systems [69]. Notably, CPET-derived parameters are associated with clinical outcomes in both HFrEF and HFpEF [70–72]. Recently, interest has focused on combining diastolic stress echocardiography and expired gas analysis (i.e., CPET) in patients presenting with unexplained dyspnea and for the evaluation of HFpEF [16,39,50,66,67,69,73]. Peak oxygen consumption (VO_2), especially percentage predicted value normalized to age, sex, and weight, is the gold standard objective marker of aerobic capacity in patients with cardiac dysfunction [69]. Previous studies have demonstrated that peak VO_2 is universally decreased in patients with HFpEF, and expired gas analysis during exercise echocardiography enables the simultaneous assessment of reduced exercise capacity [14–16,40]. In this regard, very low or relatively preserved peak VO_2 (<14 or >20 mL/min/kg) may be useful in identifying HFpEF among patients with dyspnea [39]. The factors limiting peak VO_2 (or the O_2 pathway) may vary among individual patients [14–16,30,40,74]. On the basis of the Fick principle (VO_2 = CO $\times$ arteriovenous difference in O_2 content), O_2 delivery or convection and extraction are the two physiological determinants in the O_2 pathway. Combining diastolic stress echocardiography with expired gas analysis also allows for the assessment of the CO reserve during exercise. CO can be estimated with echocardiography using the LV outflow pulse Doppler method. In healthy humans, a 6 mL/min increase in CO is required for a 1 mL/min increase in VO_2 [75]. A CO reserve limitation is determined when the observed increase in CO is <80% of the predicted value based on the change in VO_2 (Figure 6).

Peak VO_2 measurement during diastolic stress echocardiography may also be useful for evaluating the therapeutic response. Prior studies have shown improvements in functional capacity after exercise training in patients with HFpEF by demonstrating changes in peak VO_2 [76,77].

The ventilation equivalent to carbon dioxide production (V_E/VCO_2) slope represents ventilatory efficiency and is a strong prognostic marker in patients with HFrEF and HFpEF [70,78–80]. In patients with HF, ventilatory inefficiency, as evidenced by an increased V_E/VCO_2 slope, is likely to be a consequence of hemodynamic derangements during exercise or is a contributor to exercise intolerance [16,29,30,73]. Increased physiological dead space may be a primary contributor to impaired ventilatory efficiency in patients with HFpEF [29], and this could be associated with the presence of comorbid conditions including pulmonary vascular disease and chronic lung disease [16,81]. Further studies are warranted to determine the optimal use of combined exercise stress echocardiography and expired gas analysis for the diagnosis and evaluation of HFpEF.

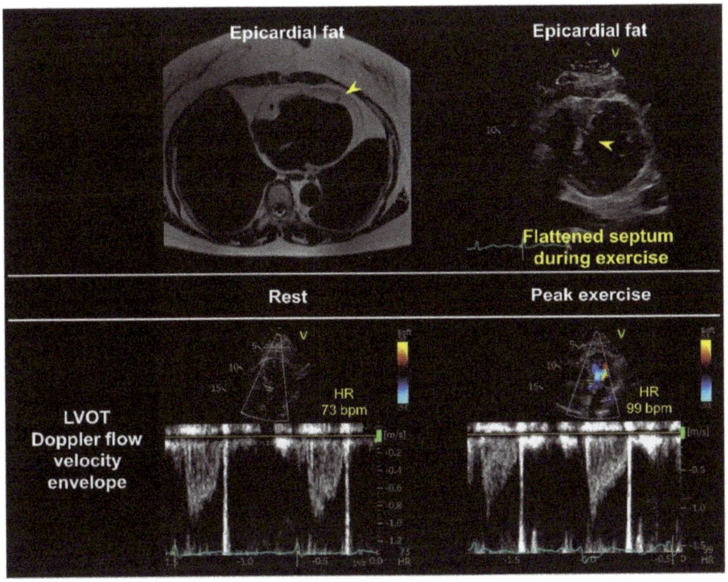

Figure 6. A case of cardiac output (CO) reserve limitation during exercise. A 79-year-old woman with obesity (body mass index, 30 kg/m^2) was referred to our echocardiographic laboratory for the evaluation of unexplained dyspnea on exertion. Her NP levels were within the normal range (N-terminal pro-brain NP, 65 pg/mL). The results of resting echocardiography were also normal; however, cardiac magnetic resonance imaging showed remarkable epicardial fat tissue (yellow arrowhead). Diastolic stress echocardiography combined with expired gas analysis showed CO reserve limitation during exercise relative to increases in VO_2 (CO, 2.9 to 3.9 L/min; VO_2, 189 to 549 mL/min; CO reserve, 48%). The septum became flattened in the parasternal short-axis view during peak ergometry exercise (yellow arrowhead), suggesting that enhanced ventricular interdependence might have contributed to the CO reserve limitation due to reduction in LV preload in addition to chronotropic incompetence. LVOT, left ventricular outflow tract.

5. Conclusions and Future Directions

Diastolic stress echocardiography plays an essential role in revealing abnormalities that develop only during exercise, and contemporary guidelines recommend its use as a diagnostic test to identify HFpEF among patients with unexplained dyspnea. Nevertheless, evidence supporting this practice remains limited and many unanswered questions and knowledge gaps remain (Table 1). Further studies are required to advance the knowledge of this method.

HFpEF is now understood as a heterogeneous syndrome, and phenotyping patients into pathophysiologically homogeneous groups may allow the personalization of new therapies [82]. Beyond resting assessments, diastolic stress echocardiography with simultaneous expired gas analysis may provide valuable information on the cardiac, pulmonary, and peripheral reserve during exercise and may improve understandings of the underlying pathophysiology and phenotypes of patients with HFpEF to facilitate better individualization of treatment.

Table 1. Key Questions and Knowledge Gaps with Respect to Diastolic Stress Echocardiography.

Key Questions	Gaps in Evidence and Future Studies Needed
Diastolic stress echocardiography allows the diagnosis of HFpEF among patients with dyspnea; however, it is unclear whether early diagnosis itself will improve the clinical outcomes.	Echocardiographic markers of congestion during exercise are associated with clinical outcomes in HFpEF, supporting the prognostic value of diastolic stress echocardiography [53,65,83,84]; however, further prospective studies are needed to determine if intervention after an early diagnosis will improve the outcomes.
No universally adopted protocols exist, and whether a multistep or ramp protocol is better remains unknown.	Patients with HFpEF are older, and a ramp protocol or a multistep protocol with low initial and incremental workload (e.g., 10 watts) may be preferred [38]. Further studies are required to develop optimal protocols.
What is the optimal workload in identifying diastolic abnormalities? It is unclear whether maximal workload is necessary.	Submaximal exercise is likely to be more feasible and equivalent to daily activities; however, few studies have examined its diagnostic value [4]. Further studies are warranted to establish the clinical value of echocardiographic indices measured during submaximal exercise.
The E/e' ratio plays a central role in diastolic stress echocardiography; however, what is the best way to address E–A fusion during exercise? What is the optimal cutoff of E/e' during exercise in patients with AF? E/e' ratio cannot be applied to patients with specific diseases, such as mitral valve diseases, mitral valve repair, or prosthetic mitral valves, or in the presence of regional wall motion abnormalities [52].	The E/e' ratio during submaximal exercise or the early recovery period can be used to diagnose HFpEF; however, evidence supporting this practice is insufficient. Data on the exercise E/e' ratio in patients with AF remain limited. Further studies are required to examine the diagnostic value of the exercise E/e' ratio, using simultaneous invasive right heart catheterization.
Identification of pulmonary hypertension during exercise is useful for diagnosing HFpEF. Pulmonary hypertension may be underestimated in some patients, such as those with severe TR or those with very high RAP during exercise. How should this be addressed?	It is unclear how the underestimation of the TR gradient in patients with severe TR should be addressed. Further studies are required. Measurements of peripheral venous pressure may be a useful alternative to RAP measurements during exercise [56,58].
What is the diagnostic value of other candidate markers of congestion during diastolic stress echocardiography, such as echocardiographic B-lines or left atrial strain [85]?	The presence of multiple B-lines may be useful in detecting pulmonary congestion that develops during exercise [63]; however, it is unclear how the data should be interpreted (e.g., the optimal cutoff value for B-lines is unknown). Further studies are warranted to establish the optimal role of the assessment of B-lines in diastolic stress echocardiography.
What is the role of expired gas analysis combined with diastolic stress echocardiography?	Simultaneous assessment of exercise capacity (peak oxygen consumption) is the major advantage of diastolic stress echocardiography [39]. Further studies are needed to determine the clinical value of combining diastolic stress echocardiography and expired gas analysis in the diagnosis of HFpEF.

A, late diastolic mitral inflow velocity; AF, atrial fibrillation; E, early diastolic mitral inflow velocity; e', early diastolic mitral annular tissue velocity; HFpEF, heart failure with preserved ejection fraction; RAP, right atrial pressure; TR, tricuspid regurgitation.

Author Contributions: Writing—Original Draft Preparation, T.H.; Writing—Review & Editing, K.K., T.K., H.I. and M.O. All authors have read and agreed to the published version of the manuscript.

Funding: Takeda Science Foundation.

Institutional Review Board Statement: Not applicable.

Informed Consent Statement: Not applicable.

Data Availability Statement: Not applicable.

Acknowledgments: Harada received the Bayer Scholarship for Cardiovascular Research. Obokata received research grants from the Fukuda Foundation for Medical Technology, Mochida Memorial Foundation for Medical and Pharmaceutical Research, Nippon Shinyaku, Takeda Science Foundation, Japanese Circulation Society, Japanese College of Cardiology, and Japan Society for the Promotion of Science KAKENHI (Grant-in-Aid for Scientific Research; grant no. 21K1607800).

Conflicts of Interest: The authors declare no conflict of interest.

References

1. Borlaug, B.A. Evaluation and management of heart failure with preserved ejection fraction. *Nat. Rev. Cardiol.* **2020**, *17*, 559–573. [CrossRef] [PubMed]
2. Dunlay, S.M.; Roger, V.L.; Redfield, M.M. Epidemiology of heart failure with preserved ejection fraction. *Nat. Rev. Cardiol.* **2017**, *14*, 591–602. [CrossRef] [PubMed]
3. Obokata, M.; Reddy, Y.N.V.; Borlaug, B.A. Diastolic Dysfunction and Heart Failure with Preserved Ejection Fraction: Understanding Mechanisms by Using Noninvasive Methods. *JACC Cardiovasc. Imaging* **2020**, *13*, 245–257. [CrossRef] [PubMed]
4. Obokata, M.; Kane, G.C.; Reddy, Y.N.V.; Olson, T.P.; Melenovsky, V.; Borlaug, B.A. Role of Diastolic Stress Testing in the Evaluation for Heart Failure with Preserved Ejection Fraction: A Simultaneous Invasive-Echocardiographic Study. *Circulation* **2017**, *135*, 825–838. [CrossRef] [PubMed]
5. Borlaug, B.A.; Nishimura, R.A.; Sorajja, P.; Lam, C.S.P.; Redfield, M.M. Exercise hemodynamics enhance diagnosis of early heart failure with preserved ejection fraction. *Circ. Heart Fail.* **2010**, *3*, 588–595. [CrossRef] [PubMed]
6. Obokata, M.; Borlaug, B.A. Stress Imaging in Heart Failure: Physiologic, Diagnostic, and Therapeutic Insights. *Circ. Cardiovasc. Imaging.* **2018**, *11*, e007785. [CrossRef] [PubMed]
7. Lancellotti, P.; Pellikka, P.A.; Budts, W.; Chaudhry, F.A.; Donal, E.; Dulgheru, R.; Edvardsen, T.; Garbi, M.; Ha, J.W.; Kane, G.C.; et al. The Clinical Use of Stress Echocardiography in Non-Ischaemic Heart Disease: Recommendations from the European Association of Cardiovascular Imaging and the American Society of Echocardiography. *J. Am. Soc. Echocardiogr.* **2017**, *30*, 101–138. [CrossRef]
8. Pieske, B.; Tschöpe, C.; De Boer, R.; Fraser, A.G.; Anker, S.D.; Donal, E.; Edelmann, F.; Fu, M.; Guazzi, M.; Lam, C.S.P.; et al. How to diagnose heart failure with preserved ejection fraction: The HFA-PEFF diagnostic algorithm: A consensus recommendation from the Heart Failure Association (HFA) of the European Society of Cardiology (ESC). *Eur. Heart J.* **2019**, *40*, 3297–3317. [CrossRef]
9. Sozzi, F.B.; Maganti, K.; Malanchini, G.; Gherbesi, E.; Tondi, L.; Ciulla, M.M.; Canetta, C.; Lombardi, F. Diastolic stress test in heart failure with preserved ejection fraction. *Eur. J. Prev. Cardiol.* **2020**, *27*, 2089–2091. [CrossRef] [PubMed]
10. Obokata, M.; Reddy, Y.N.V. The Role of Echocardiography in Heart Failure with Preserved Ejection Fraction: What Do We Want from Imaging? *Heart Fail. Clin.* **2019**, *15*, 241–256. [CrossRef]
11. Harada, T.; Kagami, K.; Kato, T.; Obokata, M. Echocardiography in the diagnostic evaluation and phenotyping of heart failure with preserved ejection fraction. *J. Cardiol.* **2021**, *11*, 3. [CrossRef] [PubMed]
12. Verbrugge, F.H.; Omote, K.; Reddy, Y.N.V.; Sorimachi, H.; Obokata, M.; Borlaug, B.A. Heart failure with preserved ejection fraction in patients with normal natriuretic peptide levels is associated with increased morbidity and mortality. *Eur. Heart J.* **2022**. Available online: http://www.ncbi.nlm.nih.gov/pubmed/35139159 (accessed on 1 March 2022). [CrossRef]
13. Obokata, M.; Nagata, Y.; Kado, Y.; Kurabayashi, M.; Otsuji, Y.; Takeuchi, M. Ventricular-Arterial Coupling and Exercise-Induced Pulmonary Hypertension During Low-Level Exercise in Heart Failure with Preserved or Reduced Ejection Fraction. *J. Card. Fail.* **2017**, *23*, 216–220. [CrossRef] [PubMed]
14. Obokata, M.; Reddy, Y.N.V.; Pislaru, S.V.; Melenovsky, V.; Borlaug, B.A. Evidence Supporting the Existence of a Distinct Obese Phenotype of Heart Failure with Preserved Ejection Fraction. *Circulation* **2017**, *136*, 6–19. [CrossRef] [PubMed]
15. Gorter, T.; Obokata, M.; Reddy, Y.; Borlaug, B. Exercise Unmasks Distinct Pathophysiologic Features of Pulmonary Vascular Disease in Heart Failure with Preserved Ejection Fraction. *Eur. Heart J.* **2018**, *39*, 2825–2835. [CrossRef] [PubMed]
16. Obokata, M.; Olson, T.P.; Reddy, Y.N.V.; Melenovsky, V.; Kane, G.C.; Borlaug, B.A. Haemodynamics, dyspnoea, and pulmonary reserve in heart failure with preserved ejection fraction. *Eur. Heart J.* **2018**, *39*, 2810–2821. [CrossRef] [PubMed]
17. Obokata, M.; Reddy, Y.N.V.; Melenovsky, V.; Kane, G.C.; Olson, T.P.; Jarolim, P.; Borlaug, B.A. Myocardial Injury and Cardiac Reserve in Patients with Heart Failure and Preserved Ejection Fraction. *J. Am. Coll. Cardiol.* **2018**, *72*, 29–40. [CrossRef] [PubMed]
18. Obokata, M.; Borlaug, B.A. The strengths and limitations of E/e' in heart failure with preserved ejection fraction. *Eur. J. Heart Fail.* **2018**, *20*, 1312–1314. [CrossRef] [PubMed]
19. Amanai, S.; Harada, T.; Kagami, K.; Yoshida, K.; Kato, T.; Wada, N.; Obokata, M. The H2FPEF and HFA-PEFF algorithms for predicting exercise intolerance and abnormal hemodynamics in heart failure with preserved ejection fraction. *Sci. Rep.* **2022**, *12*, 13. [CrossRef] [PubMed]
20. Nagueh, S.F.; Smiseth, O.A.; Appleton, C.P.; Byrd, B.F.; Dokainish, H.; Edvardsen, T.; Flachskampf, F.A.; Gillebert, T.C.; Klein, A.L.; Lancellotti, P.; et al. Recommendations for the Evaluation of Left Ventricular Diastolic Function by Echocardiography: An Update from the American Society of Echocardiography and the European Association of Cardiovascular Imaging. *J. Am. Soc. Echocardiogr.* **2016**, *29*, 277–314. [CrossRef]
21. Sharifov, O.F.; Schiros, C.G.; Aban, I.; Denney, T.S.; Gupta, H. Diagnostic accuracy of tissue Doppler index E/e' for evaluating left ventricular filling pressure and diastolic dysfunction/heart failure with preserved ejection fraction: A systematic review and meta-analysis. *J. Am. Heart Assoc.* **2016**, *5*, e002530. [CrossRef] [PubMed]
22. Reddy, Y.N.V.; Carter, R.E.; Obokata, M.; Redfield, M.M.; Borlaug, B.A. A Simple, Evidence-Based Approach to Help Guide Diagnosis of Heart Failure with Preserved Ejection Fraction. *Circulation* **2018**, *138*, 861–870. [CrossRef] [PubMed]
23. Rendón-Giraldo, J.A.; Lema, C.; Saldarriaga-Giraldo, C.I. Association between Diastolic Stress Test and H2FPEF Score. *Arch. Cardiol México.* **2021**. Available online: http://www.archivoscardiologia.com/frame_esp.php?id=388 (accessed on 1 March 2022). [CrossRef] [PubMed]

24. Tao, Y.; Wang, W.; Zhu, J.; You, T.; Li, Y.; Zhou, X. H2FPEF score predicts 1-year rehospitalisation of patients with heart failure with preserved ejection fraction. *Postgrad Med. J.* **2021**, *97*, 164–167. [CrossRef] [PubMed]
25. Sueta, D.; Yamamoto, E.; Nishihara, T.; Tokitsu, T.; Fujisue, K.; Oike, F.; Takae, M.; Usuku, H.; Takashio, S.; Arima, Y.; et al. H2FPEF Score as a Prognostic Value in HFpEF Patients. *Am. J. Hypertens.* **2019**, *32*, 1082–1090. [CrossRef] [PubMed]
26. Sun, Y.; Wang, N.; Li, X.; Zhang, Y.; Yang, J.; Tse, G.; Liu, Y. Predictive value of H2 FPEF score in patients with heart failure with preserved ejection fraction. *ESC Heart Fail.* **2021**, *8*, 1244–1252. [CrossRef] [PubMed]
27. Hwang, I.-C.; Cho, G.-Y.; Choi, H.-M.; Yoon, Y.E.; Park, J.J.; Park, J.-B.; Park, J.-H.; Lee, S.-P.; Kim, H.-K.; Kim, Y.-J. H2FPEF Score Reflects the Left Atrial Strain and Predicts Prognosis in Patients with Heart Failure with Preserved Ejection Fraction. *J. Card. Fail.* **2021**, *27*, 198–207. [CrossRef] [PubMed]
28. Borlaug, B.A.; Olson, T.P.; Lam, C.S.P.; Flood, K.S.; Lerman, A.; Johnson, B.D.; Redfield, M.M. Global cardiovascular reserve dysfunction in heart failure with preserved ejection fraction. *J. Am. Coll. Cardiol.* **2010**, *56*, 845–854. [CrossRef] [PubMed]
29. Van Iterson, E.H.; Johnson, B.D.; Borlaug, B.A.; Olson, T.P. Physiological dead space and arterial carbon dioxide contributions to exercise ventilatory inefficiency in patients with reduced or preserved ejection fraction heart failure. *Eur. J. Heart Fail.* **2017**, *19*, 1675–1685. [CrossRef] [PubMed]
30. Haykowsky, M.J.; Brubaker, P.H.; John, J.M.; Stewart, K.P.; Morgan, T.M.; Kitzman, D.W. Determinants of exercise intolerance in elderly heart failure patients with preserved ejection fraction. *J. Am. Coll. Cardiol.* **2011**, *58*, 265–274. [CrossRef]
31. Sorimachi, H.; Burkhoff, D.; Verbrugge, F.H.; Omote, K.; Obokata, M.; Reddy, Y.N.; Takahashi, N.; Sunagawa, K.; Borlaug, B.A. Obesity, venous capacitance, and venous compliance in heart failure with preserved ejection fraction. *Eur. J. Heart Fail.* **2021**, *23*, 1648–1658. [CrossRef] [PubMed]
32. Kawaguchi, M.; Hay, I.; Fetics, B.; Kass, D.A. Combined ventricular systolic and arterial stiffening in patients with heart failure and preserved ejection fraction: Implications for systolic and diastolic reserve limitations. *Circulation* **2003**, *107*, 714–720. [CrossRef] [PubMed]
33. Penicka, M.; Bartunek, J.; Trakalova, H.; Hrabakova, H.; Maruskova, M.; Karasek, J.; Kočka, V. Heart Failure with Preserved Ejection Fraction in Outpatients with Unexplained Dyspnea. A Pressure-Volume Loop Analysis. *J. Am. Coll. Cardiol.* **2010**, *55*, 1701–1710. [CrossRef] [PubMed]
34. Obokata, M.; Negishi, K.; Marwick, T.H.; Kurosawa, K.; Ishida, H.; Ito, K.; Ogawa, T.; Ando, Y.; Kurabayashi, M. Comparison of different interdialytic intervals among hemodialysis patients on their echocardiogram-based cardiovascular parameters. *Am. Heart J.* **2015**, *169*, 523–530.e2. [CrossRef] [PubMed]
35. Obokata, M.; Negishi, K.; Kurosawa, K.; Arima, H.; Tateno, R.; Ui, G.; Tange, S.; Arai, M.; Kurabayashi, M. Incremental diagnostic value of la strain with leg lifts in heart failure with preserved ejection fraction. *JACC Cardiovasc. Imaging* **2013**, *6*, 749–758. [CrossRef] [PubMed]
36. Kusunose, K.; Yamada, H.; Saijo, Y.; Nishio, S.; Hirata, Y.; Ise, T.; Yamaguchi, K.; Fukuda, D.; Yagi, S.; Soeki, T.; et al. Preload Stress Echocardiography for the Assessment of Heart Failure with Preserved Ejection Fraction. *JACC Cardiovasc. Imaging* **2022**, *15*, 375–378. [CrossRef] [PubMed]
37. Borlaug, B.A.; Jaber, W.A.; Ommen, S.R.; Lam, C.S.P.; Redfield, M.M.; Nishimura, R.A. Diastolic relaxation and compliance reserve during dynamic exercise in heart failure with preserved ejection fraction. *Heart* **2011**, *97*, 964–969. [CrossRef] [PubMed]
38. Erdei, T.; Smiseth, O.A.; Marino, P.; Fraser, A.G. A systematic review of diastolic stress tests in heart failure with preserved ejection fraction, with proposals from the EU-FP7 MEDIA study group. *Eur. J. Heart Fail.* **2014**, *16*, 1345–1361. [CrossRef] [PubMed]
39. Reddy, Y.N.V.; Olson, T.P.; Obokata, M.; Melenovsky, V.; Borlaug, B.A. Hemodynamic Correlates and Diagnostic Role of Cardiopulmonary Exercise Testing in Heart Failure with Preserved Ejection Fraction. *JACC Heart Fail.* **2018**, *6*, 665–675. [CrossRef] [PubMed]
40. Houstis, N.E.; Eisman, A.S.; Pappagianopoulos, P.P.; Wooster, L.; Bailey, C.S.; Wagner, P.D.; Lewis, G.D. Exercise Intolerance in Heart Failure with Preserved Ejection Fraction. *Circulation* **2018**, *137*, 148–161. [CrossRef]
41. Rao, V.N.; Kelsey, M.D.; Blazing, M.A.; Pagidipati, N.J.; Fortin, T.A.; Fudim, M. Unexplained Dyspnea on Exertion: The Difference the Right Test Can Make. *Circ Heart Fail.* **2022**, *15*, e008982. [CrossRef] [PubMed]
42. Kramer, B.; Massie, B.; Topic, N. Hemodynamic differences between supine and upright exercise in patients with congestive heart failure. *Circulation* **1982**, *66*, 820–825. [CrossRef] [PubMed]
43. Bhella, P.S.; Pacini, E.L.; Prasad, A.; Hastings, J.L.; Adams-Huet, B.; Thomas, J.D.; Grayburn, P.A.; Levine, B.D. Echocardiographic indices do not reliably track changes in left-sided filling pressure in healthy subjects or patients with heart failure with preserved ejection fraction. *Circ Cardiovasc. Imaging* **2011**, *4*, 482–489. [CrossRef] [PubMed]
44. Maeder, M.T.; Thompson, B.R.; Brunner-La Rocca, H.P.; Kaye, D.M. Hemodynamic basis of exercise limitation in patients with heart failure and normal ejection fraction. *J. Am. Coll. Cardiol.* **2010**, *56*, 855–863. [CrossRef] [PubMed]
45. Santos, M.; Rivero, J.; McCullough, S.D.; West, E.; Opotowsky, A.R.; Waxman, A.B.; Systrom, D.M.; Shah, A.M. E/e′ ratio in patients with unexplained dyspnea lack of accuracy in estimating left ventricular filling pressure. *Circ Heart Fail.* **2015**, *8*, 749–756. [CrossRef]
46. Hasenfuß, G.; Hayward, C.; Burkhoff, D.; Silvestry, F.E.; McKenzie, S.; Gustafsson, F.; Malek, F.; Van der Heyden, J.; Lang, I.; Petrie, M.C.; et al. A transcatheter intracardiac shunt device for heart failure with preserved ejection fraction (REDUCE LAP-HF): A multicentre, open-label, single-arm, phase 1 trial. *Lancet* **2016**, *387*, 1298–1304. [CrossRef]

47. Hammoudi, N.; Laveau, F.; Helft, G.; Cozic, N.; Barthelemy, O.; Ceccaldi, A.; Petroni, T.; Berman, E.; Komajda, M.; Michel, P.-L.; et al. Low level exercise echocardiography helps diagnose early stage heart failure with preserved ejection fraction: A study of echocardiography versus catheterization. *Clin. Res. Cardiol.* **2017**, *106*, 192–201. [CrossRef]
48. Bentivegna, E.; Luciani, M.; Martelletti, P. New Model for Non-Invasive Echocardiographic Assessment of Pulmonary-Capillary Wedge Pressure in Patients with Aortic and Mitral Regurgitation. *SN Compr. Clin. Med.* **2020**, *2*, 914–918. [CrossRef]
49. Borlaug, B.A.; Obokata, M. Is it time to recognize a new phenotype? Heart failure with preserved ejection fraction with pulmonary vascular disease. *Eur. Heart J.* **2017**, *38*, 2874–2878. [CrossRef]
50. Guazzi, M. Stress echocardiography combined with cardiopulmonary exercise testing: Opening a new window into diagnosis of heart failure with preserved ejection fraction. *Eur. J. Prev. Cardiol.* **2016**, *23*, 67–70. [CrossRef]
51. Belyavskiy, E.; Morris, D.A.; Url-Michitsch, M.; Verheyen, N.; Meinitzer, A.; Radhakrishnan, A.-K.; Kropf, M.; Frydas, A.; Ovchinnikov, A.G.; Schmidt, A.; et al. Diastolic stress test echocardiography in patients with suspected heart failure with preserved ejection fraction: A pilot study. *ESC Heart Fail.* **2019**, *6*, 146–153. [CrossRef] [PubMed]
52. Shim, C.Y.; Kim, S.-A.; Choi, D.; Yang, W.-I.; Kim, J.-M.; Moon, S.-H.; Lee, H.-J.; Park, S.; Choi, E.-Y.; Chung, N.; et al. Clinical outcomes of exercise-induced pulmonary hypertension in subjects with preserved left ventricular ejection fraction: Implication of an increase in left ventricular filling pressure during exercise. *Heart* **2011**, *97*, 1417–1424. [CrossRef] [PubMed]
53. Donal, E.; Lund, L.H.; Oger, E.; Reynaud, A.; Schnell, F.; Persson, H.; Drouet, E.; Linde, C.; Daubert, C. Value of exercise echocardiography in heart failurewith preserved ejection fraction: A substudy from the KaRen study. *Eur. Heart J. Cardiovasc. Imaging* **2016**, *17*, 106–113. [PubMed]
54. Van Riel, A.C.M.J.; Opotowsky, A.R.; Santos, M.; Rivero, J.M.; Dhimitri, A.; Mulder, B.J.M.; Bouma, B.J.; Landzberg, M.J.; Waxman, A.B.; Systrom, D.M.; et al. Accuracy of Echocardiography to Estimate Pulmonary Artery Pressures with Exercise. *Circ. Cardiovasc. Imaging* **2017**, *10*, e005711. [CrossRef] [PubMed]
55. Obokata, M.; Kane, G.C.; Sorimachi, H.; Reddy, Y.N.V.; Olson, T.P.; Egbe, A.C.; Melenovsky, V.; Borlaug, B.A. Noninvasive evaluation of pulmonary artery pressure during exercise: The importance of right atrial hypertension. *Eur. Respir J. Eur. Respir. Soc.* **2020**, *55*, 1901617. [CrossRef] [PubMed]
56. Sperry, B.W.; Campbell, J.; Yanavitski, M.; Kapadia, S.; Tang, W.H.W.; Hanna, M. Peripheral Venous Pressure Measurements in Patients with Acute Decompensated Heart Failure (PVP-HF). *Circ. Heart Fail.* **2017**, *10*, e004130. [CrossRef]
57. Vlismas, P.P.; Wiesenfeld, E.; Oh, K.T.; Murthy, S.; Vukelic, S.; Saeed, O.; Patel, S.; Shin, J.J.; Jorde, U.P.; Sims, D.B. Relation of Peripheral Venous Pressure to Central Venous Pressure in Patients with Heart Failure, Heart Transplant, and Left Ventricular Assist Device. *Am. J. Cardiol.* **2021**, *138*, 80–84. [CrossRef]
58. Yang, J.H.; Harada, T.; Choi, K.H.; Kato, T.; Kim, D.; Takama, N.; Park, T.K.; Kurabayashi, M.; Chang, S.A.; Obokata, M. Peripheral Venous Pressure-Assisted Exercise Stress Echocardiography in the Evaluation of Pulmonary Hypertension During Exercise in Patients with Suspected Heart Failure with Preserved Ejection Fraction. *Circ. Heart Fail.* **2022**. Available online: http://www.ncbi.nlm.nih.gov/pubmed/35189688 (accessed on 1 March 2022). [CrossRef]
59. Huang, D.; Dong, M.S.; Ms, S.; Zhang, M. The application of lung ultrasound in acute decompensated heart failure in heart failure with preserved and reduced ejection fraction. *Echocardiography* **2017**, *34*, 1462–1469.
60. Picano, E.; Scali, M.C.; Ciampi, Q.; Lichtenstein, D. Lung Ultrasound for the Cardiologist. *JACC Cardiovasc. Imaging* **2018**, *11*, 1692–1705. [CrossRef]
61. Platz, E.; Jhund, P.S.; Girerd, N.; Pivetta, E.; McMurray, J.J.; Peacock, W.F.; Masip, J.; Martin-Sanchez, F.J.; Miró, O.; Price, S.; et al. Expert consensus document: Reporting checklist for quantification of pulmonary congestion by lung ultrasound in heart failure. *Eur. J. Heart Fail.* **2019**, *21*, 844–851. [CrossRef] [PubMed]
62. Scali, M.C.; Zagatina, A.; Simova, I.; Zhuravskaya, N.; Ciampi, Q.; Paterni, M.; Marzilli, M.; Carpeggiani, C.; Picano, E.; Citro, R.; et al. B-lines with Lung Ultrasound: The Optimal Scan Technique at Rest and During Stress. *Ultrasound Med. Biol.* **2017**, *43*, 2558–2566. [CrossRef] [PubMed]
63. Reddy, Y.N.V.; Obokata, M.; Wiley, B.; Koepp, K.E.; Jorgenson, C.C.; Egbe, A.; Melenovsky, V.; Carter, R.E.; Borlaug, B.A. The haemodynamic basis of lung congestion during exercise in heart failure with preserved ejection fraction. *Eur. Heart J.* **2019**, *40*, 3721–3730. [CrossRef] [PubMed]
64. Platz, E.; Merz, A.; Silverman, M.; Lewis, E.; Groarke, J.D.; Waxman, A.; Systrom, D. Association between lung ultrasound findings and invasive exercise haemodynamics in patients with undifferentiated dyspnoea. *ESC Heart Fail.* **2019**, *6*, 202–220. [CrossRef] [PubMed]
65. Coiro, S.; Simonovic, D.; Deljanin-Ilic, M.; Duarte, K.; Carluccio, E.; Cattadori, G.; Girerd, N.; Ambrosio, G. Prognostic Value of Dynamic Changes in Pulmonary Congestion During Exercise Stress Echocardiography in Heart Failure with Preserved Ejection Fraction. *Circ. Heart Fail.* **2020**, *13*, e006769. [CrossRef] [PubMed]
66. Pugliese, N.R.; De Biase, N.; Gargani, L.; Mazzola, M.; Conte, L.; Fabiani, I.; Natali, A.; Dini, F.L.; Frumento, P.; Rosada, J.; et al. Predicting the transition to and progression of heart failure with preserved ejection fraction: A weighted risk score using bio-humoural, cardiopulmonary, and echocardiographic stress testing. *Eur. J. Prev. Cardiol.* **2021**, *28*, 1650–1661. [CrossRef] [PubMed]
67. D'Andrea, A.; Ilardi, F.; D'Ascenzi, F.; Bandera, F.; Benfari, G.; Esposito, R.; Malagoli, A.; Mandoli, G.E.; Santoro, C.; Russo, V.; et al. Impaired myocardial work efficiency in heart failure with preserved ejection fraction. *Eur. Heart J. Cardiovasc. Imaging* **2021**, *22*, 1312–1320. [CrossRef]

68. Kagami, K.; Harada, T.; Yamaguchi, K.; Kouno, S.; Ikoma, T.; Yoshida, K.; Kato, T.; Tomono, J.; Wada, N.; Adachi, T.; et al. Association between lung ultrasound B-lines and exercise-induced pulmonary hypertension in patients with connective tissue disease. *Echocardiography* **2021**, *38*, 1297–1306. [CrossRef] [PubMed]
69. Guazzi, M.; Bandera, F.; Ozemek, C.; Systrom, D.; Arena, R. Cardiopulmonary Exercise Testing: What Is its Value? *J. Am. Coll. Cardiol.* **2017**, *70*, 1618–1636. [CrossRef]
70. Guazzi, M.; Myers, J.; Arena, R. Cardiopulmonary exercise testing in the clinical and prognostic assessment of diastolic heart failure. *J. Am. Coll. Cardiol.* **2005**, *46*, 1883–1890. [CrossRef]
71. Nadruz, W.; West, E.; Sengeløv, M.; Santos, M.; Groarke, J.D.; Forman, D.E.; Claggett, B.; Skali, H.; Shah, A.M. Prognostic Value of Cardiopulmonary Exercise Testing in Heart Failure with Reduced, Midrange, and Preserved Ejection Fraction. *J. Am. Heart Assoc.* **2017**, *6*, e006000. [CrossRef] [PubMed]
72. Shafiq, A.; Brawner, C.A.; Aldred, H.A.; Lewis, B.; Williams, C.T.; Tita, C.; Schairer, J.R.; Ehrman, J.K.; Velez, M.; Selektor, Y.; et al. Prognostic value of cardiopulmonary exercise testing in heart failure with preserved ejection fraction. The Henry Ford HospITal CardioPulmonary EXercise Testing (FIT-CPX) project. *Am. Heart J.* **2016**, *174*, 167–172. [CrossRef]
73. Sugimoto, T.; Bandera, F.; Generati, G.; Alfonzetti, E.; Bussadori, C.; Guazzi, M. Left Atrial Function Dynamics During Exercise in Heart Failure: Pathophysiological Implications on the Right Heart and Exercise Ventilation Inefficiency. *JACC Cardiovasc. Imaging* **2017**, *10*, 1253–1264. [CrossRef] [PubMed]
74. Dhakal, B.P.; Malhotra, R.; Murphy, R.M.; Pappagianopoulos, P.P.; Baggish, A.L.; Weiner, R.B.; Houstis, N.E.; Eisman, A.S.; Hough, S.S.; Lewis, G.D. Mechanisms of exercise intolerance in heart failure with preserved ejection fraction: The role of abnormal peripheral oxygen extraction. *Circ. Heart Fail.* **2015**, *8*, 286–294. [CrossRef]
75. Abudiab, M.M.; Redfield, M.M.; Melenovsky, V.; Olson, T.P.; Kass, D.A.; Johnson, B.D.; Borlaug, B.A. Cardiac output response to exercise in relation to metabolic demand in heart failure with preserved ejection fraction. *Eur. J. Heart Fail.* **2013**, *15*, 776–785. [CrossRef] [PubMed]
76. Kitzman, D.W.; Brubaker, P.H.; Morgan, T.M.; Stewart, K.P.; Little, W.C. Exercise training in older patients with Heart failure and preserved ejection fraction: A randomized, controlled, single-blind trial. *Circ. Heart Fail.* **2010**, *3*, 659–667. [CrossRef] [PubMed]
77. Kitzman, D.W.; Brubaker, P.; Morgan, T.; Haykowsky, M.; Hundley, G.; Kraus, W.E.; Eggebeen, J.; Nicklas, B.J. Effect of caloric restriction or aerobic exercise training on peak oxygen consumption and quality of life in obese older patients with heart failure with preserved ejection fraction: A randomized clinical trial. *JAMA J. Am. Med. Assoc.* **2016**, *315*, 36–46. [CrossRef]
78. Francis, D.P.; Shamim, W.; Davies, L.C.; Piepoli, M.F.; Ponikowski, P.; Anker, S.D.; Coats, A.S. Cardiopulmonary exercise testing for prognosis in chronic heart failure: Continuous and independent prognostic value from VE/VCO^2 slope and peak VO^2. *Eur. Heart J.* **2000**, *21*, 154–161. [CrossRef] [PubMed]
79. Arena, R.; Myers, J.; Aslam, S.S.; Varughese, E.B.; Peberdy, M.A. Peak VO^2 and VE/VCO^2 slope in patients with heart failure: A prognostic comparison. *Am. Heart J.* **2004**, *147*, 354–360. [CrossRef]
80. Guazzi, M.; Myers, J.; Peberdy, M.A.; Bensimhon, D.; Chase, P.; Arena, R. Exercise oscillatory breathing in diastolic heart failure: Prevalence and prognostic insights. *Eur. Heart J.* **2008**, *29*, 2751–2759. [CrossRef] [PubMed]
81. Elbehairy, A.F.; Ciavaglia, C.E.; Webb, K.A.; Guenette, J.A.; Jensen, D.; Mourad, S.M.; Neder, J.A.; O'Donnell, D.E. Pulmonary Gas Exchange Abnormalities in Mild Chronic Obstructive Pulmonary Disease. Implications for Dyspnea and Exercise Intolerance. *Am. J. Respir. Crit. Care Med.* **2015**, *191*, 1384–1394. [CrossRef] [PubMed]
82. Shah, S.; Kitzman, D.W.; Borlaug, B.; Van Heerebeek, L.; Zile, M.; Kass, D.A.; Paulus, W.J. Phenotype-specific treatment of heart failure with preserved ejection fraction. *Circulation* **2016**, *134*, 73–90. [CrossRef] [PubMed]
83. Kosmala, W.; Przewlocka-Kosmala, M.; Rojek, A.; Mysiak, A.; Dabrowski, A.; Marwick, T.H. Association of Abnormal Left Ventricular Functional Reserve with Outcome in Heart Failure with Preserved Ejection Fraction. *JACC Cardiovasc. Imaging* **2017**, *11*, 1737–1746. [CrossRef] [PubMed]
84. Sugimoto, T.; Barletta, M.; Bandera, F.; Generati, G.; Alfonzetti, E.; Rovida, M.; Ruscone, T.G.; Rossi, A.; Cicoira, M.; Guazzi, M. Central role of left atrial dynamics in limiting exercise cardiac output increase and oxygen uptake in heart failure: Insights by cardiopulmonary imaging. *Eur. J. Heart Fail.* **2020**, *22*, 1186–1198. [CrossRef] [PubMed]
85. Marino, P.N.; Zanaboni, J.; Degiovanni, A.; Sartori, C.; Patti, G.; Fraser, A.G. Left atrial conduit flow rate at baseline and during exercise: An index of impaired relaxation in HFpEF patients. *ESC Heart Fail.* **2021**, *8*, 4334–4342. [CrossRef] [PubMed]

Journal of
*Cardiovascular
Development and Disease*

MDPI

Review

Contemporary Diagnosis and Management of Hypertrophic Cardiomyopathy: The Role of Echocardiography and Multimodality Imaging

Takeshi Kitai [1,*], Andrew Xanthopoulos [2], Shoko Nakagawa [1], Natsuko Ishii [1], Masashi Amano [1], Filippos Triposkiadis [2] and Chisato Izumi [1]

[1] National Cerebral and Cardiovascular Center, Department of Cardiovascular Medicine, Suita 564-8565, Japan; shoko-nakagawa1219@ncvc.go.jp (S.N.); ishii.natsuko@ncvc.go.jp (N.I.); m.amano@ncvc.go.jp (M.A.); izumi-ch@ncvc.go.jp (C.I.)

[2] Department of Cardiology, University Hospital of Larissa, 41110 Larissa, Greece; andrewvxanth@gmail.com (A.X.); ftriposkiadis@gmail.com (F.T.)

* Correspondence: t-kitai@kcho.jp; Tel.: +81-6-6170-1070; Fax: +81-6-6170-1917

Abstract: Hypertrophic cardiomyopathy (HCM) is an underdiagnosed genetic heart disease with an estimated prevalence of 0.2–0.5%. Although the prognosis of HCM is relatively good, with an annual general mortality of ~0.7%, some patients have an increased risk of sudden death, or of developing severe heart failure requiring heart transplantation or left ventricular (LV) assist device therapy. Therefore, earlier diagnosis and proper identification of high-risk patients may reduce disease-related morbidity/mortality by promoting timely treatment. Echocardiography is the primary imaging modality for patients with suspected HCM; it plays central roles in differential diagnosis from other causes of LV hypertrophy and in evaluating morphology, hemodynamic disturbances, LV function, and associated valvular disease. Echocardiography is also an essential tool for the continuous clinical management of patients with confirmed HCM. Other imaging modalities, such as cardiac computed tomography (CT) and cardiac magnetic resonance imaging (MRI), can supplement echocardiography in identifying high-risk as well as milder HCM phenotypes. The role of such multimodality imaging has been steadily expanding along with recent advancements in surgical techniques and minimally invasive procedures, and the emergence of novel pharmacotherapies directly targeting pathogenic molecules such as myosin inhibitors. Here we review essential knowledge surrounding HCM with a specific focus on structural and functional abnormalities assessed by imaging modalities, leading to treatment strategies.

Keywords: hypertrophic cardiomyopathy; echocardiography; multimodality imaging

1. Introduction

Hypertrophic cardiomyopathy (HCM) is a common inherited heart disease with an estimated prevalence ranging from 0.2 to 0.5% based on echocardiography screening [1–5], and it is thought that many patients are underdiagnosed [6,7]. HCM is caused by mutations of sarcomeric genes with heterogeneous clinical phenotypes, and its pathological hallmarks include non-physiological left ventricular (LV) hypertrophy not related to pressure or volume overload [1,8]. Although disease severity varies from asymptomatic or fairly symptomatic to advanced heart failure and fatal ventricular arrhythmia leading to sudden cardiac death (SCD), the general prognosis of HCM is relatively good, with a general mortality rate of about 0.7% [9–11]. Nevertheless, some patients have increased risks of SCD or of developing severe heart failure requiring heart transplantation or LV assist device therapy. Therefore, the identification of such high-risk patients is a critical issue [1,8], and earlier and prompt diagnosis leading to prognostic stratification may reduce disease-related complications by promoting optimal management. Recent advancements in the identification of pathogenic mutations in HCM have provided a new patient spectrum of genotype-positive relatives who do not have signs and symptoms of HCM. Several studies have reported that these patients have subtle abnormalities in the mitral valve apparatus or LV function.

Echocardiography is the primary modality for suspected HCM and plays a central role in excluding other causes of LV hypertrophy and in evaluating morphology, hemodynamic disturbances, and LV function [12,13]. Repeat echocardiography is also an important tool for the continuous clinical management of patients with HCM and for identifying markers associated with worse prognosis. Because preventing SCD is one of the important targets in the management of HCM, a continuous effort has been made to identify echocardiographic parameters related to SCD. The current SCD risk calculators endorsed by the European Society of Cardiology (ESC) and the American Heart Association (AHA) include echocardiographic measurements [1,8]. Recently, other imaging modalities, including cardiac computed tomography (CT) and cardiac magnetic resonance imaging (MRI), have been employed to supplement and support echocardiography with the identification of the high-risk HCM phenotype as well as with the identification of milder spectrum or early stages of HCM. In addition, the role of multimodality imaging has been steadily expanding, with recent advancements in medical therapy directly targeting pathogenic molecules. In this article, we review essential knowledge of HCM, with a specific focus on structural and functional abnormalities assessed by imaging modalities, leading to treatment strategies.

2. Diagnosis and Variation of Hypertrophy

The diagnostic criteria for HCM are currently as follows: prominent LV hypertrophy without other causes of hypertrophy, a maximum LV wall thickness of $\geq$15 mm, or a maximum LV wall thickness of $\geq$13 mm for patients with a first-degree relative with confirmed HCM [1,8]. The pattern and the distribution of LV hypertrophy are highly variable. The interventricular septum is commonly affected, but LV hypertrophy can also be isolated to the LV free wall, apex, and anterolateral wall. Asymmetric hypertrophy is considered one of the hallmarks of HCM, defined as a septal-to-posterior wall thickness ratio of $\geq$1.3 in normotensive patients or $\geq$1.5 in hypertensive patients. However, some patients with hypertension can have asymmetric hypertrophy, so this definition is not necessarily specific to HCM [13].

In addition to the hypertrophic LV wall, HCM is characterized by heterogeneous clinical expression, in which some patients may present with severe symptoms of dyspnea, chest pain, or syncope, while other patients may remain asymptomatic. Structural abnormalities, such as left ventricular outflow tract (LVOT) or mid-ventricular obstruction (MVO), left ventricular apical aneurysm, systolic anterior motion of the mitral valve, and other mitral valve apparatus abnormalities are often related to the symptoms and complications of HCM.

Assessment of LV Wall Hypertrophy

Echocardiography is the primary imaging modality in the screening, diagnosis, prognostic stratification, and follow-up of HCM patients [1,8,14]. Comprehensive echocardiographic evaluations are recommended for the initial disease screening. As a first step for the diagnosis of HCM, careful assessment of LV wall thickness from the base to the apex is essential. LV wall thickness is recommended to be measured at end-diastole and preferably in parasternal short axis views, but it is important not to include RV trabeculations while measuring the septal wall thickness. The LV wall thickness measured at any site of the LV end-diastole is defined as maximal diastolic LV wall thickness. Although two-dimensional (2D) echocardiography is the first-line modality for diagnosing HCM, it may fail to diagnose some HCM phenotypes, such as localized hypertrophy of LV segments. Even localized mild hypertrophy is still at risk for disease complications like SCD. In patients with poor echocardiographic images, cardiovascular magnetic resonance (CMR) imaging is useful to detect the site and extent of LV hypertrophy. In addition to the LV wall, CMR can provide high-resolution moving images of systolic anterior motion (SAM) of the mitral valve, LVOT flow turbulence, mitral regurgitation, and abnormalities in papillary muscles.

The patterns of hypertrophy vary. Originally, Maron et al. proposed the following four-type classification based on the location of LV hypertrophy: type I, hypertrophy involving the basal anteroseptum; type II, hypertrophy involving the whole septum; type III, hypertrophy involving the whole septum and at least one region among the anterior, posterior, or lateral wall; and type IV, other localization involving the posterior, apex, or lateral wall (Figure 1) [15]. Although this classification is the most popular and clinically useful, the localization of the thickened wall changes depending on the cross section of the short axis view in echocardiography. This results from the helical arrangement of the muscle fibers in the LV (Figure 2). Syed et al. proposed the following five-phenotype classification: type A, a predominant mid-septal convexity toward the LV cavity, with the cavity often having a crescent shape (reverse curvature septum HCM); type B, a generally ovoid LV cavity, with the septum being concave to the LV cavity and a prominent basal septal bulge (sigmoid septum HCM); type C, an overall straight septum that is neither predominantly convex nor concave toward the LV cavity (neutral septum HCM); type D, predominant apical distribution of hypertrophy (apical HCM); and type E, predominant hypertrophy at the mid-ventricular level (mid-ventricular HCM) [16]. Helmy proposed another classification based on clinical presentation: pattern 1, septal hypertrophy alone; pattern 2, septum and adjacent segments' hypertrophy, but not apical hypertrophy; pattern 3, apical in combination with other LV segments' hypertrophy; and pattern 4, apical hypertrophy alone [17]. These differences are likely determined by the underlying genetic substrate, but the data are currently insufficient to confirm this hypothesis.

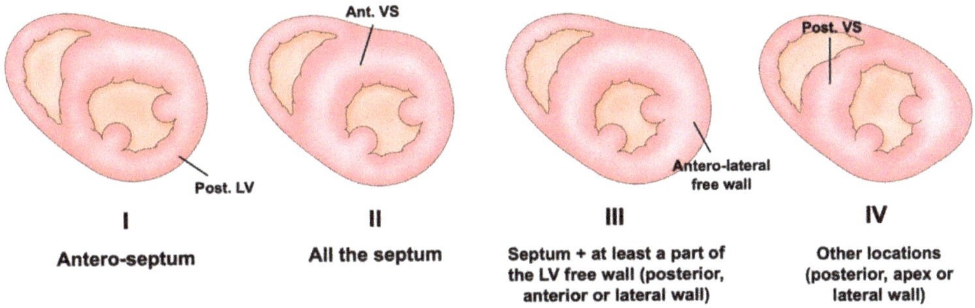

Figure 1. The classical four phenotypes of Maron's classification based on the location and degree of hypertrophy. Post. = posterior; LV = left ventricle; Ant. = anterior; VS = ventricular septum.

Although the diagnosis of HCM primarily depends on unphysiological LV hypertrophy, LV hypertrophy can also be caused by other conditions, such as hypertensive heart disease, athlete heart, aortic stenosis, cardiac amyloidosis, Fabry disease, and sigmoid septum leading to isolated basal hypertrophy. Although maximal LV wall thickness greater than 15 mm is favorable for the diagnosis of HCM and unusually observed in the other conditions, this is not specific for HCM. In addition to the clinical information such as symptoms, heart murmur, family history, and genetic testing, multimodality imaging is useful for the differential diagnosis. For example, a cardiac magnetic resonance late gadolinium enhancement imaging (CMR-LGE) pattern of patchy distribution in middle segment is a typical finding in HCM. On the other hand, low QRS voltage in ECG, apical sparing pattern in longitudinal strain echo imaging, and ^{99m}Tc-pyrophosphate (PYP) scintigraphy are characteristics of the cardiac amyloidosis. Although differentiation from athlete's heart is sometimes challenging, the absence of LGE and reduction in extracellular volume by T1 mapping in CMR are favorable for the diagnosis of athlete's heart [18].

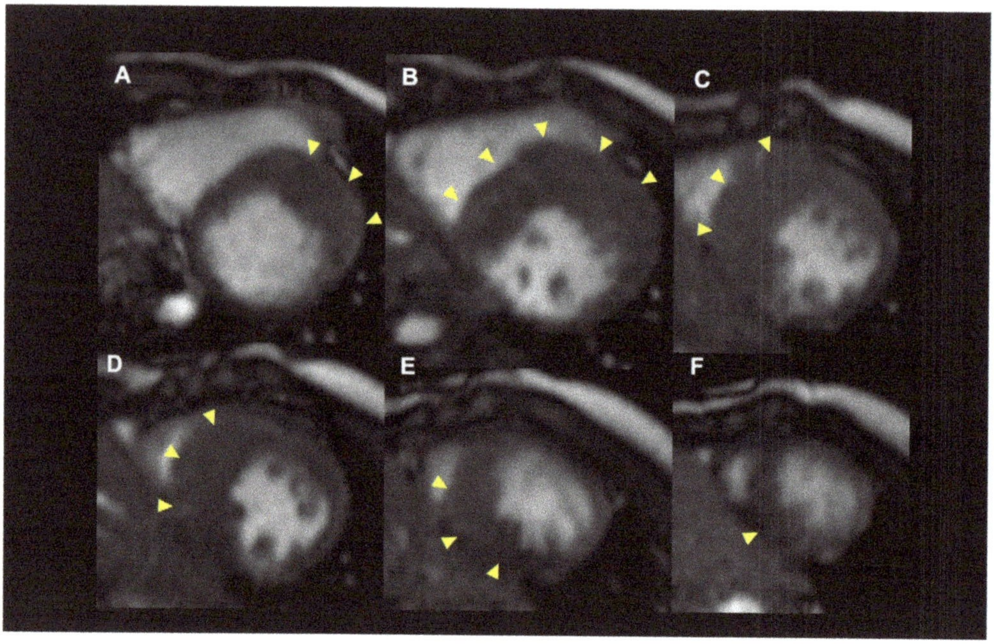

Figure 2. A representative case in which the hypertrophied region is changing along with the helical structure of myocardial fibers. The arrowheads indicate the location of hypertrophy. LV short axis views from the basal (**A**) to the apex (**F**).

3. Various Types of Left Ventricular Structural Abnormality

3.1. Left Ventricular Outflow Obstruction (LVOTO)

In addition to the aforementioned classifications, mainly based on the location of LV hypertrophy, functional and hemodynamical classifications also exist. An obstructive HCM is defined as a significant intraventricular pressure gradient of $\geq$30 mmHg. One-third of patients with HCM have significant obstructions at rest, one-third are latent obstructive after provocative maneuvers (Valsalva/standing/exercise), and one-third are truly non-obstructive (Figure 3) [8,19,20]. Intraventricular obstruction, such as that in the LVOT and mid-ventricle, is dynamic and may vary depending on loading conditions; additionally, it is associated with symptoms and heart failure progression even in patients with latent obstruction. Further, 38% of patients who have resting obstruction have symptoms, compared to 20% of patients with provocative obstruction and 10% of patients without obstruction [8]. LVOT obstruction (LVOTO) represents an important predictor of heart failure progression and poor outcomes in HCM, especially in females [21]. Therefore, provocative maneuvers are mandatory in all patients, especially symptomatic patients without significant obstructions at rest [13]. In addition to gradient provocation, exercise echocardiography is recommended in all symptomatic patients with resting intraventricular gradients of <50 mmHg or in asymptomatic patients when provocation is relevant for their management and for risk stratification [13,22].

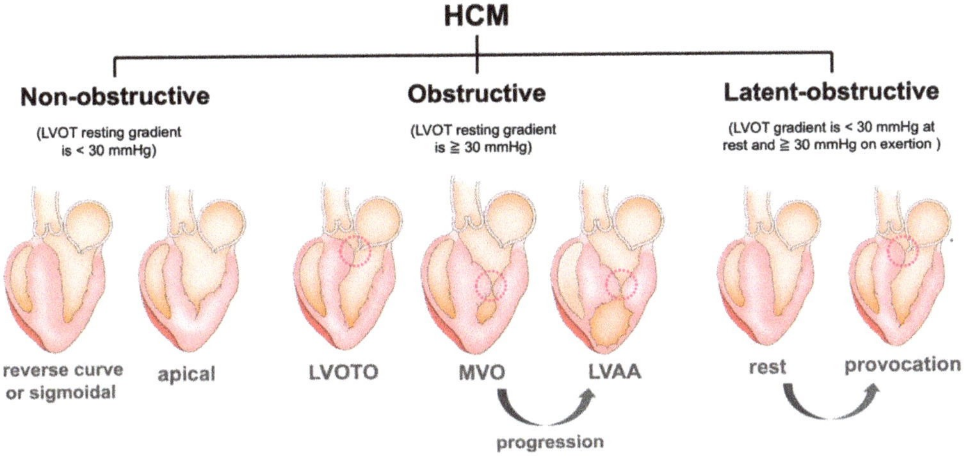

Figure 3. Schematic diagram of the different variants of HCM based on hemodynamic (obstructive vs. non-obstructive) classification. HCM = hypertrophic cardiomyopathy, LVOT = left ventricular outflow tract, LVOTO = left ventricular outflow tract obstruction, MVO = mid-ventricular obstruction, and LVAA = left ventricular apical aneurysm.

Accelerated color flow Doppler imaging helps to detect the presence of obstruction, and continuous-wave Doppler imaging is useful in measuring the peak gradient. In cases with turbulence of the color Doppler flow in the LVOT, it is recommended to interrogate the flow using a pulse-wave Doppler, starting in the LV apex or mid-ventricle and advancing the velocity sample box toward the LVOT and aortic valve to confirm aliasing of velocities at the LVOT level. The Doppler envelope typically has a late systolic peak or a mid-systolic temporary drop in cases of more severe obstruction. Care should be taken to avoid the mitral regurgitation (MR) jet velocity, which can overestimate obstruction severity [13]. The duration and shape of the jet should be considered to avoid measuring the MR jet instead of the obstruction flow. The MR jet starts with isovolumic relaxation, resulting in a longer systolic ejection period than the LVOT profile. The MR jet envelope typically has a mid-systolic peak and a more rounded appearance, with a peak velocity of about ≥6 m/s. A continuous sweep from LVOT flow toward MR flow can differentiate the two different Doppler profiles, as the flows will be displayed almost simultaneously adjacent.

The mechanism of obstruction is multifactorial. The obstruction was initially considered to be related to systolic contraction of the hypertrophied basal ventricular septum, which would then encroach into the LVOT with a resultant suction, or Venturi force, which would pull the mitral valve leaflets into the LVOT and produce further obstruction. Although isolated basal ventricular septal bulge is fairly common in older patients and can cause LVOTO, a ventricular septal bulge alone is usually not a significant cause of LVOTO. Rather, concomitant abnormalities of the mitral valve apparatus leading to SAM of the mitral valve play a central role by narrowing the LVOT [23]. Recent advances in imaging modality have enabled a deeper understanding of the complex way that the mitral valve apparatus contributes to dynamic LVOT obstruction.

Significant LVOTO is another risk factor for symptoms, progression of heart failure, and mortality in patients with HCM [19]. Hemodynamically significant LVOTO is considered as a gradient of ≥50 mmHg. Although pharmacological therapy is effective to improve symptoms and reduce pressure gradient, residual LVOTO > 50 mmHg with drug-refractory symptoms is considered to be an indication for invasive septal reduction therapies, including surgical myectomy or percutaneous transluminal septal myocardial ablation (PTSMA) [1,8]. Although clinical outcomes are comparable between PTSMA and surgical septal myectomy, the choice of septal reduction therapy should be individualized based on the patient's age, surgical risk, anatomical consideration, and extent of the hypertrophy, in addition to the patient's preference [24]. Progress in cardiac imaging has provided useful intervention strategies in cases of PTSMA (Figures 4 and 5). In particular, the importance of CT in the diagnosis and management of HCM has been increasingly recognized. In addition to the intervention strategies for PTSMA, advanced CT imaging can offer evaluation of coronary artery disease, distribution of LV hypertrophy, presence or absence of LVOTO or MVO, and left ventricular apical aneurysm.

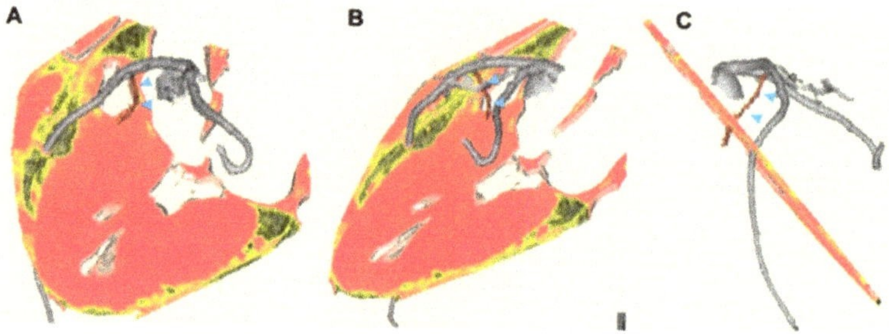

Figure 4. Three-dimensional CT images for the assessment of appropriate septal branch coronary artery for patients with significant left ventricular outflow tract obstruction planned for PTSMA. The arrowheads indicate the septal branch. CT = computed tomography, PTSMA = percutaneous transluminal septal myocardial alcohol ablation. D-dimensional views of the first major septal branch from different angles (**A**–**C**).

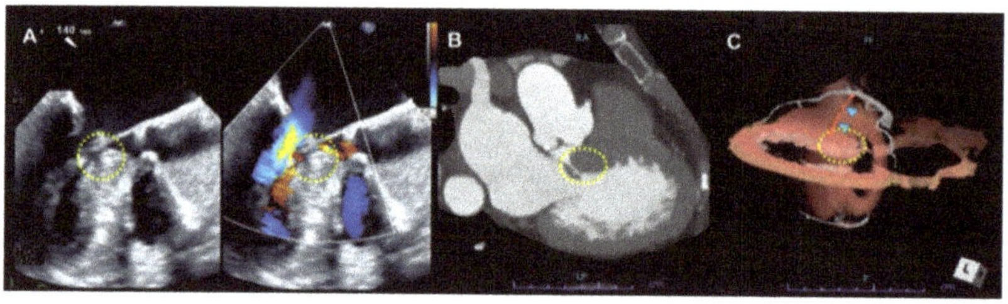

Figure 5. A representative case of LVOT obstruction. Transesophageal echocardiography (**A**), CT images for LVOT obstruction (**B**), and a target septal branch for PTSMA (**C**).

3.2. *Systolic Anterior Motion (SAM) of the Mitral Valve and Anomaly in the Mitral Valve Apparatus*

One of the morphological features observed in the mitral valve apparatus that contributes to LVOTO is the SAM of the mitral valve [14]. The detection of SAM is classically done by M-mode echocardiography findings such as mid-systolic notching of the aortic valve and contact of the anterior mitral valve to the basal ventricular septum. There is less traction on the anterior leaflet, which is pulled into the LVOT in early systole by drag forces generated by the LV, thereby causing obstruction [25]. In the presence of SAM, failure of mitral valve leaflet coaptation can cause MR directing laterally and posteriorly.

The severity of SAM is defined as mild when there is no mitral leaflet-septal contact, with a 10-mm minimum distance between the mitral valve and the ventricular septum. Severe SAM is defined as mitral leaflet-septal contact of >30%. SAM and LVOT obstruction are less common in other causes of LV hypertrophy, such as hypertensive heart disease and amyloidosis, which suggests that primary abnormalities of the mitral valve, specific to HCM, predispose individuals to develop SAM and LVOT obstruction. The displaced papillary muscle is typically hypertrophied and is compounding the obstruction by causing greater LVOT area reduction [1,26].

In patients with HCM, the mitral valve leaflet may be intrinsically normal. Rather, there may be abnormalities in the surrounding structures in the mitral valve apparatus, including elongation of the mitral chordae and anterior displacement of hypertrophied papillary muscles. Prominent displacement of papillary muscle directly into the mitral valve leaflet can be a cause of LVOTO. In the initial screening echocardiography for HCM patients, assessment of the mitral valve apparatus should be focused; leaflet morphology and coaptation, the severity of mitral regurgitation (MR), and the regurgitant jet direction should all be assessed. In patients with SAM, MR often coexists and is directed laterally and posteriorly. MR due to SAM predominates during mid- and late systole, and the severity of MR is proportional to the ventricular load and LV contractility that affect the severity of LVOTO. However, it is important to also diagnose other causes of mitral regurgitation, such as degenerative mitral valve prolapse, especially in cases with consideration of surgical or catheter intervention.

3.3. *Mid-Ventricular Obstruction (MVO) and Left Ventricular Apical Aneurysm (LVAA)*

The site of obstruction is usually located in the LVOT, but it can also be present in the mid-ventricle or close to the apex due to the hypertrophied LV wall and/or papillary muscles abutting against the septum. Similar to the detection of LVOTO, color Doppler and pulse-wave Doppler are often used to identify the anatomic site of obstruction, and careful assessments of the whole LV (apex/mid-ventricular/LVOT) should be routinely conducted [13,14]. The gradient due to MVO also has significant variability, which relates to changes in loading conditions and contractility [27]. Significant obstruction can be detected only after provocation. The presence of MVO increases the risk of left ventricular apical aneurysms (LVAAs).

Patients with HCM and LVAAs are at risk for SCD or ventricular arrhythmias, and thromboembolic events in cases of apical thrombus. HCM with LVAAs larger than 4 cm is reported to be associated with increased risk of SCD, with a mortality rate of 3.4% per year [28]. Aneurysms can be visualized by echocardiography, but CT or MRI are particularly useful for the detection of apical aneurysms and thrombi (Figure 6) [13,14].

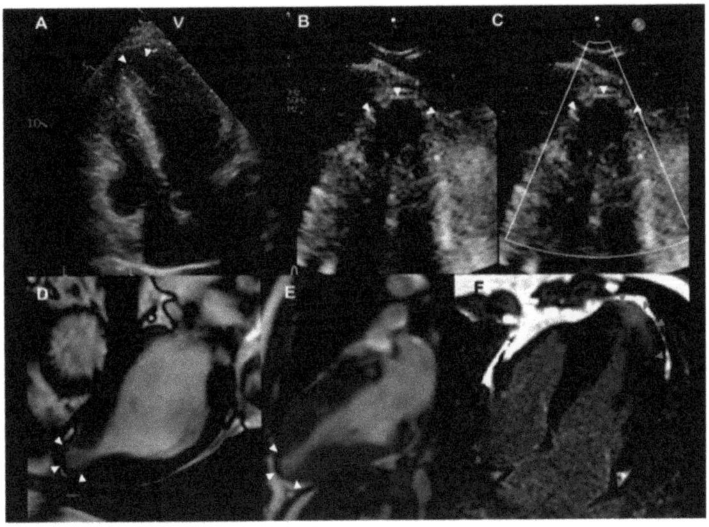

Figure 6. Representative cases with left ventricular apical aneurysm. Transthoracic echocardiography (**A–C**) and cardiac magnetic resonance imaging (**D–F**). Yellow arrowheads indicate apical aneurysms and red arrowheads indicate late gadolinium enhancement.

3.4. Reduced LV Function (Dilated Phase/End-Stage/Advanced Stage)

The clinical course of HCM is heterogeneous. Compared with the increased understanding of SCD risk stratification strategies, the risk factor of progressive heart failure remains unknown, although heart failure is responsible for approximately 60% of HCM-related deaths [29,30].

Left ventricular ejection fraction (LVEF) is typically preserved or supranormal in patients with HCM. However, LVEF is inadequate to evaluate systolic function in HCM. Patients with HCM usually have small LVs and reduced LV volumes, and LVEF can overestimate systolic function. A significant impairment of longitudinal LV systolic function is reported in patients with HCM who had preserved LVEF [31]. In a study including more than 3000 patients with HCM, abnormal global longitudinal strain (GLS) was associated with ventricular arrythmia [32]. Therefore, LVEF only decreases in the late-stage in a small subset of patients, less than approximately 15% [8]; this stage is referred to as the dilated phase, advanced stage, or end-stage [33–35]. An LVEF value of <50% indicates the end-stage or dilated phase of HCM [36,37], but data regarding optimal LVEF cut-off values for defining end-stage HCM are scarce. Extensive late gadolinium enhancement (LGE), defined as $\geq$15% of total LV mass, is reported to indicate the progression to end-stage HCM [38]. Nevertheless, longitudinal follow-up studies to identify risk factors and characteristics related to adverse LV remodeling are still warranted.

4. Risk of Sudden Cardiac Death

HCM is generally a low-event-rate disease, but SCD represents the most devastating complication of its natural history. It has been reported that the estimated overall incidence of SCD is 0.5–1.0% per year, compared with 0.2% in the general population, 2.0–3.0% in high-risk patients, including carriers of complex genotypes, and 4.7% in the presence of LV apical aneurysms [39]. Potential mediators for SCD include myocardial fibrosis, microvascular ischemia, and extensive disarray with disorganized myocyte arrangement. At present, there is no evidence-based pharmacological treatment for SCD prevention in HCM; the implantable cardioverter defibrillator (ICD) represents the only effective treatment for reducing SCD risk in high-risk individuals [1,8,40]. Therefore, risk stratification is important to assess those at risk of SCD; however, it remains challenging [41,42].

4.1. Risk Scores

The HCM Risk-SCD is a clinical risk prediction model for SCD based on a cohort of 3675 patients with HCM, providing 5-year risk analyses of SCD [43]. The HCM Risk-SCD uses seven variables: maximum LV wall thickness, LA size, LVOT gradient at rest as a continuum in addition to age, family history of SCD, non-sustained ventricular tachycardia (NSVT), and unexplained syncope. The 2014 ESC guidelines incorporated the HCM Risk-SCD model to classify patients as low-risk (5-year risk of SCD, <4%), intermediate-risk (5-year risk of SCD, 4–6%), or high-risk (5-year risk of SCD, >6%). ICD implantation was recommended as class IIB or IIA in the aforementioned groups.

In a validation study of 1629 patients with HCM in the United States, the risk of SCD calculated by the ESC risk score was significantly lower than the actual event rate. Only 11% of 35 patients who had an SCD event were considered high-risk, which indicated that ICD was recommended, whereas 60% of the patients who experienced a clinical SCD event were low-risk, and ICD was not recommended [44,45]. On the other hand, Nakagawa et al. validated the Risk-SCD model in 370 Japanese patients with HCM and reported the supportive results, in particular for those with LVEF $\geq$ 50% [46]. In addition, a recent meta-analysis of 7291 patients showed that the prevalence of SCD endpoints was about 1% in low-risk patients, 2.4% in intermediate-risk patients, and 8.4% in high-risk patients, according to the HCM Risk-SCD score groups. Most SCD endpoints (68%) occurred in patients with an estimated 5-year risk of $\geq$4% [47], suggesting that the HCM Risk-SCD model provided reasonable risk estimations able to guide ICD therapy. However, there are no existing randomized trials or statistically validated prospective prediction models that guide ICD implantation in patients with HCM so far. In addition to the aforementioned risk scores, some HCM patients begin in an intermediate-risk group based on this current risk stratification, and additional echocardiographic parameters may be used to determine ICD implantation as a primary prevention. For example, patients with severe LV hypertrophy (MWT >30 mm) have a 3-fold higher risk for ventricular arrhythmia [9,48], and LVOT obstruction at rest increases the absolute risk of SCD from 0.9% to 1.5% [49]. Additionally, LV apical aneurysm, disarray, and myocardial fibrosis might be valuable to include in the risk score assessment for SCD.

4.2. Role of Cardiac MRI for SCD Risk Stratification

While echocardiography is the first-line imaging modality in providing anatomical and functional details in patients with HCM, cardiac MRI (CMR) can often improve both the diagnosis and prognostic stratification, especially when echocardiography images are inadequate. CMR can provide excellent anatomical data regarding the distribution of myocardial fibrosis, assessed as LGE and extracellular volume [13]. Several studies have assessed the positive correlation between LGE and risk of SCD [38,50]. LGE exceeding 15% of the whole LV has been associated with a 2-fold increased risk in low-risk patients [51]. A combined use of global extracellular volume and ESC-SCD risk score has been reported to have better performance than LGE [52]. Additionally, CMR may help to detect right ventricular hypertrophy in HCM [53]. CMR can also provide a more detailed assessment of the multiple abnormalities in the mitral valve complex, including papillary muscle and chordal morphology and anatomy [54]. The information from the combined use of echocardiography and CMR is particularly useful to enhance our understanding of the mechanism of SAM and LVOT obstruction, leading to a better strategy for patients who are candidates for invasive septal reduction therapy. The risk of microvascular dysfunction has been suggested to be attributable to hypertrophy in HCM. Stress-induced perfusion detected by CMR or myocardial perfusion imaging-gated SPECT images are reported to be useful to detect microvascular disruption in patients with HCM [55,56].

4.3. Novel Echocardiographic Technique

Novel echocardiographic techniques are also useful to differentiate HCM from other causes of LV hypertrophy and to identify patients at high-risk of SCD or development of HF. Three-dimensional (3D) echocardiography has some advantages over standard 2D echocardiography, offering more information, such as the distribution and the extent of hypertrophy, the quantitative LV wall mass, and the mechanism of dynamic LV obstruction [14]. Furthermore, LV volumes, mass, and ejection fraction derived from 3D echocardiography have a stronger correlation than those obtained using CMR [13].

Myocardial deformation imaging can offer additional prognostic implications. A significant reduction in LV systolic velocity by tissue Doppler imaging (TDI) (<4 cm/s at the lateral site) has been reported as an independent predictor of death or hospitalization for worsening heart failure [57]. In addition, impairment of LV-GLS was associated with poor cardiovascular outcomes [32].

Speckle-tracking strain echocardiography can be used to assess mechanical and/or electrical dispersion, which may reflect heterogeneous contraction. Mechanical dispersion is defined as the standard deviation of time from Q/R wave onset on an electrocardiogram (ECG) to the peak negative strain in 16 LV segments [58]. A recent study has reported that mechanical dispersion was associated with malignant ventricular arrhythmias in cardiomyopathies and relates to fibrosis detected by CMR in patients with HCM [59–62].

5. Role of Pharmacological Therapy

Pharmacological interventions currently do not directly target the core molecular mechanism of HCM but are recommended to control symptoms, intraventricular pressure gradient, arrhythmia, and/or anticoagulation if needed [1,8].

Non-vasodilating β-blockers, such as bisoprolol, metoprolol, atenolol, propranolol, and nadolol, are usually the first-line therapy in symptomatic obstructive HCM [40]. Particularly, β-blockers are effective in patients with latent obstruction, although those with resting obstruction also respond [63]. β-blockers also have anti-arrhythmic effects. Specifically, propranolol was associated with a reduction in mortality in the pediatric population, especially in high doses [64]. In another study, sotalol was associated with a reduction in suppressing supraventricular and ventricular arrhythmias [65]. Calcium channel blocker (CCB) is sometimes used as an alternative in patients who are intolerant or have contraindications to β-blockers, with a class IB for verapamil and IIA for diltiazem. As the second-line agent, some class IA antiarrhythmic drugs, such as disopyramide or cibenzoline, can be an option when non-vasodilating β-blockers or verapamil therapy is ineffective. These drugs have negative inotropic effects and can decrease resting and provoked LV obstruction [40,66,67]. However, anticholinergic side effects may limit their use, and their efficacy may decrease over time.

Amiodarone is employed as an arrhythmic control agent to reduce ventricular arrhythmic burden as well as the ICD shocks, often in combination with β-blockers. Drugs such as dihydropyridine CCB, nitrates, digoxin, angiotensin-converting enzyme (ACE)-inhibitors, and angiotensin II receptor blockers (ARBs) have risks associated with worsening intraventricular gradient, and it is recommended that they be avoided in patients with HOCM.

New Drugs

The aforementioned traditional medical therapy is known to be effective in relieving symptoms; however, there is no evidence for any improvement in the natural course of the disease progression. Therefore, considerable efforts have been made to develop molecular approaches aimed at the core mechanism of the disease. Recently, a new pharmacological treatment was developed using a novel myosin inhibitor, mavacamten. This treatment was designed to reversibly inhibit β-myosin from binding to actin and to promote the super-relaxed conformation [68]; its effect includes an improvement in clinical outcomes, as well as a reduction of morbidity and mortality. In a phase-2 PIONEER-HCM study, mavacamten was associated with significantly decreased LVOT pressure gradient, increased peak VO_2, and symptomatic benefits in patients with HCM [69]. A recent phase-3 EXPLORER-HCM multicenter, double-blind, placebo-controlled study evaluated the efficacy and safety of mavacamten in 251 symptomatic patients with obstructive HCM. Patients were randomly assigned to oral mavacamten or a matching placebo once daily for 30 weeks. Dose titration was individualized from 2.5 mg to 15 mg to achieve the target reduction in the LVOT gradient (<30 mmHg) and the target mavacamten plasma concentration (350–700 ng/mL). Patients who received mavacamten were associated with an increase in peak VO_2 (≥3.0 mL/kg/min) or peak VO_2 (≥1.5 mL/kg/min), with NYHA improvement as a primary endpoint (37% vs. 17%, $p = 0.005$). In addition, patients treated with mavacamten were associated with reduced LVOT gradient and improved heart failure biomarkers, symptoms, exercise performance, and health status [70]. Mavacamten was associated with reduced LV wall thickness and LA volumes, and it improved diastolic parameters compared with baseline [71]. Based on these promising results, mavacamten has a potential to change the clinical practice in the management of HCM.

6. Role of Genetic Testing

HCM is one the most common genetic cardiovascular diseases. At present, more than 1400 mutations in 11 or more genes have been identified in patients with HCM, with the majority encoding proteins of the cardiac sarcomere. Affected genes include β-myosin heavy chain (*MYH*), myosin-binding protein C (*MYBPC3*), cardiac troponin T (*TNNT2*) and I (*TNNI3*), α-tropomyosin (*TPM1*), actin (*ACTC1*), titin (*TTN*), and myosin light chains (*MYL3*) [14]. Types of mutations vary and include deletions, insertions, missense, and splice site mutations. These known mutations are inherited in an autosomal dominant manner. However, not all HCM patients have detectable pathogenic mutations, and mutations in other genes outside of the sarcomeric myofilaments have also been implicated in HCM. Previous studies have reported that patients with sarcomere mutations were associated with an increased risk of developing heart failure compared with patients with non-sarcomere mutation or negative results from genetic testing [72–74].

The identification of pathogenic mutations enables us to screen first-degree relatives who are at risk of developing HCM. Although several studies have reported that genotype-positive relatives without LV hypertrophy had subtle changes in myocardial function or the mitral valve apparatus [75], the clinical course of these patients is favorable. In a recent series of 203 individuals, only 10% converted to a true HCM phenotype, and none experienced cardiac events [76]. In another study from the Framingham and Jackson Heart Study cohorts, 11.2% of participants with sarcomere gene variants carried at least one rare non-synonymous sarcomere variant, and 0.6% of participants carried mutations considered to be pathogenic based on conservative criteria [77]. Interestingly, many of these participants were not diagnosed with HCM, although the sarcomere variants indicated an increased risk of future cardiovascular events [77].

7. Conclusions and Future Perspective

Over the past 20 years, the pathophysiological understanding and clinical management of HCM have changed significantly. In particular, the introduction of ICD for SCD prevention is a paradigm for disease management. Although the SCD-risk model is proposed by existing guidelines, more precise risk stratification models are still needed. In addition to prevention for SCD, risk stratification for progression of heart failure or dilated HCM remains inconclusive.

The combined use of novel imaging techniques has the potential to identify several structural or functional abnormalities related to adverse events in HCM, leading to future gene-directed approaches, as well as assessment of the effect of novel pharmacological management on the disease progression and outcomes. In addition, further mechanistic studies are warranted for a deeper understanding of the phenotype–genotype linkage; such studies have the potential to lead to the development of novel specific therapeutic approaches for HCM.

Author Contributions: T.K., A.X., S.N. and N.I. wrote original draft, and M.A., F.T. and C.I. provided reviews and editing. All authors have read and agreed to the published version of the manuscript.

Funding: This research received no external funding.

Conflicts of Interest: The authors declare no conflict of interest.

References

1. Elliott, P.M.; Anastasakis, A.; Borger, M.A.; Borggrefe, M.; Cecchi, F.; Charron, P.; Hagege, A.A.; Lafont, A.; Limongelli, G.; Mahrholdt, H.; et al. 2014 ESC Guidelines on Diagnosis and Management of Hypertrophic Cardiomyopathy: The Task Force for the Diagnosis and Management of Hypertrophic Cardiomyopathy of the European Society of Cardiology (ESC). *Eur. Heart J.* **2014**, *35*, 2733–2779. [CrossRef] [PubMed]
2. Maron, B.J.; Rowin, E.J.; Maron, M.S. Global Burden of Hypertrophic Cardiomyopathy. *JACC Heart Fail.* **2018**, *6*, 376–378. [CrossRef] [PubMed]
3. Semsarian, C.; Ingles, J.; Maron, M.S.; Maron, B.J. New Perspectives on the Prevalence of Hypertrophic Cardiomyopathy. *J. Am. Coll. Cardiol.* **2015**, *65*, 1249–1254. [CrossRef] [PubMed]
4. Maron, B.J.; Gardin, J.M.; Flack, J.M.; Gidding, S.S.; Kurosaki, T.T.; Bild, D.E. Prevalence of Hypertrophic Cardiomyopathy in a General Population of Young Adults. Echocardiographic Analysis of 4111 Subjects in the CARDIA Study. Coronary Artery Risk Development in (Young) Adults. *Circulation* **1995**, *92*, 785–789. [CrossRef]
5. Hada, Y.; Sakamoto, T.; Amano, K.; Yamaguchi, T.; Takenaka, K.; Takahashi, H.; Takikawa, R.; Hasegawa, I.; Takahashi, T.; Suzuki, J. Prevalence of Hypertrophic Cardiomyopathy in a Population of Adult Japanese Workers as Detected by Echocardiographic Screening. *Am. J. Cardiol.* **1987**, *59*, 183–184. [CrossRef]
6. Maron, M.S.; Hellawell, J.L.; Lucove, J.C.; Farzaneh-Far, R.; Olivotto, I. Occurrence of Clinically Diagnosed Hypertrophic Cardiomyopathy in the United States. *Am. J. Cardiol.* **2016**, *117*, 1651–1654. [CrossRef]
7. Maron, B.J. Clinical Course and Management of Hypertrophic Cardiomyopathy. *N. Engl. J. Med.* **2018**, *379*, 655–668. [CrossRef]

8. Gersh, B.J.; Maron, B.J.; Bonow, R.O.; Dearani, J.A.; Fifer, M.A.; Link, M.S.; Naidu, S.S.; Nishimura, R.A.; Ommen, S.R.; Rakowski, H.; et al. G, American Association for Thoracic S, American Society of E, American Society of Nuclear C, Heart Failure Society of A, Heart Rhythm S. ACCF/AHA guideline for the diagnosis and treatment of hypertrophic cardiomyopathy: A report of the American College of Cardiology Foundation/American Heart Association Task Force on Practice Guidelines; Society for Cardiovascular A, Interventions and Society of Thoracic S. *Circulation* **2011**, *124*, e783–e831.
9. Spirito, P.; Autore, C.; Formisano, F.; Assenza, G.E.; Biagini, E.; Haas, T.S.; Bongioanni, S.; Semsarian, C.; Devoto, E.; Musumeci, B.; et al. Risk of Sudden Death and Outcome in Patients with Hypertrophic Cardiomyopathy with Benign Presentation and Without Risk Factors. *Am. J. Cardiol.* **2014**, *113*, 1550–1555. [CrossRef]
10. Maron, B.J.; Rowin, E.J.; Casey, S.A.; Haas, T.S.; Chan, R.H.; Udelson, J.E.; Garberich, R.F.; Lesser, J.R.; Appelbaum, E.; Manning, W.J.; et al. Risk Stratification and Outcome of Patients with Hypertrophic Cardiomyopathy >=60 Years of Age. *Circulation* **2013**, *127*, 585–593. [CrossRef]
11. Rowin, E.J.; Hausvater, A.; Link, M.S.; Abt, P.; Gionfriddo, W.; Wang, W.; Rastegar, H.; Estes, N.A.M.; Maron, M.S.; Maron, B.J. Clinical Profile and Consequences of Atrial Fibrillation in Hypertrophic Cardiomyopathy. *Circulation* **2017**, *136*, 2420–2436. [CrossRef] [PubMed]
12. Afonso, L.C.; Bernal, J.; Bax, J.J.; Abraham, T.P. Echocardiography in Hypertrophic Cardiomyopathy: The Role of Conventional and Emerging Technologies. *JACC Cardiovasc. Imaging* **2008**, *1*, 787–800. [CrossRef] [PubMed]
13. Cardim, N.; Galderisi, M.; Edvardsen, T.; Plein, S.; Popescu, B.A.; D'Andrea, A.; Bruder, O.; Cosyns, B.; Davin, L.; Donal, E.; et al. Role of Multimodality Cardiac Imaging in the Management of Patients with Hypertrophic Cardiomyopathy: An Expert Consensus of the European Association of Cardiovascular Imaging Endorsed by the Saudi Heart Association. *Eur. Heart J. Cardiovasc. Imaging* **2015**, *16*, 280. [CrossRef] [PubMed]
14. Williams, L.K.; Frenneaux, M.P.; Steeds, R.P. Echocardiography in Hypertrophic Cardiomyopathy Diagnosis, Prognosis, and Role in Management. *Eur. J. Echocardiogr.* **2009**, *10*, iii9–iii14. [CrossRef] [PubMed]
15. Maron, B.J.; Gottdiener, J.S.; Epstein, S.E. Patterns and Significance of Distribution of Left Ventricular Hypertrophy in Hypertrophic Cardiomyopathy. A Wide Angle, Two Dimensional Echocardiographic Study of 125 Patients. *Am. J. Cardiol.* **1981**, *48*, 418–428. [CrossRef]
16. Syed, I.S.; Ommen, S.R.; Breen, J.F.; Tajik, A.J. Hypertrophic Cardiomyopathy: Identification of Morphological Subtypes by Echocardiography and Cardiac Magnetic Resonance Imaging. *JACC Cardiovasc. Imaging* **2008**, *1*, 377–379. [CrossRef]
17. Helmy, S.M.; Maauof, G.F.; Shaaban, A.A.; Elmaghraby, A.M.; Anilkumar, S.; Shawky, A.H.; Hajar, R. Hypertrophic Cardiomyopathy: Prevalence, Hypertrophy Patterns, and Their Clinical and ECG Findings in a Hospital at Qatar. *Heart Views* **2011**, *12*, 143–149. [CrossRef]
18. Swoboda, P.P.; McDiarmid, A.K.; Erhayiem, B.; Broadbent, D.A.; Dobson, L.E.; Garg, P.; Ferguson, C.; Page, S.P.; Greenwood, J.P.; Plein, S. Assessing Myocardial Extracellular Volume by T1 Mapping to Distinguish Hypertrophic Cardiomyopathy from Athlete's Heart. *J. Am. Coll. Cardiol.* **2016**, *67*, 2189–2190. [CrossRef]
19. Maron, M.S.; Olivotto, I.; Betocchi, S.; Casey, S.A.; Lesser, J.R.; Losi, M.A.; Cecchi, F.; Maron, B.J. Effect of Left Ventricular Outflow Tract Obstruction on Clinical Outcome in Hypertrophic Cardiomyopathy. *N. Engl. J. Med.* **2003**, *348*, 295–303. [CrossRef]
20. Maron, M.S.; Rowin, E.J.; Olivotto, I.; Casey, S.A.; Arretini, A.; Tomberli, B.; Garberich, R.F.; Link, M.S.; Chan, R.H.M.; Lesser, J.R.; et al. Contemporary Natural History and Management of Nonobstructive Hypertrophic Cardiomyopathy. *J. Am. Coll. Cardiol.* **2016**, *67*, 1399–1409. [CrossRef]
21. Olivotto, I.; Maron, M.S.; Adabag, A.S.; Casey, S.A.; Vargiu, D.; Link, M.S.; Udelson, J.E.; Cecchi, F.; Maron, B.J. Gender-Related Differences in the Clinical Presentation and Outcome of Hypertrophic Cardiomyopathy. *J. Am. Coll. Cardiol.* **2005**, *46*, 480–487. [CrossRef] [PubMed]
22. Rowin, E.J.; Maron, B.J.; Olivotto, I.; Maron, M.S. Role of Exercise Testing in Hypertrophic Cardiomyopathy. *JACC Cardiovasc. Imaging* **2017**, *10*, 1374–1386. [CrossRef] [PubMed]
23. Levine, R.A.; Vlahakes, G.J.; Lefebvre, X.; Guerrero, J.L.; Cape, E.G.; Yoganathan, A.P.; Weyman, A.E. Papillary Muscle Displacement Causes Systolic Anterior Motion of the Mitral Valve. Experimental Validation and Insights into the Mechanism of Subaortic Obstruction. *Circulation* **1995**, *91*, 1189–1195. [CrossRef]
24. Veselka, J.; Krejci, J.; Tomasov, P.; Zemanek, D. Long-term survival after alcohol septal ablation for hypertrophic obstructive cardiomyopathy: A comparison with general population. *Eur. Heart J.* **2014**, *35*, 2040–2045. [CrossRef]
25. Ibrahim, M.; Rao, C.; Ashrafian, H.; Chaudhry, U.; Darzi, A.; Athanasiou, T. Modern Management of Systolic Anterior Motion of the Mitral Valve. *Eur. J. Cardiothorac. Surg.* **2012**, *41*, 1260–1270. [CrossRef]
26. Yu, E.H.; Omran, A.S.; Wigle, E.D.; Williams, W.G.; Siu, S.C.; Rakowski, H. Mitral Regurgitation in Hypertrophic Obstructive Cardiomyopathy: Relationship to Obstruction and Relief with Myectomy. *J. Am. Coll. Cardiol.* **2000**, *36*, 2219–2225. [CrossRef]
27. Kizilbash, A.M.; Heinle, S.K.; Grayburn, P.A. Spontaneous Variability of Left Ventricular Outflow Tract Gradient in Hypertrophic Obstructive Cardiomyopathy. *Circulation* **1998**, *97*, 461–466. [CrossRef]
28. Rowin, E.J.; Maron, B.J.; Haas, T.S.; Garberich, R.F.; Wang, W.; Link, M.S.; Maron, M.S. Hypertrophic Cardiomyopathy with Left Ventricular Apical Aneurysm: Implications for Risk Stratification and Management. *J. Am. Coll. Cardiol.* **2017**, *69*, 761–773. [CrossRef]
29. Autore, C.; Musumeci, M.B. The Natural History of Hypertrophic Cardiomyopathy. *Eur. Heart J. Suppl.* **2020**, *22*, L11–L14. [CrossRef]

30. Maron, B.J.; Rowin, E.J.; Casey, S.A.; Maron, M.S. How Hypertrophic Cardiomyopathy Became a Contemporary Treatable Genetic Disease with Low Mortality: Shaped by 50 Years of Clinical Research and Practice. *JAMA Cardiol.* **2016**, *1*, 98–105. [CrossRef]
31. Haland, T.F.; Hasselberg, N.E.; Almaas, V.M.; Dejgaard, L.A.; Saberniak, J.; Leren, I.S.; Berge, K.E.; Haugaa, K.H.; Edvardsen, T. The Systolic Paradox in Hypertrophic Cardiomyopathy. *Open Heart* **2017**, *4*, e000571. [CrossRef] [PubMed]
32. Tower-Rader, A.; Mohananey, D.; To, A.; Lever, H.M.; Popovic, Z.B.; Desai, M.Y. Prognostic Value of Global Longitudinal Strain in Hypertrophic Cardiomyopathy: A Systematic Review of Existing Literature. *JACC Cardiovasc. Imaging* **2019**, *12*, 1930–1942. [CrossRef] [PubMed]
33. Olivotto, I.; Cecchi, F.; Poggesi, C.; Yacoub, M.H. Patterns of Disease Progression in Hypertrophic Cardiomyopathy: An Individualized Approach to Clinical Staging. *Circ. Heart Fail.* **2012**, *5*, 535–546. [CrossRef] [PubMed]
34. Musumeci, M.B.; Russo, D.; Limite, L.R.; Canepa, M.; Tini, G.; Casenghi, M.; Francia, P.; Adduci, C.; Pagannone, E.; Magrì, D.; et al. Long-Term Left Ventricular Remodeling of Patients with Hypertrophic Cardiomyopathy. *Am. J. Cardiol.* **2018**, *122*, 1924–1931. [CrossRef]
35. Maron, B.J.; Spirito, P. Implications of Left Ventricular Remodeling in Hypertrophic Cardiomyopathy. *Am. J. Cardiol.* **1998**, *81*, 1339–1344. [CrossRef]
36. Harris, K.M.; Spirito, P.; Maron, M.S.; Zenovich, A.G.; Formisano, F.; Lesser, J.R.; Mackey-Bojack, S.; Manning, W.J.; Udelson, J.E.; Maron, B.J. Prevalence, Clinical Profile, and Significance of Left Ventricular Remodeling in the End-Stage Phase of Hypertrophic Cardiomyopathy. *Circulation* **2006**, *114*, 216–225. [CrossRef]
37. Kubo, T.; Gimeno, J.R.; Bahl, A.; Steffensen, U.; Steffensen, M.; Osman, E.; Thaman, R.; Mogensen, J.; Elliott, P.M.; Doi, Y.; et al. Prevalence, Clinical Significance, and Genetic Basis of Hypertrophic Cardiomyopathy with Restrictive Phenotype. *J. Am. Coll. Cardiol.* **2007**, *49*, 2419–2426. [CrossRef]
38. Chan, R.H.; Maron, B.J.; Olivotto, I.; Pencina, M.J.; Assenza, G.E.; Haas, T.; Lesser, J.R.; Gruner, C.; Crean, A.M.; Rakowski, H.; et al. Prognostic Value of Quantitative Contrast-Enhanced Cardiovascular Magnetic Resonance for the Evaluation of Sudden Death Risk in Patients with Hypertrophic Cardiomyopathy. *Circulation* **2014**, *130*, 484–495. [CrossRef]
39. Elliott, P.M.; Gimeno, J.R.; Thaman, R.; Shah, J.; Ward, D.; Dickie, S.; Tome Esteban, M.T.; McKenna, W.J. Historical Trends in Reported Survival Rates in Patients with Hypertrophic Cardiomyopathy. *Heart* **2006**, *92*, 785–791. [CrossRef]
40. Ammirati, E.; Contri, R.; Coppini, R.; Cecchi, F.; Frigerio, M.; Olivotto, I. Pharmacological Treatment of Hypertrophic Cardiomyopathy: Current Practice and Novel Perspectives. *Eur. J. Heart Fail.* **2016**, *18*, 1106–1118. [CrossRef]
41. Elliott, P.M.; Poloniecki, J.; Dickie, S.; Sharma, S.; Monserrat, L.; Varnava, A.; Mahon, N.G.; McKenna, W.J. Sudden Death in Hypertrophic Cardiomyopathy: Identification of High Risk Patients. *J. Am. Coll. Cardiol.* **2000**, *36*, 2212–2218. [CrossRef]
42. Weissler-Snir, A.; Allan, K.; Cunningham, K.; Connelly, K.A.; Lee, D.S.; Spears, D.A.; Rakowski, H.; Dorian, P. Hypertrophic Cardiomyopathy-Related Sudden Cardiac Death in Young People in Ontario. *Circulation* **2019**, *140*, 1706–1716. [CrossRef] [PubMed]
43. O'Mahony, C.; Jichi, F.; Pavlou, M.; Monserrat, L.; Anastasakis, A.; Rapezzi, C.; Biagini, E.; Gimeno, J.R.; Limongelli, G.; McKenna, W.J.; et al. IA Novel Clinical Risk Prediction Model for Sudden Cardiac Death in Hypertrophic Cardiomyopathy (HCM Risk-SCD). *Eur. Heart J.* **2014**, *35*, 2010–2020. [CrossRef]
44. Maron, B.J.; Casey, S.A.; Chan, R.H.; Garberich, R.F.; Rowin, E.J.; Maron, M.S. Independent Assessment of the European Society of Cardiology Sudden Death Risk Model for Hypertrophic Cardiomyopathy. *Am. J. Cardiol.* **2015**, *116*, 757–764. [CrossRef] [PubMed]
45. Fraiche, A.; Wang, A. Hypertrophic Cardiomyopathy: New Evidence since the 2011 American Cardiology of Cardiology Foundation and American Heart Association Guideline. *Curr. Cardiol. Rep.* **2016**, *18*, 70. [CrossRef] [PubMed]
46. Nakagawa, S.; Okada, A.; Nishimura, K.; Hamatani, Y.; Amano, M.; Takahama, H.; Amaki, M.; Hasegawa, T.; Kanzaki, H.; Kusano, K.; et al. Validation of the 2014 European Society of Cardiology Sudden Cardiac Death Risk Prediction Model Among Various Phenotypes in Japanese Patients with Hypertrophic Cardiomyopathy. *Am. J. Cardiol.* **2018**, *122*, 1939–1946. [CrossRef]
47. O'Mahony, C.; Akhtar, M.M.; Anastasiou, Z.; Guttmann, O.P.; Vriesendorp, P.A.; Michels, M.; Magrì, D.; Autore, C.; Fernández, A.; Ochoa, J.P.; et al. Effectiveness of the 2014 European Society of Cardiology Guideline on Sudden Cardiac Death in Hypertrophic Cardiomyopathy: A Systematic Review and Meta-Analysis. *Heart* **2019**, *105*, 623–631. [CrossRef]
48. Spirito, P.; Bellone, P.; Harris, K.M.; Bernabo, P.; Bruzzi, P.; Maron, B.J. Magnitude of Left Ventricular Hypertrophy and Risk of Sudden Death in Hypertrophic Cardiomyopathy. *N. Engl. J. Med.* **2000**, *342*, 1778–1785. [CrossRef]
49. Popescu, B.A.; Rosca, M.; Schwammenthal, E. Dynamic Obstruction in Hypertrophic Cardiomyopathy. *Curr. Opin. Cardiol.* **2015**, *30*, 468–474. [CrossRef]
50. Wang, W.; Lian, Z.; Rowin, E.J.; Maron, B.J.; Maron, M.S.; Link, M.S. Prognostic Implications of Nonsustained Ventricular Tachycardia in High-Risk Patients with Hypertrophic Cardiomyopathy. *Circ. Arrhythmia Electrophysiol.* **2017**, *10*, e004604. [CrossRef]
51. Chan, R.H.; Maron, B.J.; Olivotto, I.; Assenza, G.E.; Haas, T.S.; Lesser, J.R.; Gruner, C.; Crean, A.M.; Rakowski, H.; Rowin, E.; et al. Significance of Late Gadolinium Enhancement at Right Ventricular Attachment to Ventricular Septum in Patients with Hypertrophic Cardiomyopathy. *Am. J. Cardiol.* **2015**, *116*, 436–441. [CrossRef]
52. Avanesov, M.; Münch, J.; Weinrich, J.; Well, L.; Säring, D.; Stehning, C.; Tahir, E.; Bohnen, S.; Radunski, U.K.; Muellerleile, K.; et al. Prediction of the Estimated 5-Year Risk of Sudden Cardiac Death and Syncope or Non-Sustained Ventricular Tachycardia in

Patients with Hypertrophic Cardiomyopathy Using Late Gadolinium Enhancement and Extracellular Volume CMR. *Eur. Radiol.* **2017**, *27*, 5136–5145. [CrossRef] [PubMed]
53. Maron, M.S.; Hauser, T.H.; Dubrow, E.; Horst, T.A.; Kissinger, K.V.; Udelson, J.E.; Manning, W.J. Right Ventricular Involvement in Hypertrophic Cardiomyopathy. *Am. J. Cardiol.* **2007**, *100*, 1293–1298. [CrossRef] [PubMed]
54. Nagueh, S.F.; Bierig, S.M.; Budoff, M.J.; Desai, M.; Dilsizian, V.; Eidem, B.; Goldstein, S.A.; Hung, J.; Maron, M.S.; Ommen, S.R.; et al. American Society of Echocardiography Clinical Recommendations for Multimodality Cardiovascular Imaging of Patients with Hypertrophic Cardiomyopathy: Endorsed by the American Society of Nuclear Cardiology, Society for Cardiovascular Magnetic Resonance, and Society of Cardiovascular Computed Tomography. *J. Am. Soc. Echocardiogr.* **2011**, *24*, 473–498. [CrossRef]
55. Petersen, S.E.; Jerosch-Herold, M.; Hudsmith, L.E.; Robson, M.D.; Francis, J.M.; Doll, H.A.; Selvanayagam, J.B.; Neubauer, S.; Watkins, H. Evidence for microvascular dysfunction in hypertrophic cardiomyopathy: New insights from multiparametric magnetic resonance imaging. *Circulation* **2007**, *115*, 2418–2425. [CrossRef]
56. Loong, C.Y.; Reyes, E.; Underwood, S.R. Significant inducible perfusion abnormality in an asymptomatic patient with hypertrophic cardiomyopathy demonstrated by radionuclide myocardial perfusion imaging. *Heart* **2003**, *89*, 989. [CrossRef] [PubMed]
57. Kitaoka, H.; Kubo, T.; Okawa, M.; Takenaka, N.; Sakamoto, C.; Baba, Y.; Hayashi, K.; Yamasaki, N.; Matsumura, Y.; Doi, Y.L. Tissue Doppler Imaging and Plasma BNP Levels to Assess the Prognosis in Patients with Hypertrophic Cardiomyopathy. *J. Am. Soc. Echocardiogr.* **2011**, *24*, 1020–1025. [CrossRef] [PubMed]
58. Take, Y.; Morita, H.; Toh, N.; Nishii, N.; Nagase, S.; Nakamura, K.; Kusano, K.F.; Ohe, T.; Ito, H. Identification of High-Risk Syncope Related to Ventricular Fibrillation in Patients with Brugada Syndrome. *Heart Rhythm* **2012**, *9*, 752–759. [CrossRef] [PubMed]
59. Haland, T.F.; Almaas, V.M.; Hasselberg, N.E.; Saberniak, J.; Leren, I.S.; Hopp, E.; Edvardsen, T.; Haugaa, K.H. Strain Echocardiography Is Related to Fibrosis and Ventricular Arrhythmias in Hypertrophic Cardiomyopathy. *Eur. Heart J. Cardiovasc. Imaging* **2016**, *17*, 613–621. [CrossRef] [PubMed]
60. Sarvari, S.I.; Haugaa, K.H.; Anfinsen, O.G.; Leren, T.P.; Smiseth, O.A.; Kongsgaard, E.; Amlie, J.P.; Edvardsen, T. Right Ventricular Mechanical Dispersion Is Related to Malignant Arrhythmias: A Study of Patients with Arrhythmogenic Right Ventricular Cardiomyopathy and Subclinical Right Ventricular Dysfunction. *Eur. Heart J.* **2011**, *32*, 1089–1096. [CrossRef]
61. Haugaa, K.H.; Smedsrud, M.K.; Steen, T.; Kongsgaard, E.; Loennechen, J.P.; Skjaerpe, T.; Voigt, J.U.; Willems, R.; Smith, G.; Smiseth, O.A.; et al. Mechanical Dispersion Assessed by Myocardial Strain in Patients After Myocardial Infarction for Risk Prediction of Ventricular Arrhythmia. *JACC Cardiovasc. Imaging* **2010**, *3*, 247–256. [CrossRef] [PubMed]
62. Haugaa, K.H.; Goebel, B.; Dahlslett, T.; Meyer, K.; Jung, C.; Lauten, A.; Figulla, H.R.; Poerner, T.C.; Edvardsen, T. Risk Assessment of Ventricular Arrhythmias in Patients with Nonischemic Dilated Cardiomyopathy by Strain Echocardiography. *J. Am. Soc. Echocardiogr.* **2012**, *25*, 667–673. [CrossRef] [PubMed]
63. Nistri, S.; Olivotto, I.; Maron, M.S.; Ferrantini, C.; Coppini, R.; Grifoni, C.; Baldini, K.; Sgalambro, A.; Cecchi, F.; Maron, B.J. Beta Blockers for Prevention of Exercise-Induced Left Ventricular Outflow Tract Obstruction in Patients with Hypertrophic Cardiomyopathy. *Am. J. Cardiol.* **2012**, *110*, 715–719. [CrossRef] [PubMed]
64. Ostman-Smith, I.; Wettrell, G.; Riesenfeld, T. A Cohort Study of Childhood Hypertrophic Cardiomyopathy: Improved Survival Following High-Dose Beta-Adrenoceptor Antagonist Treatment. *J. Am. Coll. Cardiol.* **1999**, *34*, 1813–1822. [CrossRef]
65. Tendera, M.; Wycisk, A.; Schneeweiss, A.; Poloński, L.; Wodniecki, J. Effect of Sotalol on Arrhythmias and Exercise Tolerance in Patients with Hypertrophic Cardiomyopathy. *Cardiology* **1993**, *82*, 335–342. [CrossRef]
66. Sherrid, M.V.; Barac, I.; McKenna, W.J.; Elliott, P.M.; Dickie, S.; Chojnowska, L.; Casey, S.; Maron, B.J. Multicenter Study of the Efficacy and Safety of Disopyramide in Obstructive Hypertrophic Cardiomyopathy. *J. Am. Coll. Cardiol.* **2005**, *45*, 1251–1258. [CrossRef]
67. Adler, A.; Fourey, D.; Weissler-Snir, A.; Hindieh, W.; Chan, R.H.; Gollob, M.H.; Rakowski, H. Safety of Outpatient Initiation of Disopyramide for Obstructive Hypertrophic Cardiomyopathy Patients. *J. Am. Heart Assoc.* **2017**, *6*. [CrossRef]
68. Anderson, R.L.; Trivedi, D.V.; Sarkar, S.S.; Henze, M.; Ma, W.; Gong, H.; Rogers, C.S.; Gorham, J.M.; Wong, F.L.; Morck, M.M.; et al. Deciphering the Super Relaxed State of Human Beta-Cardiac Myosin and the Mode of Action of Mavacamten from Myosin Molecules to Muscle Fibers. *Proc. Natl. Acad. Sci. USA* **2018**, *115*, E8143–E8152. [CrossRef]
69. Heitner, S.B.; Jacoby, D.; Lester, S.J.; Owens, A.; Wang, A.; Zhang, D.; Lambing, J.; Lee, J.; Semigran, M.; Sehnert, A.J. Mavacamten Treatment for Obstructive Hypertrophic Cardiomyopathy: A Clinical Trial. *Ann. Intern. Med.* **2019**, *170*, 741–748. [CrossRef]
70. Olivotto, I.; Oreziak, A.; Barriales-Villa, R.; Abraham, T.P.; Masri, A.; Garcia-Pavia, P.; Saberi, S.; Lakdawala, N.K.; Wheeler, M.T.; Owens, A.; et al. Mavacamten for Treatment of Symptomatic Obstructive Hypertrophic Cardiomyopathy (Explorer-HCM): A Randomised, Double-Blind, Placebo-Controlled, phase 3 Trial. *Lancet* **2020**, *396*, 759–769. [CrossRef]
71. Saberi, S.; Cardim, N.; Yamani, M.; Schulz-Menger, J.; Li, W.; Florea, V.; Sehnert, A.J.; Kwong, R.Y.; Jerosch-Herold, M.; Masri, A.; et al. Mavacamten Favorably Impacts Cardiac Structure in Obstructive Hypertrophic Cardiomyopathy: Explorer-HCM Cardiac Magnetic Resonance Substudy Analysis. *Circulation* **2021**, *143*, 606–608. [CrossRef] [PubMed]
72. Fujita, T.; Fujino, N.; Anan, R.; Tei, C.; Kubo, T.; Doi, Y.; Kinugawa, S.; Tsutsui, H.; Kobayashi, S.; Yano, M.; et al. Sarcomere Gene Mutations Are Associated with Increased Cardiovascular Events in Left Ventricular Hypertrophy: Results from Multicenter Registration in Japan. *JACC Heart Fail.* **2013**, *1*, 459–466. [CrossRef] [PubMed]

73. Li, Q.; Gruner, C.; Chan, R.H.; Care, M.; Siminovitch, K.; Williams, L.; Woo, A.; Rakowski, H. Genotype-Positive Status in Patients with Hypertrophic Cardiomyopathy Is Associated with Higher Rates of Heart Failure Events. *Circ. Cardiovasc. Genet.* **2014**, *7*, 416–422. [CrossRef] [PubMed]
74. Olivotto, I.; Girolami, F.; Ackerman, M.J.; Nistri, S.; Bos, J.M.; Zachara, E.; Ommen, S.R.; Theis, J.L.; Vaubel, R.A.; Re, F.; et al. Myofilament Protein Gene Mutation Screening and Outcome of Patients with Hypertrophic Cardiomyopathy. *Mayo Clin. Proc.* **2008**, *83*, 630–638. [CrossRef]
75. Maron, M.S.; Olivotto, I.; Harrigan, C.; Appelbaum, E.; Gibson, C.M.; Lesser, J.R.; Haas, T.S.; Udelson, J.E.; Manning, W.J.; Maron, B.J. Mitral Valve Abnormalities Identified by Cardiovascular Magnetic Resonance Represent a Primary Phenotypic Expression of Hypertrophic Cardiomyopathy. *Circulation* **2011**, *124*, 40–47. [CrossRef] [PubMed]
76. Maurizi, N.; Michels, M.; Rowin, E.J.; Semsarian, C.; Girolami, F.; Tomberli, B.; Cecchi, F.; Maron, M.S.; Olivotto, I.; Maron, B.J. Clinical Course and Significance of Hypertrophic Cardiomyopathy Without Left Ventricular Hypertrophy. *Circulation* **2019**, *139*, 830–833. [CrossRef]
77. Bick, A.G.; Flannick, J.; Ito, K.; Cheng, S.; Vasan, R.S.; Parfenov, M.G.; Herman, D.S.; DePalma, S.R.; Gupta, N.; Gabriel, S.B.; et al. Burden of Rare Sarcomere Gene Variants in the Framingham and Jackson Heart Study Cohorts. *Am. J. Hum. Genet.* **2012**, *91*, 513–519. [CrossRef]

Journal of
Cardiovascular Development and Disease

MDPI

Article

Diagnostic Accuracy of Global Longitudinal Strain for Detecting Exercise Intolerance in Patients with Ischemic Heart Disease

Sisi Zhang [1,†], Yujian Liu [1,†], Luying Jiang [1,2], Zhaozhao Wang [1], Wanjun Liu [1,*] and Houjuan Zuo [1,*]

1 Division of Cardiology, Department of Internal Medicine, Tongji Hospital, Tongji Medical College, Huazhong University of Science and Technology, Wuhan 430030, China
2 Hubei Key Laboratory of Genetics and Molecular Mechanisms of Cardiologic Disorders, Wuhan 430030, China
* Correspondence: wjliu@tjh.tjmu.edu.cn (W.L.); zuohoujuan@126.com (H.Z.)
† These authors contributed equally to this work.

Abstract: Objective: Global longitudinal strain (GLS) is a sensitive and reproducible predictive factor in patients with ischemic heart disease (IHD), although its correlation with exercise tolerance is unknown. We aimed to identify the correlation between global longitudinal strain (GLS) and cardiopulmonary exercise testing (CPX) parameters and assess the prognostic implications and accuracy of GLS in predicting exercise intolerance in populations with ischemic heart disease (IHD) using CPET criteria. Methods: Prospectively, 108 patients with IHD underwent CPX and 2D speckle-tracking echocardiography. Correlation between GLS and multiple CPX variables was assessed using Spearman's correlation analysis and univariate regression analysis. A receiver operating characteristic (ROC) curve analysis was performed on GLS to detect exercise intolerance. Results: GLS was correlated with peak oxygen uptake (peak VO_2; r = −0.438, p = 0.000), %PPeak VO_2 (−0.369, p = 0.000), peak metabolic equivalents (METs@peak; r = −0.438, $p < 0.01$), and the minute ventilation–carbon dioxide production (VE/VCO_2) slope (r = 0.257, $p < 0.01$). Weak-to-moderate correlations were also identified for the respiratory exchange rate at the anaerobic threshold (RER@AT), end-tidal carbon dioxide at the anaerobic threshold ($PETCO_2$@AT), oxygen consumption at the anaerobic threshold (VO_2@AT), carbon dioxide production at the anaerobic threshold (VCO_2@AT), and metabolic equivalents at the anaerobic threshold (METs@AT; $p < 0.01$). On multivariate analysis, the results showed that age, the BMI, and GLS are independent predictors for reduced exercise capacity in patients with IHD ($p < 0.01$). The area under the ROC curve value of GLS for identifying patients with a peak VO_2 of <14 mL/kg/min was 0.73 (p = 0.000). Conclusion: As a sensitive echocardiographic assessment of patients with ischemic heart disease, global longitudinal strain is an independent predictor of reduced exercise capacity and has a sensitivity of 74.2% and a specificity of 66.7% to detect exercise intolerance.

Keywords: 2D speckle-tracking echocardiography; global longitudinal strain; cardiopulmonary exercise testing; exercise intolerance; ischemic heart disease

1. Introduction

Catheter coronary angiography (CCA), the traditional gold standard for diagnosing coronary artery disease (CAD), identifies visual obstructive lesions [1]. Despite its advantages, the widespread clinical application of CCA remains limited due to the relative risk, technical dependence, and substantial equipment costs. Furthermore, two-thirds of females and one-third of males with stable ischemic heart disease (IHD) have no obstructive CAD on CCA [2], which is associated with worse outcomes. Conventional echocardiography predominantly depends on assessing the left ventricle (LV) ejection fraction (EF) and abnormal wall motion. However, since regional wall motion abnormalities (WMAs) are not evident at rest in approximately 50% of patients, transthoracic echocardiography (TTE) is not diagnostically informative in patients with IHD [3–6]. Two-dimensional speckle-tracking echocardiographic (2D-STE) imaging is a novel, effective method to measure myocardial deformation and provides a comprehensive quantitative assessment of cardiac function. In patients with ST-elevation myocardial infarction (STEMI), 2D longitudinal strain allows a more objective assessment of myocardial regional and global kinetic injuries and the severity of CAD [7].

Cardiopulmonary exercise testing (CPX) is another non-invasive test that can assess cardiovascular, respiratory, and skeletal physiology. Compared to traditional electrocardiogram (ECG) stress testing, CPX gas exchange variables, such as peak oxygen pulse (O_2 pulse), peak oxygen uptake (peak VO_2), peak carbon dioxide exertion (peak VCO_2), anaerobic threshold (AT), VO_2/WR, and respiratory equivalent during anaerobic threshold (VE/VCO_2), provide more sensitive and specific information to detect the onset of ischemia, mortality, and hospitalization [8–11].

Previous studies have failed to identify the correlation between the EF and peak VO_2, except for diastolic function and right ventricular (RV) function [12–14]. However, these studies predominantly focused on patients with heart failure (HF), and there have been no studies on the correlation between the exercise capacity determined with CPET and 2D-STE in patients with IHD. This study aims to identify and evaluate this correlation to assess whether GLS can predict the exercise capacity and cardiorespiratory fitness (CRF) of these patients.

2. Materials and Methods

2.1. Study Population

This prospective study was conducted at Tongji Hospital, Tongji Medical College, and Huazhong University of Science and Technology from November 2021 to May 2022.

A total of 108 patients with stable IHD, which also means chronic coronary syndromes (CCS), as defined by the European Society for Cardiology (ESC) guidelines in 2019. The patients were treated through either percutaneous coronary intervention (PCI) or optimal medical therapy following coronary stenosis on cardiac catheterization examination. They also underwent conventional 2D-ECG and symptom-limited CPX within 1 day. Comorbidities and hematological examinations were recorded. The exclusion criteria were patients with acute myocardial infarction or unstable angina in the previous 6 months, reduced LVEF (<40%), intermittent claudication, mitral stenosis, aortic valve disease, atrial fibrillation, and premature ventricular complexes; patients with abnormal resting regional wall motion on ECG; and patients with suboptimal-quality images to assess strain.

2.2. Cardiopulmonary Exercise Testing

All patients underwent symptom-limited CPX on a CARDIOVIT CS-200 (Schiller, Barr, Switzerland) on the same day before/after 2D-STE, and the procedure complied with the American Heart Association (AHA) statement concerning exercise Standards for Testing and Training [15,16]. The test was performed using modified Bruce protocols via cycle ergometry with a gradual increase in the work rate within 1 min. The increased value was tailored based on the individual's physical conditioning and exercise tolerance, resulting in a test duration of 8 to 12 min until the subject could no longer maintain a consistent pedaling frequency [17]. A 12-lead ECG and oxygen saturation were monitored continuously during the test, with blood pressure measured every 2 min. Peak VO_2 was the average value of the highest 20 s at the last stage of the exercise test and was expressed as absolute (L/min) or relative (mL/kg/min). The VE/VCO_2 slope was calculated using linear regression during exercise (y = mx + b, m = slope), while the anaerobic threshold (AT) was determined using the V-slope technique [18,19]. The following formula was used to calculate the percentage of predicted peak VO_2 (%PPeak VO_2): %PPeak VO_2 = achieved peak VO_2/predicted peak VO_2 obtained using the Wasserman equation $\times$ 100 [20]. A %PPeak VO_2 of <80% is considered the best stratification of patients with functional impairment (New York

Heart Association Class II or higher) compared with those without limitations [21]. The slope of the relationship between the rise in VO_2 over the rate of increase in the work rate ($\triangle VO_2/\triangle$work rate) was expressed as follows: $\triangle VO_2/\triangle$work rate = (peak VO_2 − unloaded VO_2)/[(T − 0.75) × S], where T is the time of incremental exercise and S is the slope of work rate incremental in watts per minute [22].

2.3. *Conventional Echocardiography*

Standardized transesophageal echocardiogram (TEE) examinations were performed using Vivid E9 Ultrasound systems (GE Healthcare Vingmed Ultrasound AS, Horten, Norway) under the guidelines of the American Society of Echocardiography [23]. The electrocardiogram (ECG) data included left end-diastolic dimensions (LVEDD), the LVEF (calculated according to Simpson's method), peak early diastolic filling (E) and late diastolic filling (A) velocities, the E/A ratio, and early and late diastolic septal mitral annular velocities (E′ and A′, respectively), obtained from the pulsed-wave tissue ratio [24].

2.4. *Two-Dimensional Speckle-Tracking Echocardiography (2D-STE)*

As previously described, a strain specialist blind to the clinical data of the patients performed longitudinal strain assessments of the LV from three apical views (4-chamber, 2-chamber, and 3-chamber) using EchoPAC (GE Healthcare Vingmed Ultrasound AS) [24]. The endocardial border and myocardium were automatically tracked throughout the cardiac cycle. A region of interest was traced along the endocardial border from an end-systolic frame, and the thickness of the region of interest was adjusted to include the maximum wall thickness. The mean peak longitudinal systolic strain of all LV segments from the three apical views was used to calculate GLS and generated a 17-segment bull's-eye display (Figure 1). GLS values were presented as negative values. According to a previous report, the normal value of GLS is ≤ -17.6 [25].

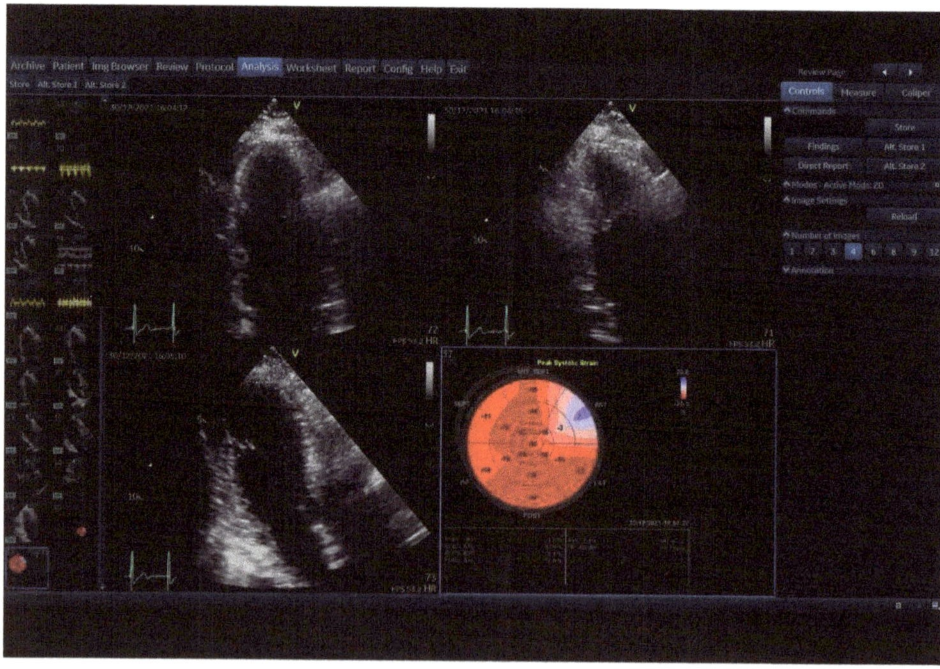

Figure 1. Two-dimensional speckle-tracking echocardiography (2D STE) analysis shows the result of global longitudinal strain (GLS) on a bull's-eye depiction acquired by EchoPAC.

2.5. Statistical Analysis

Continuous data were presented as the mean ± SD or the median (interquartile range, IQR). Categorical variables were expressed as numbers and percentages. Student's *t*-test and the Mann–Whitney test were performed for quantitative variables, while Pearson's chi-square test and Fisher's exact test were performed for categorical variables to compare the differences between the two groups (normal GLS group vs. impaired GLS group). Correlations between GLS and multiple CPX variables were performed using Spearman's correlation analysis. The significant variables ($p < 0.05$) from the univariate analysis were included in the multiple stepwise regression analysis for assessing independent correlations to peak VO_2. Receiver operating characteristic (ROC) curves were generated, and area under the curve (AUC) values were calculated to determine the discrimination value of GLS to predict a peak VO_2 of <14 mL/kg/min. A *p*-value of <0.05 was considered statistically significant. All data were analyzed using SPSS Statistics software. (SPSS 18, SPSS Inc., Chicago, IL, USA).

3. Results

3.1. Patients' Baseline Characteristics

Of the 108 patients included in the study, 56.5% (n = 61) had impaired GLS (>−17.6), while 43.5% (n = 47) had normal GLS (≤−17.6). The baseline characteristics of the two groups are presented in Table 1. No significant differences were found between the two groups except for angiotensin-converting enzyme inhibitor/angiotensin receptor blocker (ACEI/ARB) usage.

Table 1. Baseline characteristics stratified by a GLS median of −17.6%.

Variable	GLS ≥ −17.6 (n = 61)	GLS < −17.6 (n = 47)	*p*-Value
Age (years)	57.21 ± 10.89	60.96 ± 5.95	0.025
Gender (%)			
Male	39 (63.93)	28 (59.57)	0.643
Female	22 (36.07)	19 (40.43)	0.643
Height (cm)	164.74 ± 7.19	163.12 ± 7.64	0.262
Weight (kg)	163.12 ± 7.64	66.29 ± 11.20	0.1
BMI (kg/m^2)	25.65 ± 2.97	24.80 ± 3.03	0.145
Comorbidities (%)			
Hypertension	31 (50.82)	30 (63.83)	0.176
Diabetes	18 (29.51)	13 (27.66)	0.833
Dyslipidemia	24 (39.34)	13 (27.66)	0.205
SBP (mmHg)	135.79 ± 28.73	142.04 ± 15.52	0.151
DBP (mmHg)	73.74 ± 15.21	73.55 ± 9.36	0.942
HR (bpm)	101.33 ± 13.30	98.28 ± 12.24	0.224
Medications (%)			
β-Blocker	38 (62.30)	24 (51.06)	0.242
ACE inhibitors/ARB	22 (36.07)	26 (55.32)	0.046 *
Statin	57 (93.44)	47 (100.00)	0.074
Aspirin	57 (93.44)	44 (93.62)	0.971
Clopidogrel	55 (90.16)	46 (97.87)	0.107
CCB	14 (22.95)	14 (29.79)	0.422
Serum marker			
Creatinine (umol/L)	82.03 ± 23.00	76.82 ± 20.28	0.233
CK (mmol/L)	258.11 ± 802.31	96.77 ± 42.57	0.15
Cholesterol (mmol/L)	4.39 ± 1.30	4.05 ± 1.12	0.155
Glucose (mmol/L)	6.320 (5.4, 8.4)	6.510 (5.9, 8.2)	0.479

Table 1. *Cont.*

Variable	GLS ≥ −17.6 (*n* = 61)	GLS < −17.6 (*n* = 47)	*p*-Value
HDL (mmol/L)	1.050 (0.9, 1.3)	1.080 (0.9, 1.2)	0.942
LDL (mmol/L)	2.67 ± 1.03	2.35 ± 0.94	0.111
Lipoprotein (a) (mmol/L)	40.12 ± 47.97	45.81 ± 57.46	0.59
Triglycerides (mmol/L)	1.560 (1.0, 2.7)	1.600 (0.9, 2.7)	0.829
Hemoglobin (g/L)	137.49 ± 16.41	135.30 ± 16.79	0.507
NT-proBNP	315.26 ± 789.62	286.42 ± 1077.99	0.898
IHD (%)			
Non-PCI	27 (44.26)	28 (59.57)	0.115
PCI	34 (55.74)	19 (40.43)	0.115

Abbreviations: GLS, global longitudinal strain; BMI, body mass index; SBP, systolic blood pressure; DBP, diastolic blood pressure; HR, heart rate; ACE, angiotensin-converting enzyme; ARB, angiotensin II receptor blockers; CCB, calcium channel blocker; CK, creatine kinase; HDL, high-density lipoprotein; LDL, low-density lipoprotein; NT-proBNP, N-terminal pro-B-type natriuretic peptide; IHD, ischemic heart disease; PCI, percutaneous intervention. * $p < 0.05$.

3.2. ECG and CPX data

ECG and CPX parameters between the two groups are shown in Table 2. Compared with the impaired GLS group, patients with normal GLS exhibited significantly higher VO_2/kg@AT, Load@AT, VCO_2/kg@AT, RER@AT, metabolic equivalents (METs)@AT, VO_2/kg@peak, VCO_2/kg@peak, RER@peak, and %PPeak VO_2, which indicated a better exercise capacity. TEE data were similar across both groups.

Table 2. Echocardiographic characteristics, global longitudinal strain, and primary CPET variables between groups.

Variables	GLS ≥ −17.6 (*n* = 61)	GLS < −17.6 (*n* = 47)	*p*-Value
GLS (%)	−14.68 ± 2.16	−19.61 ± 1.45	0.000
LVEDD (mm)	47.68 ± 4.84	47.14 ± 4.68	0.568
LVEF (%)	0.580 (0.5,0.6)	0.630 (0.6, 0.7)	0.003
E (cm/s)	71.53 ± 24.19	71.02 ± 19.26	0.911
A (cm/s)	83.96 ± 24.05	75.27 ± 20.77	0.061
E/A	0.94 ± 0.44	0.96 ± 0.28	0.796
E′ (cm/s)	5.84 ± 1.76	6.23 ± 1.58	0.254
A′ (cm/s)	9.58 ± 2.28	9.64 ± 2.43	0.909
RER@ AT	1.02 ± 0.07	1.05 ± 0.06	0.030 *
VO_2/kg@ AT (mL/kg/min)	11.32 ± 1.92	12.22 ± 1.59	0.010 *
Load@ AT (w)	52.52 ± 19.90	52.91 ± 13.11	0.908
VE@ AT (L/min)	24.80 ± 5.04	24.27 ± 4.42	0.573
VE/kg@ AT (mL/kg/min)	351.52 ± 73.47	368.50 ± 55.74	0.19
VCO_2/kg@ AT (mL/kg/min)	11.57 ± 2.13	12.83 ± 2.08	0.003 **
HR@ AT (beats)	101.33 ± 13.30	98.28 ± 12.24	0.224
Metabolic equivalents@ AT (Mets)	3.24 ± 0.55	3.50 ± 0.45	0.009 **
RER@ peak	1.21 ± 0.09	1.24 ± 0.08	0.028 *
VO_2/kg@ peak (mL/kg/min)	17.01 ± 3.22	19.19 ± 3.42	0.001 **
VO_2 peak/predicted	0.66 ± 0.14	0.76 ± 0.09	0.000 **
Load@ peak (w)	88.39 ± 30.73	92.60 ± 24.83	0.446

Table 2. *Cont.*

Variables	GLS ≥ −17.6 (*n* = 61)	GLS < −17.6 (*n* = 47)	*p*-Value
VE@ peak (L/min)	43.79 ± 10.89	45.82 ± 11.88	0.358
VE/kg@ peak (mL/kg/min)	622.35 ± 159.42	691.72 ± 145.81	0.022 *
VCO_2/kg@ peak (mL/kg/min)	20.65 ± 4.55	24.01 ± 5.30	0.001 **
HR@ peak (beats)	123.97 ± 18.77	126.09 ± 21.18	0.584
Metabolic equivalents@ peak (Mets)	4.86 ± 0.92	5.49 ± 0.97	0.001
VE/VCO_2 slope	28.91 ± 5.83	26.65 ± 5.98	0.051
dVO_2/d Work rate (mL/min/watt)	9.19 ± 1.77	9.72 ± 1.64	0.112
FEV1 (L)	2.44 ± 0.70	2.47 ± 0.61	0.8
FVC (L)	3.05 ± 0.79	3.13 ± 0.80	0.622
FEV1/FVC (%)	0.80 ± 0.09	0.80 ± 0.10	0.978
VC max	3.19 ± 0.79	3.23 ± 0.78	0.784

Abbreviations: LVEDD, left ventricular end-diastolic diameter; LVEF, left ventricular ejection fraction; RER, respiratory exchange ratio; AT, anaerobic threshold; VO_2, oxygen uptake; VCO_2, ventilatory carbon dioxide; HR, heart rate; VE, exercise ventilation; FEV1, forced expiratory volume in 1 s; FVC, forced vital capacity; VC, vital capacity. * $p < 0.05$, ** $p < 0.01$.

3.3. Correlation of GLS with CPX Variables

The Pearson correlation of GLS with CPX data (Table 3) revealed that GLS is inversely related to some of the analyzed CPX variables, including RER@peak (r = −0.341, p < 001), VO_2/kg@peak (r = −0.432, $p < 0.01$), METs@peak (r = −0.438, $p < 0.01$), VE/kg@peak (r = −0.328, $p < 0.01$), and %PPeak VO_2 (r = −0.37, $p < 0.01$), and directly related to VE/VCO_2slope (r = 0.257, $p < 0.01$); see Figure 2. Correlations were also found for RER@AT, PETCO_2@AT, VO_2/kg@AT, VCO_2/kg@AT, and METs@AT ($p < 0.01$). The EF value showed no significant correlation with any of the analyzed CPET variables (Table 3).

Table 3. Correlations between numerical parameters of CPX with the left ventricular ejection fraction (LVEF) and global longitudinal strain (GLS).

Values	GLS		EF	
	r	*p*-Value	r	*p*-Value
dVO_2/dWR (mL/min/W)	−0.177	0.067	−0.023	0.82
VE @AT (L/min)	0.007	0.944	−0.064	0.526
HR @AT (bpm)	0.151	0.118	−0.007	0.445
Load @AT (watts)	−0.04	0.682	0.037	0.711
RER@ AT	−0.305	0.001 **	0.081	0.421
PETCO_2 @AT (mmHg)	−0.274	0.004 **	0.187	0.062
PETO_2 @AT (mmHg)	0.047	0.63	−0.086	0.394
Systolic BP@A (mmHg)	−0.077	0.431	0.144	0.151
Diastolic BP@AT (mmHg)	0.019	0.848	0.028	0.784
VE/kg @AT (mL/kg/min)	−0.158	0.102	0.097	0.335
VO_2/kg @AT (mL/kg/min)	−0.267	0.005 **	0.202	0.042
VCO_2/kg @AT (mL/kg/min)	−0.335	0.000 **	0.192	0.054
Metabolic equivalents (METs)@ AT	−0.271	0.005 **	0.205	0.04
VE @peak (L/min)	−0.2	0.038	−0.077	0.445
HR @peak (bpm)	−0.098	0.313	−0.087	0.39
Load @peak (watts)	−0.151	0.118	−0.025	0.808
RER@ peak	−0.341	0.000 **	0.016	0.875
PETCO_2 @peak (mmHg)	−0.244	0.011	0.078	0.438
PETO_2 @peak (mmHg)	0.035	0.717	−0.126	0.209

Table 3. *Cont.*

Values	GLS		EF	
	r	*p*-Value	r	*p*-Value
Systolic BP@peak (mmHg)	−0.167	0.085	0.131	0.19
Diastolic BP@peak (mmHg)	−0.093	0.339	−0.031	0.762
VE/kg @peak (mL/kg/min)	−0.328	0.001 **	0.035	0.725
VO_2/kg @peak (mL/kg/min)	−0.432	0.000 **	0.075	0.459
VCO_2/kg @peak (mL/kg/min)	−0.456	0.000 **	0.068	0.499
Metabolic equivalents (METs)@ peak	−0.438	0.000 **	0.076	0.448
VE/VCO_2slope	0.257	0.007 **	−0.242	0.015
%PPeak VO_2 (%)	−0.369	0.000 **	0.135	0.178
VC max (L)	−0.087	0.369	−0.045	0.655
FEV1 (L)	−0.024	0.808	−0.009	0.931
FVC (L)	−0.1	0.308	0.004	0.966
FEV1/FVC (%)	0.116	0.238	−0.019	0.852

Abbreviations: dVO_2/dWR: oxygen-consumption-to-work-rate ratio; VE, exercise ventilation; HR, heart rate; RER, respiratory exchange ratio; AT, anaerobic threshold; $PETCO_2$, end-tidal carbon dioxide; $PETO_2$, end-tidal partial pressures of oxygen; BP, blood pressure; VO_2, oxygen uptake; VCO_2, ventilatory carbon dioxide; FEV1, forced expiratory volume in 1 s; FVC, forced vital capacity; VC, vital capacity. ** $p < 0.01$.

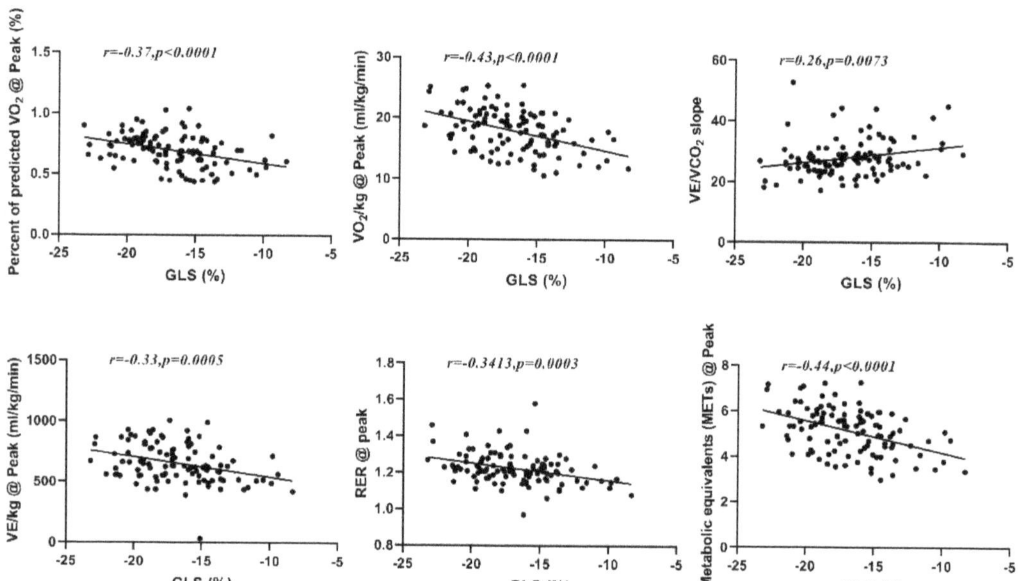

Figure 2. Correlation between GLS and %PPeak VO_2, peak VO_2, VE/VCO_2slope, peak VE, peak RER, and peak METs.

On univariate analysis, the results showed that age ($p < 0.01$) and GLS ($p < 0.01$) appear to be associated with reduced exercise tolerance in subjects with IHD, while on multivariate analysis, age, the BMI, and GLS were independent predictors of reduced exercise capacity (Table 4).

Table 4. Univariate and multivariate predictors to predict reduced exercise capacity (peak VO_2) in patients with IHD.

Variables	Univariate Analysis			Multivariate Analysis		
	OR	95%CI	*p*-Value	OR	95%CI	*p*-Value
Gender	4	1.258–12.72	0.019	3.998	0.766–20.859	0.1
Age	0.869	0.791–0.954	<0.01	0.793	0.684–0.919	<0.01
BMI	0.824	0.681–0.997	0.047	0.663	0.487–0.903	<0.01
EF	0.975	0.010–97.809	0.991	0.028	0.000–4.464	0.167
GLS	0.737	0.606–0.896	<0.01	0.618	0.445–0.859	<0.01
LV	0.946	0.844–1.060	0.34	0.876	0.731–1.05	0.152

Abbreviations: BMI, body mass index; EF, ejection fraction; GLS, global longitudinal strain; LV, left ventricular; OR, odds ratio; CI, confidence interval.

The area under the ROC curve (AUC) value for GLS in the detection of peak VO_2 of <14 mL/kg/min was 0.73 (95% confidence interval (CI) 0.6–0.86), with a sensitivity of 74.2% and a specificity of 66.7%, for a cut-off GLS value of −15.2% ($p = 0.000$); see Figure 3.

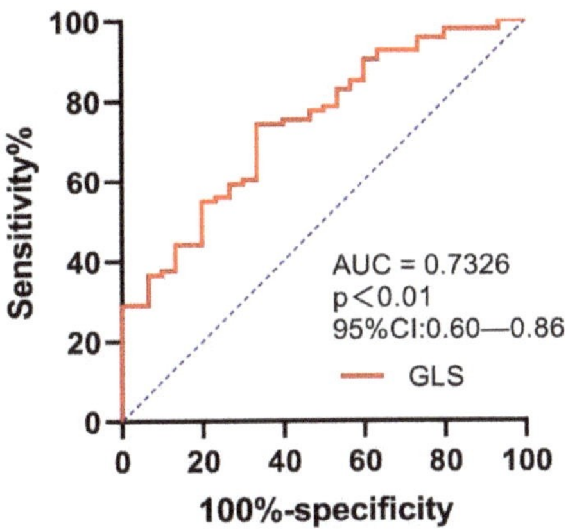

Figure 3. ROC curve for evaluating the ability of GLS in predicting VO_2 of <14 mL/kg/min.

4. Discussion

To the best of our knowledge, this is the first study to describe the relationship between GLS and CPX parameters in the population with IHD. The study highlights weak-to-moderate correlations between GLS and functional CPX parameters and further demonstrates that GLS can detect reduced exercise capacity in these patients.

The non-invasive detection of ischemia for non-obstructive CAD remains a clinical challenge. Previous studies have recognized GLS as one of the most sensitive and reproducible indicators of ischemia and have shown that GLS is superior to the EF in detecting an early reduction in contractile function [26]. The LVEF is not correlated with functional capacity [27]. Most evidence on the association between exercise tolerance and cardiac strain has predominantly focused on patients with HF [28]. However, this relationship has not been investigated and demonstrated in patients with IHD. GLS has emerged as a promising parameter of exercise capacity [29]. This study is the first to show the correlation between GLS and exercise capacity in patients with IHD, which has not been investigated in prior studies of 2D-STE and CPX after a coronary angiogram. More than half of the patients referred for coronary angiography are reported to have normal or non-obstructive CAD, and compared to optimal medical treatment, revascularization is only beneficial in patients with severe ischemia [30,31]. Further coronary angiograms should be considered for symptomatic patients with cardiac dysfunction of reduced peak VO_2 (<70% of predicted) on CPET. Furthermore, revascularization does not improve the peak VO_2 for patients with multivessel disease, suggesting that CPET plays a vital role in characterizing the functional consequences of myocardial ischemia [32]. Hence, a more sensitive index for coronary revascularization is needed.

Patients with IHD frequently have reduced exercise capacity, even when the conventional parameters of left ventricular function, such as ejection fraction (LVEF), are within the normal range. In addition, the role of disability, particularly in the context of exercise intolerance, is not fully understood. GLS is associated with the extent of viable myocardial tissue in patients with chronic IHD, where the load has less of an impact. Since sub-endocardial fibers are more sensitive to ischemia, numerous studies have demonstrated that GLS is more accurate at detecting early myocardial disturbances caused by ischemia compared with the EF value [3,25]. Previous research has suggested that GLS is related to the ability to exercise through poor contractile reservation during exercise [33]. Peak VO_2 and VE/VCO_2 slope are critical parameters in the detection of obstructive CAD, and in this study, patients with normal GLS had a higher peak VO_2 (19.19 ± 3.42 mL/kg/min vs. 17.01 ± 3.22 mL/kg/min), and compared with the resting EF, GLS showed a relationship with peak VO_2 ($r = -0.432$, $p < 0.01$) and the VE/VCO_2 slope ($r = 0.257$, $p = 0.000$). Moreover, multivariable analysis demonstrated that GLS is independently associated with reduced peak VO_2. Thus, reduced GLS may be an effective indicator of exercise intolerance in this group of patients.

Peak VO_2, defined as cardiorespiratory fitness (CRF), is a vital clinical sign of all-cause and cardiovascular mortality in patients with cardiovascular diseases, as well as in healthy individuals [34]. Reduced peak VO_2 is recognized as an independent risk factor for adverse cardiovascular events in populations with IHD. The correlations between GLS and exercise capacity identified in this study further highlight the potential importance of early detection of LV dysfunction in individuals with IHD with exercise intolerance.

Ng et al. reported that GLS at rest was -16.3 ± 2.4 in patients with CAD vs. -19.1 ± 2.9 in patients with non-significant CAD [35]. Similar results were obtained by Biering-Sørensen et al. [36], Gaibazzi et al. [37], Evensen et al. [38], and Shimoni et al. [39]. In this study, the cut-off value of GLS to detect a peak VO_2 of <14 mL/min/kg was -15.2, with a sensitivity of 74.2% and a specificity of 66.7%. Collectively, these findings indicate the quantifiable and prognostic significance of GLS as a suitable alternative to evaluate patients with reduced exercise capacity.

The value of using CPX in detecting macrovascular ischemia has been previously reported [9]. However, the direct measurement of CPX requires specialized equipment and trained personnel to accurately interpret the results. In addition, patients may be unable or unwilling to undergo this testing. Thus, CPX remains underused in China. Simultaneously, despite numerous attempts to develop surrogates and regression models based on non-experimental test data to predict peak VO_2, the models are not specific enough to classify CRF as routine practice. Hence, determination of the relationship between GLS and exercise intolerance could potentially allow the prediction of CRF of patients with IHD based solely on ECG-derived GLS. The exercise intolerance prediction results from this study extend the findings of Maia et al. [40] regarding GLS measured in patients with systolic heart failure. In this study, the GLS cut-off value for detecting a peak VO_2 of <14 mL/min/kg was -15.2. Therefore, GLS could be a valuable tool to discriminate patients with normal exercise capacity from those with reduced exercise capacity.

4.1. Limitations

Despite the valuable findings of this study, there are several significant limitations that should also be considered. First, as a single-center study, the small size of the population in the study may limit the generalizability of the findings. Second, more than 50% of the participants in both experimental groups were taking β-receptor blocker medication, a primary treatment for IHD, which significantly lowers the peak VO_2 in CPX. Further studies should be conducted on subjects using 3D STE.

4.2. Conclusions

The study presented the value of GLS measured with 2D speckle-tracking echocardiograph in patients with IHD. The assessment of GLS was able to detect exercise intolerance and identify what has a poor prognosis.

Author Contributions: S.Z. and Y.L. designed the research. L.J. and Z.W. performed the data analysis. W.L. and H.Z. contributed to the revision and finalized the manuscript. All authors have read and agreed to the published version of the manuscript.

Funding: This research received no external funding.

Institutional Review Board Statement: The study was conducted in accordance with the Declaration of Helsinki, and approved by the Institutional Ethical Committee of the Union Hospital, Tongji Medical College, Huazhong University of Science and Technology, Wuhan, China (TJ-IRB20220314).

Informed Consent Statement: Written informed consent for participation was obtained from the individuals for publication.

Data Availability Statement: Data is unavailable due to privacy or ethical restrictions.

Conflicts of Interest: The authors declare that the research was conducted in the absence of any commercial or financial relationships that could be construed as a potential conflict of interest.

References

1. DeRouen, T.A.; Murray, J.A.; Owen, W. Variability in the analysis of coronary arteriograms. *Circulation* **1977**, *55*, 324–328. [CrossRef] [PubMed]
2. Sedlak, T.L.; Lee, M.; Izadnegahdar, M.; Merz, C.N.; Gao, M.; Humphries, K.H. Sex differences in clinical outcomes in patients with stable angina and no obstructive coronary artery disease. *Am. Heart J.* **2013**, *166*, 38–44. [CrossRef] [PubMed]
3. Choi, J.O.; Cho, S.W.; Song, Y.B.; Cho, S.J.; Song, B.G.; Lee, S.C.; Park, S.W. Longitudinal 2D strain at rest predicts the presence of left main and three vessel coronary artery disease in patients without regional wall motion abnormality. *Eur. J. Echocardiogr. J. Work. Group Echocardiogr. Eur. Soc. Cardiol.* **2009**, *10*, 695–701. [CrossRef]
4. Fleischmann, K.E.; Lee, R.T.; Come, P.C.; Goldman, L.; Cook, E.F.; Weissman, M.A.; Johnson, P.A.; Lee, T.H. Impact of Valvular Regurgitation and Ventricular Dysfunction on Long-Term Survival in Patients with Chest Pain. *Am. J. Cardiol.* **1997**, *80*, 1266–1272. [CrossRef] [PubMed]
5. Savonitto, S.; Ardissino, D.; Granger, C.B.; Morando, G.; Prando, M.D.; Mafrici, A.; Cavallini, C.; Melandri, G.; Thompson, T.D.; Vahanian, A.; et al. Prognostic value of the admission electrocardiogram in acute coronary syndromes. *Jama* **1999**, *281*, 707–713. [CrossRef] [PubMed]
6. Elhendy, A.; van Domburg, R.T.; Bax, J.J.; Roelandt, J.R. Significance of resting wall motion abnormalities in 2-dimensional echocardiography in patients without previous myocardial infarction referred for pharmacologic stress testing. *J. Am. Soc. Echocardiogr. Off. Publ. Am. Soc. Echocardiogr.* **2000**, *13*, 1–8. [CrossRef]
7. Zito, C.; Longobardo, L.; Citro, R.; Galderisi, M.; Oreto, L.; Carerj, M.L.; Manganaro, R.; Cusmà-Piccione, M.; Todaro, M.C.; Di Bella, G.; et al. Ten Years of 2D Longitudinal Strain for Early Myocardial Dysfunction Detection: A Clinical Overview. *BioMed Res. Int.* **2018**, *2018*, 8979407. [CrossRef]
8. Chaudhry, S.; Arena, R.; Wasserman, K.; Hansen, J.E.; Lewis, G.D.; Myers, J.; Chronos, N.; Boden, W.E. Exercise-induced myocardial ischemia detected by cardiopulmonary exercise testing. *Am. J. Cardiol.* **2009**, *103*, 615–619. [CrossRef]
9. Belardinelli, R.; Lacalaprice, F.; Carle, F.; Minnucci, A.; Cianci, G.; Perna, G.; D'Eusanio, G. Exercise-induced myocardial ischaemia detected by cardiopulmonary exercise testing. *Eur. Heart J.* **2003**, *24*, 1304–1313. [CrossRef]
10. Edvardsen, T.; Skulstad, H.; Aakhus, S.; Urheim, S.; Ihlen, H. Regional myocardial systolic function during acute myocardial ischemia assessed by strain Doppler echocardiography. *J. Am. Coll. Cardiol.* **2001**, *37*, 726–730. [CrossRef]
11. Zuo, H.J.; Yang, X.T.; Liu, Q.G.; Zhang, Y.; Zeng, H.S.; Yan, J.T.; Wang, D.W.; Wang, H. Global Longitudinal Strain at Rest for Detection of Coronary Artery Disease in Patients without Diabetes Mellitus. *Curr. Med. Sci.* **2018**, *38*, 413–421. [CrossRef] [PubMed]
12. Salerno, G.; D'Andrea, A.; Bossone, E.; Scarafile, R.; Riegler, L.; Di Salvo, G.; Gravino, R.; Pezzullo, E.; Limongelli, G.; Romano, M.; et al. Association between right ventricular two-dimensional strain and exercise capacity in patients with either idiopathic or ischemic dilated cardiomyopathy. *J. Cardiovasc. Med.* **2011**, *12*, 625–634. [CrossRef] [PubMed]
13. Hummel, Y.M.; Bugatti, S.; Damman, K.; Willemsen, S.; Hartog, J.W.; Metra, M.; Sipkens, J.S.; van Veldhuisen, D.J.; Voors, A.A. Functional and hemodynamic cardiac determinants of exercise capacity in patients with systolic heart failure. *Am. J. Cardiol.* **2012**, *110*, 1336–1341. [CrossRef] [PubMed]
14. Franciosa, J.A.; Park, M.; Levine, T.B. Lack of correlation between exercise capacity and indexes of resting left ventricular performance in heart failure. *Am. J. Cardiol.* **1981**, *47*, 33–39. [CrossRef]

15. Fletcher, G.F.; Ades, P.A.; Kligfield, P.; Arena, R.; Balady, G.J.; Bittner, V.A.; Coke, L.A.; Fleg, J.L.; Forman, D.E.; Gerber, T.C.; et al. Exercise standards for testing and training: A scientific statement from the American Heart Association. *Circulation* **2013**, *128*, 873–934. [CrossRef]
16. Fletcher, G.F.; Balady, G.J.; Amsterdam, E.A.; Chaitman, B.; Eckel, R.; Fleg, J.; Froelicher, V.F.; Leon, A.S.; Piña, I.L.; Rodney, R.; et al. Exercise standards for testing and training: A statement for healthcare professionals from the American Heart Association. *Circulation* **2001**, *104*, 1694–1740. [CrossRef]
17. Myers, J.; Bellin, D. Ramp exercise protocols for clinical and cardiopulmonary exercise testing. *Sport. Med.* **2000**, *30*, 23–29. [CrossRef]
18. Beaver, W.L.; Wasserman, K.; Whipp, B.J. A new method for detecting anaerobic threshold by gas exchange. *J. Appl. Physiol.* **1986**, *60*, 2020–2027. [CrossRef]
19. Bard, R.L.; Gillespie, B.W.; Clarke, N.S.; Egan, T.G.; Nicklas, J.M. Determining the best ventilatory efficiency measure to predict mortality in patients with heart failure. *J. Heart Lung Transplant. Off. Publ. Int. Soc. Heart Transplant.* **2006**, *25*, 589–595. [CrossRef]
20. Coates, A.L. *Principles of Exercise Testing and Interpretation. By K. Wasserman, J.E. Hansen, D.V. Sue, and B.J. Whipp. Philadelphia: Lea & Febiger, 1987*; Wiley Online Library: Hoboken, NJ, USA, 1987; Volume 3, p. 378. [CrossRef]
21. Patel, V.; Critoph, C.H.; Elliott, P.M. Mechanisms and medical management of exercise intolerance in hypertrophic cardiomyopathy. *Curr. Pharm. Des.* **2015**, *21*, 466–472. [CrossRef]
22. Balady, G.J.; Arena, R.; Sietsema, K.; Myers, J.; Coke, L.; Fletcher, G.F.; Forman, D.; Franklin, B.; Guazzi, M.; Gulati, M.; et al. Clinician' Guide to Cardiopulmonary Exercise Testing in Adults. *Circulation* **2010**, *122*, 191–225. [CrossRef] [PubMed]
23. Lang, R.M.; Badano, L.P.; Mor-Avi, V.; Afilalo, J.; Armstrong, A.; Ernande, L.; Flachskampf, F.A.; Foster, E.; Goldstein, S.A.; Kuznetsova, T.; et al. Recommendations for cardiac chamber quantification by echocardiography in adults: An update from the American Society of Echocardiography and the European Association of Cardiovascular Imaging. *J. Am. Soc. Echocardiogr. Off. Publ. Am. Soc. Echocardiogr.* **2015**, *28*, 1–39.e14. [CrossRef] [PubMed]
24. Duncan, A.E.; Kateby Kashy, B.; Sarwar, S.; Singh, A.; Stenina-Adognravi, O.; Christoffersen, S.; Alfirevic, A.; Sale, S.; Yang, D.; Thomas, J.D.; et al. Hyperinsulinemic Normoglycemia Does Not Meaningfully Improve Myocardial Performance during Cardiac Surgery: A Randomized Trial. *Anesthesiology* **2015**, *123*, 272–287. [CrossRef] [PubMed]
25. Yingchoncharoen, T.; Agarwal, S.; Popović, Z.B.; Marwick, T.H. Normal ranges of left ventricular strain: A meta-analysis. *J. Am. Soc. Echocardiogr. Off. Publ. Am. Soc. Echocardiogr.* **2013**, *26*, 185–191. [CrossRef]
26. Ponikowski, P.; Voors, A.A.; Anker, S.D.; Bueno, H.; Cleland, J.G.F.; Coats, A.J.S.; Falk, V.; González-Juanatey, J.R.; Harjola, V.P.; Jankowska, E.A.; et al. 2016 ESC Guidelines for the diagnosis and treatment of acute and chronic heart failure: The Task Force for the diagnosis and treatment of acute and chronic heart failure of the European Society of Cardiology (ESC)Developed with the special contribution of the Heart Failure Association (HFA) of the ESC. *Eur. Heart J.* **2016**, *37*, 2129–2200. [CrossRef]
27. Arena, R.; Guazzi, M.; Cahalin, L.P.; Myers, J. Revisiting cardiopulmonary exercise testing applications in heart failure: Aligning evidence with clinical practice. *Exerc. Sport Sci. Rev.* **2014**, *42*, 153–160. [CrossRef]
28. Kou, S.; Suzuki, K.; Akashi, Y.J.; Mizukoshi, K.; Takai, M.; Izumo, M.; Shimozato, T.; Hayashi, A.; Ohtaki, E.; Osada, N.; et al. Global longitudinal strain by two-dimensional speckle tracking imaging predicts exercise capacity in patients with chronic heart failure. *J. Echocardiogr.* **2011**, *9*, 64–72. [CrossRef]
29. Shimoni, O.; Korenfeld, R.; Goland, S.; Meledin, V.; Haberman, D.; George, J.; Shimoni, S. Subclinical Myocardial Dysfunction in Patients Recovered from COVID-19 Disease: Correlation with Exercise Capacity. *Biology* **2021**, *10*, 1201. [CrossRef]
30. Boden, W.E.; O'Rourke, R.A.; Teo, K.K.; Hartigan, P.M.; Maron, D.J.; Kostuk, W.J.; Knudtson, M.; Dada, M.; Casperson, P.; Harris, C.L.; et al. Optimal medical therapy with or without PCI for stable coronary disease. *N. Engl. J. Med.* **2007**, *356*, 1503–1516. [CrossRef]
31. Patel, M.R.; Peterson, E.D.; Dai, D.; Brennan, J.M.; Redberg, R.F.; Anderson, H.V.; Brindis, R.G.; Douglas, P.S. Low diagnostic yield of elective coronary angiography. *N. Engl. J. Med.* **2010**, *362*, 886–895. [CrossRef]
32. Engstrøm, T.; Kelbæk, H.; Helqvist, S.; Høfsten, D.E.; Kløvgaard, L.; Holmvang, L.; Jørgensen, E.; Pedersen, F.; Saunamäki, K.; Clemmensen, P.; et al. Complete revascularisation versus treatment of the culprit lesion only in patients with ST-segment elevation myocardial infarction and multivessel disease (DANAMI-3—PRIMULTI): An open-label, randomised controlled trial. *Lancet* **2015**, *386*, 665–671. [CrossRef] [PubMed]
33. Hasselberg, N.E.; Haugaa, K.H.; Sarvari, S.I.; Gullestad, L.; Andreassen, A.K.; Smiseth, O.A.; Edvardsen, T. Left ventricular global longitudinal strain is associated with exercise capacity in failing hearts with preserved and reduced ejection fraction. *Eur. Heart J. Cardiovasc. Imaging* **2015**, *16*, 217–224. [CrossRef] [PubMed]
34. Conraads, V.M.; Pattyn, N.; De Maeyer, C.; Beckers, P.J.; Coeckelberghs, E.; Cornelissen, V.A.; Denollet, J.; Frederix, G.; Goetschalckx, K.; Hoymans, V.Y.; et al. Aerobic interval training and continuous training equally improve aerobic exercise capacity in patients with coronary artery disease: The SAINTEX-CAD study. *Int. J. Cardiol.* **2015**, *179*, 203–210. [CrossRef] [PubMed]
35. Ng, A.C.; Sitges, M.; Pham, P.N.; da Tran, T.; Delgado, V.; Bertini, M.; Nucifora, G.; Vidaic, J.; Allman, C.; Holman, E.R.; et al. Incremental value of 2-dimensional speckle tracking strain imaging to wall motion analysis for detection of coronary artery disease in patients undergoing dobutamine stress echocardiography. *Am. Heart J.* **2009**, *158*, 836–844. [CrossRef]

36. Biering-Sørensen, T.; Hoffmann, S.; Mogelvang, R.; Zeeberg Iversen, A.; Galatius, S.; Fritz-Hansen, T.; Bech, J.; Jensen, J.S. Myocardial strain analysis by 2-dimensional speckle tracking echocardiography improves diagnostics of coronary artery stenosis in stable angina pectoris. *Circ. Cardiovasc. Imaging* **2014**, *7*, 58–65. [CrossRef]
37. Gaibazzi, N.; Pigazzani, F.; Reverberi, C.; Porter, T.R. Rest global longitudinal 2D strain to detect coronary artery disease in patients undergoing stress echocardiography: A comparison with wall-motion and coronary flow reserve responses. *Echo Res. Pract.* **2014**, *1*, 61–70. [CrossRef]
38. Evensen, K.; Sarvari, S.I.; Rønning, O.M.; Edvardsen, T.; Russell, D. Carotid artery intima-media thickness is closely related to impaired left ventricular function in patients with coronary artery disease: A single-centre, blinded, non-randomized study. *Cardiovasc. Ultrasound* **2014**, *12*, 39. [CrossRef]
39. Shimoni, S.; Gendelman, G.; Ayzenberg, O.; Smirin, N.; Lysyansky, P.; Edri, O.; Deutsch, L.; Caspi, A.; Friedman, Z. Differential effects of coronary artery stenosis on myocardial function: The value of myocardial strain analysis for the detection of coronary artery disease. *J. Am. Soc. Echocardiogr. Off. Publ. Am. Soc. Echocardiogr.* **2011**, *24*, 748–757. [CrossRef]
40. Maia, R.J.C.; Brandão, S.C.S.; Leite, J.; Parente, G.B.; Pinheiro, F.; Araújo, B.T.S.; Aguiar, M.I.R.; Martins, S.M.; Brandão, D.C.; Andrade, A.D. Global Longitudinal Strain Predicts Poor Functional Capacity in Patients with Systolic Heart Failure. *Arq. Bras. De Cardiol.* **2019**, *113*, 188–194. [CrossRef]

Journal of
Cardiovascular Development and Disease

MDPI

Article

The Prognostic Value of Pulmonary Venous Flow Reversal in Patients with Significant Degenerative Mitral Regurgitation

Alon Shechter [1,2,3,*], Steele C. Butcher [4], Robert J. Siegel [3,5], Jenan Awesat [1,2], Merry Abitbol [1,2], Mordehay Vaturi [1,2], Alex Sagie [1,2], Ran Kornowski [1,2], Yaron Shapira [1,2] and Idit Yedidya [1,2]

1 Department of Cardiology, Rabin Medical Center, Petach Tikva 4941492, Israel
2 Faculty of Medicine, Tel Aviv University, Tel Aviv 69978, Israel
3 Department of Cardiology, Smidt Heart Institute, Cedars-Sinai Medical Center, Los Angeles, CA 90048, USA
4 Department of Cardiology, Royal Perth Hospital, Perth, WA 6000, Australia
5 David Geffen School of Medicine, University of California Los Angeles, Los Angeles, CA 90095, USA
* Correspondence: alon.shechter@cshs.org or alonshechter@gmail.com;
Tel.: +1-(310)-423-2726; Fax: +1-(310)-423-0166

Abstract: *Background*: The prognostic significance of pulmonary venous (PV) flow reversal in degenerative mitral regurgitation (dMR) is not well-established. *Objective*: We aimed to assess whether reversed PV flow is associated with adverse outcomes in patients with significant dMR. *Methods*: We retrospectively analyzed consecutive patients referred to a tertiary center for evaluation of dMR of greater than moderate degree, who had normal sinus rhythm, had a left ventricular ejection fraction of above 60%, and did not suffer from any other major valvular disorders. The primary outcome was the combined rate of all-cause mortality, mitral intervention, or new-onset atrial fibrillation (AF) at 5 years following index echocardiogram. Secondary outcomes included individual components of the primary outcome. *Results*: Overall, 135 patients (median age 68 (IQR, 58–74) years; 93 (68.9%) males; 89 (65.9%) with severe MR) met the inclusion criteria and were followed for 115.2 (IQR, 60.0–155.0) months. Patients with a reversed PV flow pattern (PVFP) (n = 34) more often presented with severe MR compared to those with a normal (n = 49) and non-reversed PVFP (n = 101) (RR = 2.03 and 1.59, respectively, all $p < 0.001$). At 5 years, they experienced the highest cumulative incidence of the primary outcome (80.2% vs. 59.2% and 67.3%, $p = 0.008$ and 0.018, respectively). Furthermore, a reversed PVFP was independently associated with a higher risk of the primary outcome compared to normal PVFP (HR 2.53, 95% CI 1.21–5.31, $p = 0.011$) and non-reversed PVFP (HR 2.14, 95% CI 1.12–4.10, $p = 0.022$). Conclusion: PV flow reversal is associated with a worse 5-year composite of mortality, mitral intervention, or AF in patients with significant dMR.

Keywords: degenerative mitral regurgitation; pulmonary veins; atrial fibrillation; prognosis

1. Introduction

Degenerative mitral regurgitation (dMR) is the second-most common form of chronic mitral regurgitation (MR) in developed nations [1]. Affecting 15 out of every 1000 adult Americans in the year 2000 [1], the disease constitutes a significant health and economic burden at an advanced stage. Timely valvular intervention is therefore of paramount importance. Previous retrospective studies have identified atrial fibrillation (AF) and left atrial (LA) dilation as predictors of increased mortality among dMR patients, both conservatively managed [2,3] and surgically treated [3,4]. Serving as the mechanistic link between MR and atrial aberrations [5,6] is LA remodeling, the manifestations of which may include abnormal pulmonary venous (PV) flow pattern (PVFP). Already considered to be supportive evidence of severe MR [7], a reversed PVFP likely signifies a worse disease state which may adversely affect prognosis. Using a contemporary cohort of real-world patients, we assessed whether pulmonary venous flow reversal was associated with worse clinical outcomes in patients with significant chronic dMR.

2. Methods

2.1. Study Population and Outcomes

This is a single-center, retrospective analysis of consecutive patients with dMR of greater than moderate grade who were referred to transesophageal echocardiography (TEE) at Rabin Medical Center (RMC), Israel, between May 1995 and June 2017.

Inclusion criteria comprised the following: 1. absence of documented AF or flutter prior to the TEE; 2. normal left ventricular (LV) systolic function, defined as an LV ejection fraction (LVEF) of above 60% on the transthoracic echocardiogram (TTE) part of the index examination; and 3. an isolated degenerative mitral pathology not accompanied by other valvular disorders of greater than mild-to-moderate grade. Patients that underwent any previous valvular intervention, as well as those without complete baseline data (importantly, the documentation of PVFP bilaterally) were excluded. Follow-up duration spanned the timeframe between the date of echocardiogram and either death or 30 April 2020.

The primary outcome was defined as the composite of all-cause mortality, any form of invasive mitral intervention, and new-onset AF or flutter during the first 5 years of follow-up, excluding arrhythmic events in the first post-interventional month. Secondary outcomes included single components of the primary outcome.

Data regarding endpoints were retrieved using Ofek Software (dbMotion, Pittsburg, PA, USA), which is a web-based medical chart platform shared by most of Israel's public medical providers. Atrial arrythmias were ascertained by inspecting patient files for any mention of obvious AF or flutter on a 12-lead electrocardiogram (ECG) and/or an irregular ventricular electrical activity without discernible P waves on a 30-s strip [8].

The study was conducted in accordance with the Declaration of Helsinki and received Institutional Review Board (IRB) approval. The requirement for informed consent was waived due to the study's retrospective nature.

2.2. Echocardiographic Assessment

All echocardiograms were performed and interpreted by level-III-trained sonographers and echocardiologists. Echo systems used included Vivid 3 Premium and Vivid E95 (General Electric, Milwaukee, WN, USA), Agilent 5500 (Agilent, Santa Clara, CA, USA), HP 77020 (Hewlett Packard, Andover, MA, USA), and IE33 and EPIQ (Philips, Amsterdam, The Netherlands). Diagnostic measurements and conclusions made at each study were based on criteria set forth by the relevant American Society of Echocardiography guidelines [8,9]. Mitral valve assessment incorporated standard multiple views. Regurgitation severity was determined based on the integration of qualitative and semiquantitative measures, whenever possible. A diagnosis of degenerative mitral valve (MV) disease required the visualization of leaflet prolapse, signified by a $\geq$2 mm atrial displacement of the leaflet tip from the mitral annular level at end-systole. Pulmonary veins (PVs) were assessed bilaterally. After verification of tangentiality by color Doppler, the flow at each PV was sampled by a pulsed-wave (PW) Doppler beam placed within 1 cm of the PV ostia. Normal PVFP was defined by a peak systolic (S) velocity to peak diastolic (D) velocity ratio of 1 and above (Figure 1); conversely, PVFP reversal was characterized by an S to D ratio of below zero. Blunted PVFP, considered a form of non-reversed PVFP, was further identified by an S to D ratio between zero and below 1. Overall flow was determined according to the lowest S to D ratio observed. Pulmonary arterial systolic pressure (PASP) assessment was based on the peak systolic pressure gradient measured across the tricuspid valve and the estimated right atrial pressure (RAP) using the diameter and respiratory collapsibility of the inferior vena cava (IVC), both during the TTE part of each study. Global right ventricular (RV) function was evaluated qualitatively. All reports were blindly scrutinized for integrity by two physicians (A.Shechter and I.Y.).

(**A**)

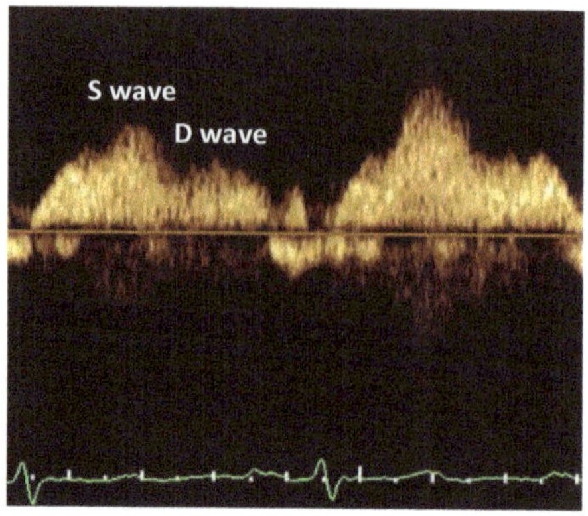

(**B**)

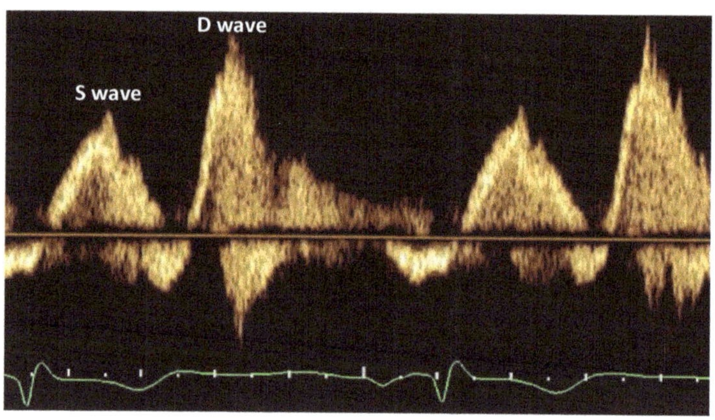

(**C**)

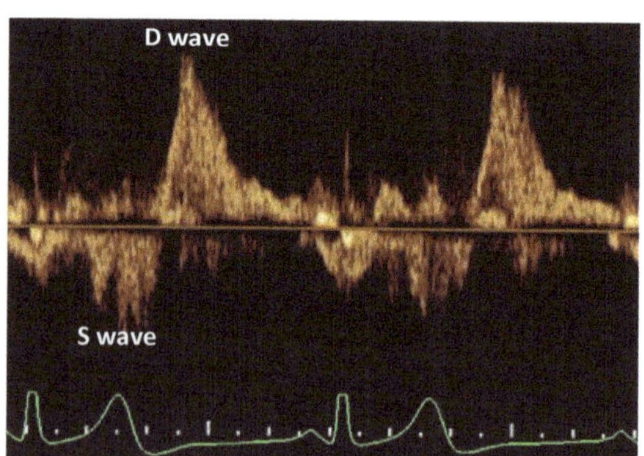

Figure 1. Pulmonary Venous Flow Patterns as Imaged on Transesophageal Echocardiogram. Normal pattern is signified by a peak systolic (S) to peak diastolic (D) flow velocities ratio of $\geq$1. Abnormal pattern may include either a blunted or a reversed S wave, manifested by an S/D ratio of <1 or <0, respectively. (**A**) Normal Flow Pattern. (**B**) Blunted Flow Pattern. (**C**) Reversed Flow Pattern.

2.3. Statistical Analysis

The study cohort was split into three main groups according to baseline PVFP, namely normal, reversed, and non-reversed, with the latter comprising patients exhibiting either normal or blunted flow patterns in the PVs. In each group, continuous variables were expressed as means and standard deviations (SDs) or as medians and interquartile ranges (IQRs). Categorical variables were reported as frequencies and percentages. Between-group comparison of continuous variables with normal distribution was performed using Student's t test, while that of continuous variables demonstrating non-normal distribution was performed using the Mann–Whitney U test. Categorical variables were compared using Pearson's chi-squared test or Fisher's exact test. Importantly, only two groups were compared at a time.

The risk for the development of the primary outcome according to PVFP was graphically displayed using the Kaplan–Meier method, with comparisons of cumulative survival across strata conducted using the log rank test. To identify independent associations between the primary outcome and baseline variables, particularly different forms of PVFP, univariable Cox regression analysis was employed, after which parameters showing a p-value of <0.1 were integrated into a multivariable model.

Patients with missing data were censored from the relevant analyses. A two-sided p-value of <0.05 was considered to represent statistical significance. All analyses were performed using SPSS^{TM} Statistic for Windows software, version 24 (IBM Corporation, Armonk, NY, USA).

3. Results

3.1. Baseline Characteristics of the Study Population

Out of 485 patients that underwent TEE for an evaluation of chronic dMR at RMC between May 1995 and June 2017, a total of 135 met the study inclusion criteria (Figure 2). The median follow-up duration was 115.2 (IQR, 60.0–155.0) months. Three patients — two in the normal PVFP group and one in the reversed PVFP group—were lost to follow-up after a median of 20.0 months.

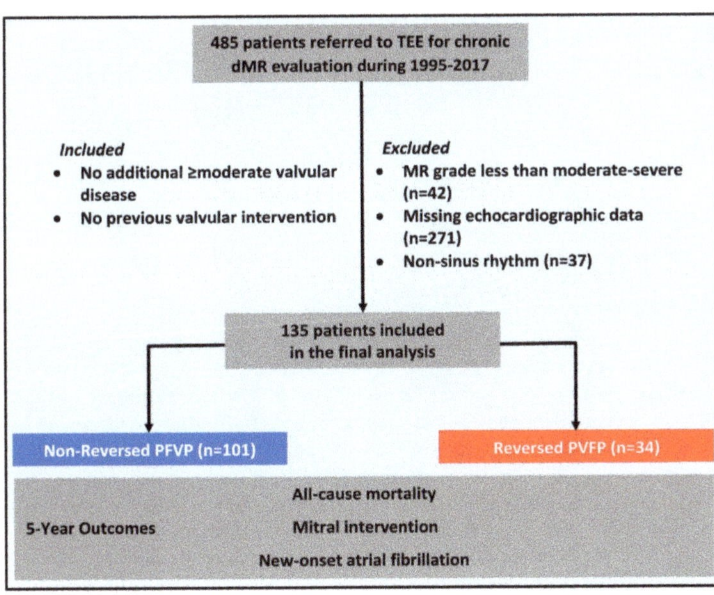

Figure 2. Study Flow Chart. dMR = degenerative mitral regurgitation; LV = left ventricle; NSR = normal sinus rhythm; PVFP = pulmonary venous flow pattern.

Baseline clinical and echocardiographic characteristics of the study cohort are presented in Tables 1 and 2, respectively. Notably, the patients were mostly male (n = 93, 68.9%) and the median age was 68 (IQR, 58–74) years. Additionally, more than half (n = 70, 56.5%) were hypertensive. MR was concluded as severe in 89 (65.9%) cases and prolapse mainly involved the posterior leaflet alone (n = 94, 69.5%), followed by both leaflets (n = 26, 19.3%) and the anterior leaflet only (n = 15, 11.1%).

Table 1. Baseline Clinical Characteristics of the Study Population.

	Total Cohort (N = 135)	Normal PVFP (N = 49)	Reversed PVFP (N = 34)	Non-Reversed PVFP (N = 101)	*p*-Value Normal vs. Reversed	*p*-Value Non-Reversed vs. Reversed
Demographic Data						
Age (years)	68 (58–74)	68 (58–73)	69 (56–76)	68 (58–74)	0.636	0.941
Male sex	93 (68.9)	31 (63.3)	24 (64.7)	70 (70.3)	1.000	0.542
Comorbidities						
BMI						
Median (kg/m^2)	25.0 (22.5–27.2)	25.7 (23.2–28.9)	23.1 (20.5–25.3)	26.0 (23.0–27.9)	0.007	0.001
$\geq$30 kg/m^2	11 (10.8)	6 (18.2)	0 (0.0)	11 (15.1)	0.026	0.027
BSA (m^2)	1.82 (1.69–1.98)	1.80 (1.70–1.93)	1.80 (1.59–1.93)	1.85 (1.70–2.00)	0.628	0.323
Hypertension	70 (56.5)	26 (61.9)	15 (45.5)	55 (60.4)	0.155	0.137
Diabetes Mellitus	12 (9.7)	7 (16.7)	0 (0.0)	12 (13.2)	0.016	0.035
Functional Status						
NYHA Class					0.063	0.010
I	34 (34.7)	14 (37.8)	6 (24.0)	28 (38.4)		
II	38 (38.8)	14 (37.8)	8 (32.0)	30 (41.1)		
III	23 (23.5)	9 (24.3)	8 (32.0)	15 (20.5)		
IV	3 (3.1)	0 (0.0)	3 (12.0)	0 (0.0)		
II and Above	64 (65.3)	23 (62.2)	19 (76.0)	45 (61.6)	0.427	0.193
Medications						
Beta blockers	37 (30.1)	13 (31.0)	6 (18.2)	31 (34.4)	0.207	0.081
RAS inhibitors	53 (43.1)	20 (47.6)	14 (43.1)	39 (43.3)	0.654	0.928
MRAs	5 (4.1)	2 (4.8)	0 (0.0)	5 (5.6)	0.501	0.323

Data are presented as number (percentage) or median (interquartile range), where appropriate. BMI = body mass index; BSA = body surface area; MRA = mineralocorticoid receptor antagonist; NYHA = New York Heart Association; PVFP = pulmonary venous flow pattern; RAS = renin–angiotensin system.

3.2. Pulmonary Venous Flow Pattern

Overall, 49 (36.3%) patients exhibited a normal flow pattern in the PVs on both sides and 86 (63.7%) patients had an abnormal PVFP on at least one side. Among the latter, 34 (25.2%) were diagnosed with a reversed PVFP and 52 (38.5%) had a blunted PVFP. The proportion of PV flow reversal was considerably higher among individuals with severe MR compared to those with moderate-to-severe MR (31/89; 34.8% vs. 3/46; 6.5%, $p < 0.001$).

Compared to patients with normal or non-reversed PVFP, those with reversed PVFP were less likely to be obese and diabetic (Table 1). While similarly symptomatic overall (n = 19, 76.0%), they exhibited greater functional impairment, expressed by the New York Heart Association (NYHA) classification, which was statistically significant when comparing the non-reversed and reversed PV flow groups. Lastly, patients with a reversed PVFP had the highest prevalence of severe MR (91.2%), as well as increased PASP values (Table 2). No significant differences were noted in other clinical and echocardiographic parameters, including LV end-systolic diameter, LA dimensions, and prolapse site.

Table 2. Baseline Echocardiographic Parameters.

	Total Cohort (N = 135)	Normal PVFP (N = 49)	Reversed PVFP (N = 34)	Non-Reversed PVFP (N = 101)	*p*-Value Normal vs. Reversed	*p*-Value Non-Reversed vs. Reversed
Mitral Regurgitation						
MR Severity					<0.001	<0.001
Moderate-to-Severe	46 (34.1)	27 (55.1)	3 (8.8)	43 (42.6)		
Severe	89 (65.9)	22 (44.9)	31 (91.2)	58 (57.4)		
MR PISA EROA						
Median (cm^2)	0.48 (0.36–0.63)	0.38 (0.30–0.49)	0.60 (0.48–0.69)	0.43 (0.33–0.54)	0.001	0.005
≥0.4 cm^2	40 (66.7)	9 (42.9)	16 (88.9)	24 (57.1)	0.003	0.017
MR PISA RVol						
Median (mL)	71 (55–88)	60 (45–81)	81 (70–94)	68 (51–77)	0.042	0.029
≥60 mL	39 (73.6)	10 (50.0)	16 (94.1)	23 (63.9)	0.003	0.022
Prolapses Site					0.563	
Anterior	15 (11.1)	10 (20.4)	4 (11.8)	11 (10.9)	0.301	1.000
Posterior	94 (69.5)	31 (63.3)	23 (67.6)	71 (70.3)	0.681	0.771
Both	26 (19.3)	8 (16.3)	7 (20.6)	19 (18.8)	0.620	0.820
Left Heart Dimensions						
LV ESD						
Median (mm)	32 (28–37)	30 (27–37)	35 (30–39)	31 (27–37)	0.056	0.070
≥40 mm	21 (15.6)	7 (14.3)	5 (14.7)	16 (15.8)	1.000	0.874
LA Diameter						
Median (mm)	45 (40–50)	45 (40–50)	46 (40–52)	44 (40–49)	0.452	0.321
>55 mm	8 (5.9)	2 (4.1)	3 (8.8)	5 (5.0)	0.396	0.415
LA Area						
Median (cm^2)	26 (22–31)	24 (21–28)	27 (23–33)	25 (22–31)	0.057	0.387
>20 cm^2	103 (76.3)	33 (67.3)	26 (76.5)	77 (76.2)	0.367	0.978
Right Heart						
RV Dysfunction	2 (1.5)	1 (2.0)	0 (0.0)	2 (2.0)	1.000	1.000
PASP						
Median (mmHg)	39 (30–50)	32 (26–40)	44 (34–55)	38 (30–48)	0.001	0.115
≥50 mmHg	26 (19.3)	4 (8.2)	8 (23.5)	18 (17.8)	0.063	0.465

Data are presented as number (percentage), median (interquartile range), or mean ± standard deviation, where appropriate. EF = ejection fraction; EROA = effective regurgitant orifice area; ESD = end-systolic diameter; LA = left atrial; LV = left ventricular; MR = mitral regurgitation; PASP = pulmonary arterial systolic pressure; PISA = proximal isovelocity surface area; PVFP = pulmonary venous flow pattern; RV = right ventricular; RVol = regurgitant volume.

3.3. Outcomes

After 5 years of follow-up, 11 (8.1%) patients died, 87 (64.4%) underwent mitral intervention, and 22 (16.3%) developed AF or flutter (Table 3). Intervention types included, in decreasing frequency, the following: surgical repair (n = 60, 69%); surgical replacement (n = 19, 21.8%); and transcatheter edge-to-edge repair (TEER) using the MitraClip system (Abbott Vascular Inc, Santa Clara, CA, USA) (n = 8, 9.2%).

The primary outcome, a composite of all three separate endpoints, was reported in 98 (72.6%) patients and proved significantly more frequent in those with reversed PVFP at baseline (88.2% compared to 59.2% in the normal PVFP group and 67.3% in the non-reversed PVFP group, $p = 0.004$ and $p = 0.018$, respectively). This was reflected in significantly shorter event-free survival durations within the reversed PVFP group (16.0 ± 20.1 vs. 38.4 ± 25.9 and 34.9 ± 25.8 months, respectively, all log rank $p < 0.001$) (Figure 3). Notably, PV flow reversal was also associated with an increased cumulative incidence of the primary outcome when compared to a blunted PVFP (88.2% vs. 75.0%, $p = 0.022$). By contrast, patients with PV flow blunting experienced a non-statistically higher rate of the primary outcome compared to that of patients with a normal PVFP (75.9% vs. 59.2%, $p = 0.137$) (Supplemental Figure S1).

Table 3. Outcomes at 5 Years.

	Total Cohort (N = 135)	Normal PVFP (N = 49)	Reversed PVFP (N = 34)	Non-Reversed PVFP (N = 101)	*p*-Value	
					Normal vs. Reversed	Non-Reversed vs. Reversed
All-Cause Mortality, Mitral Intervention, or New-Onset Atrial Fibrillation	98 (72.6)	29 (59.2)	30 (88.2)	68 (67.3)	0.004	0.018
All-Cause Mortality	11 (8.1)	2 (4.1)	2 (5.9)	9 (8.9)	1.000	0.730
Mitral Intervention	87 (64.4)	25 (51.0)	29 (85.3)	58 (57.4)	0.001	0.003
New-Onset Atrial Fibrillation	22 (16.3)	4 (8.2)	4 (11.8)	18 (17.8)	0.711	0.408

Data are presented as number (percentage). PVFP = pulmonary venous flow pattern.

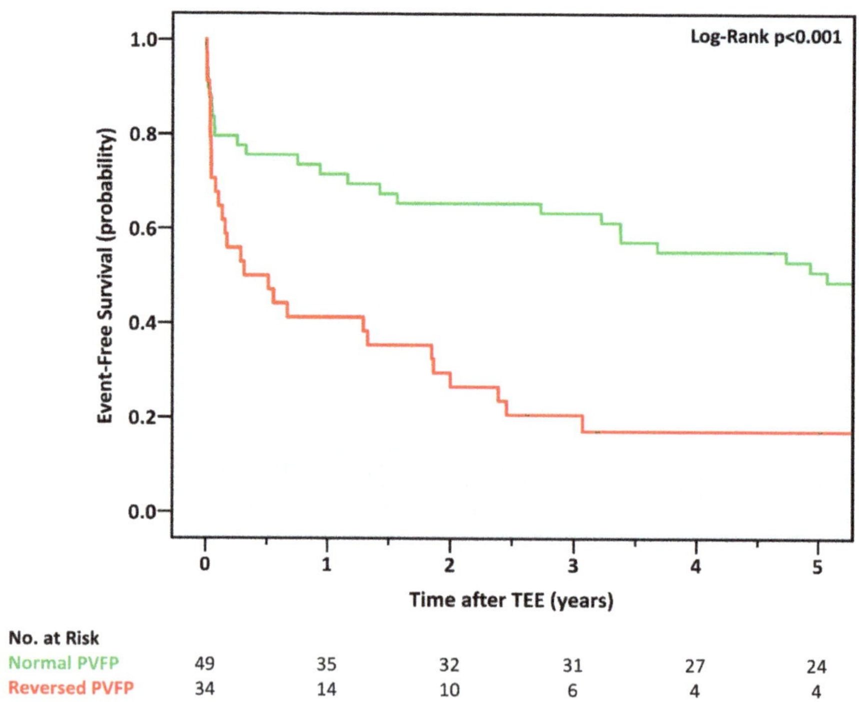

(A)

Figure 3. *Cont.*

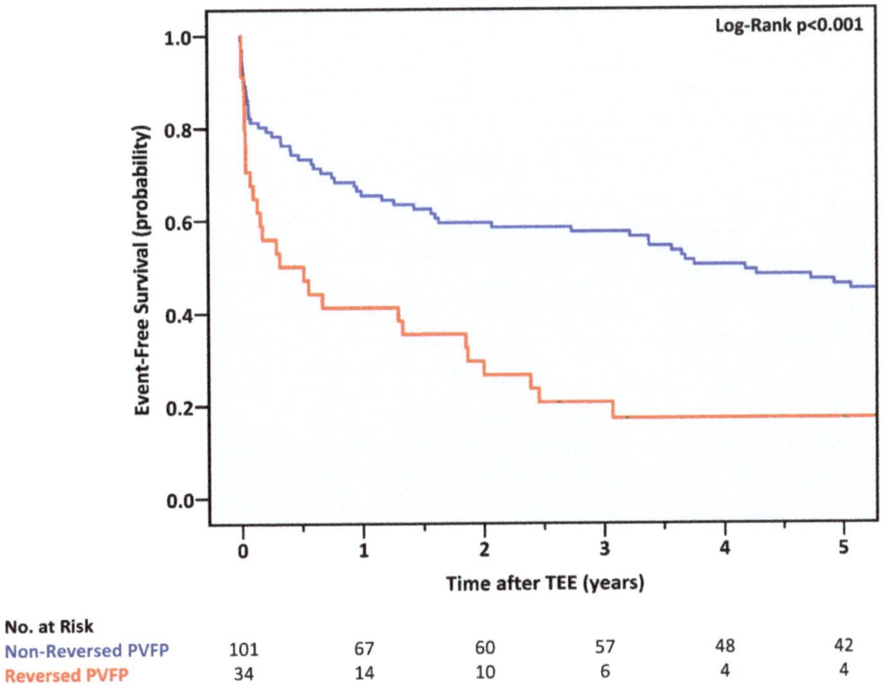

(**B**)

Figure 3. Five-Year Cumulative Incidence of the Combined Outcome of All-Cause Mortality, Mitral Intervention, or New-Onset Atrial Fibrillation According to Pulmonary Venous Flow Pattern at Baseline. PVFP = pulmonary venous flow pattern; TEE = transesophageal echocardiogram. (**A**) Normal vs. Reversed Pulmonary Venous Flow Pattern. (**B**) Non-Reversed vs. Reversed Pulmonary Venous Flow Pattern.

According to a Cox proportional hazard model, presented in Supplemental Table S1 (univariable analysis) and in Table 4 (multivariable analysis), a reversed PVFP independently predicted an increased risk for the primary outcome compared to both normal PVFP (HR 2.53, 95% CI 1.21–5.31, $p = 0.011$) and non-reversed PVFP (HR 2.14, 95% CI 1.12–4.10, $p = 0.022$).

Table 4. Multivariable Cox Proportional Hazard Model for the Combined Outcomes of All-Cause Mortality, Mitral Intervention, or New-Onset Atrial Fibrillation at 5 Years.

	HR (95% CI)	*p*-Value
NYHA Class (per 1 class rise)	1.43 (1.09–1.87)	0.010
LV ESD ≥40 mm	2.11 (0.94–4.73)	0.069
LA Diameter (continuous)	1.47 (1.07–2.03)	0.018
RV Dysfunction	1.30 (0.17–9.92)	0.800
Severe MR	1.53 (0.85–2.75)	0.161
Posterior Prolapse Site	1.78 (0.98–3.23)	0.056
PVFP		
Abnormal (vs. Normal)	1.62 (0.93–2.84)	0.091
Reversed (vs. Normal)	2.53 (1.21–5.31)	0.011
Reversed (vs. Non-Reversed)	2.14 (1.12–4.10)	0.022

CI = confidence interval; EF = ejection fraction; ESD = end-systolic diameter; HR = hazard ratio; LA = left atrial; LV = left ventricular; MR = mitral regurgitation; NYHA = New York Heart Association; PVFP = pulmonary venous flow pattern; RV = right ventricular.

Of the secondary outcomes, mitral interventions (but not deaths and AF or flutter) occurred earlier and more frequently during 5 years of follow-up in patients with reversed PVFP compared to patients with normal or non-reversed PVFP (Table 3). After multivariable analysis, PV flow reversal at baseline arose as an independent risk factor for mitral intervention, but not for mortality or new-onset AF (Supplemental Table S2).

4. Discussion

Our study examined the prognostic utility of PV flow reversal, as observed on TEE, in patients with significant dMR, normal LV systolic function, and normal sinus rhythm. Based on a retrospective, single-center analysis of 135 consecutive cases, we observed the following: 1. a reversed PVFP was evident in approximately one-quarter of the cohort and among almost all patients with severe MR; 2. its presence was associated with a more severe MR and a higher pulmonary arterial pressure, as well as with a lower functional status at baseline; 3. patients with PV flow reversal experienced a higher cumulative incidence of deaths, mitral interventions, or new-onset AF during 5 years of follow-up compared to those with either normal, non-reversed, or blunted PV flow patterns; and 4. PV flow reversal independently predicted a higher risk for mitral interventions and the composite of the three separate endpoints, more than doubling the risk for both compared to normal and non-reversed PVFP.

As a surrogate of altered LA hemodynamics [10], abnormal flow in PVs has been previously shown to manifest in disease states characterized by elevated LA filling pressures, such as MV disorders [5], AF [11], diastolic dysfunction [12], and atrioventricular (AV) dissociation [13]. In MR, a reversed PVFP could also represent a direct effect of the regurgitant jet which, depending on the exact location of the underlying pathology, may be situated against the PV ostia [14]. As both filling pressures and the regurgitant jet are not exclusively determined by the mere severity of the valvular disease, PV flow abnormalities, while highly specific, are not 100% sensitive to significant MR. This could explain the less-than 100% prevalence of reversed PVFP in our cohort, particularly among patients with severe MR.

In line with prior studies that have linked a reversed PV flow with severe MR [15], a larger proportion of patients in our study exhibiting this finding had severe MR compared to patients with a normal flow pattern, and vice versa. However, the hazardous association between reversed PVFP and outcomes remained after controlling for MR grade, suggesting that PV flow reversal may serve not only as a diagnostic criterion for severe dMR, but also as a prognostic marker in both moderate-to-severe and severe dMR. Theoretically, the worse prognosis experienced by patients with dMR and a reversed PVFP may have been not only the result of the more advanced valvular disease, but also a reflection of an accompanying atrial myopathy, a condition well-described in the literature [16,17], which could by itself lead to reduced cardiac output, elevated pulmonary vascular pressure, and thromboembolism [18]. Furthermore, patients with PV flow reversal may have experienced a more pronounced diastolic dysfunction, which also could contribute to a less favorable prognosis. While this last notion could not be fully ascertained by echocardiography due to the presence of significant MV disease, altered PVFP has previously been correlated with diastolic dysfunction using right heart catheterization [19], and in our study was indeed associated with LA dilation and pulmonary hypertension, both of which are mutually related to LA pathology and LV stiffness [20]. Still, the fact that PV flow reversal demonstrated an independent prognostic ability according to a comprehensive multivariable analysis that considered all of the above-mentioned parameters may suggest a dominant role for MR grade in that regard nonetheless.

On a final note, our findings may have therapeutic implications, particularly among dMR patients who do not fulfill current practice guideline criteria for intervention [8,21]. As mentioned, the worse 5-year outcomes observed within the reversed PVFP group encompassed both patients with severe MR and normal LV function, as well as patients with less than severe (i.e., moderate-to-severe) MR. Although regurgitation severity is also a function of loading conditions and may thus fluctuate, and while MR severity, rather than PVFP, may have been the driving force for the higher event rate in our cohort, a reversed PVFP was independently associated with the primary outcome and with mitral interventions. In view of its prognostic impact, PV flow reversal may warrant earlier intervention in patients with significant dMR. Future research may assess the implication of integrating this finding in the decision-making process when caring for dMR patients.

5. Limitations

A single-center, retrospective design may undermine the external validity of the study results. Nevertheless, we employed the largest cohort to date of significant dMR patients with normal LV function and sinus rhythm that were specifically assessed for PVFP. Moreover, baseline patient characteristics were apparently comparable to those presented by previous reports of dMR populations [22] and echocardiographic reports were blindly assessed. Regarding conceptual matters, death causes and mitral intervention indications, as well as additional indices of atrial myopathy (such as indexed volume and serum natriuretic peptides) and of diastolic function (including invasive hemodynamic parameters), were not explored, thus impairing the ability to identify the exact pathogenic correlations and consequences of a deranged PVFP. Additionally, AF diagnoses were mostly based on surface ECGs and not continuous tracings, the use of which could have led to more accurate estimates of arrhythmic burden. During the protracted timeframe of the study, practice guidelines changed, potentially affecting the interpretation of baseline observations and the definition of downstream events. However, all patients were assessed concomitantly and exposed to similar methodologies, arguably making any interaction with such an evolution non-significant. Lastly, echocardiographic assessments of MR and PVFP may be prone to operator-dependent errors and patient-specific features, such as hemodynamic status. Nevertheless, we noted a significant association between MR severity and PVFP anomaly and deliberately included both moderate-to-severe and severe MR cases, keeping in mind the possibility of shifting severity of the valvular disease.

6. Conclusions

In our single-center experience, patients with significant dMR, normal LV systolic function, and normal sinus rhythm experienced earlier, more frequent composite events of death, mitral intervention, or new-onset AF at 5 years when faced with a reversed PVFP. Furthermore, PV flow reversal was independently associated with more than twice the risk for the composite outcome compared to normal and non-reversed flow patterns, regardless of MR severity, LA diameter, or pulmonary arterial systolic pressure.

Supplementary Materials: The following supporting information can be downloaded at: https://www.mdpi.com/article/10.3390/jcdd10020049/s1, Figure S1: Five-Year Cumulative Incidence of the Combined Outcome of All-Cause Mortality, Mitral Intervention, or New-Onset Atrial Fibrillation According to Detailed Pulmonary Venous Flow Pattern at Baseline; Table S1: Univariable Cox Proportional Hazard Model for the Combined Outcome of All-Cause Mortality, Mitral Intervention, or New-Onset Atrial Fibrillation at 5 Years; Table S2: Cox Proportional Hazard Model for the Separate Outcomes at 5 Years.

Author Contributions: Conceptualization, I.Y.; methodology, A.S. (Alon Shechter), M.V., A.S. (Alex Sagie), Y.S. and I.Y.; formal analysis, A.S. (Alon Shechter) and S.C.B.; writing—original draft preparation, A.S. (Alon Shechter); writing—review and editing, A.S. (Alon Shechter), S.C.B., R.J.S., J.A., M.A., M.V., A.S. (Alex Sagie), R.K., Y.S. and I.Y. All authors have read and agreed to the published version of the manuscript.

Funding: This research received no external funding.

Institutional Review Board Statement: The study was conducted in accordance with the Declaration of Helsinki, and approved by the Institutional Review Board of Rabin Medical Center (protocol code 0488-17-RMC, date of approval 28 December 2017).

Informed Consent Statement: Patient consent was waived due to the study's retrospective nature.

Data Availability Statement: The data underlying this article will be shared on reasonable request to the corresponding author.

Conflicts of Interest: The authors declare no conflict of interest.

Abbreviations

LA = Left atrium
MR = Mitral regurgitation
dMR = Degenerative MR
PV = Pulmonary vein/venous
PVFP = Pulmonary venous flow pattern

References

1. de Marchena, E.; Badiye, A.; Robalino, G.; Junttila, J.; Atapattu, S.; Nakamura, M.; De Canniere, D.; Salerno, T. Respective Prevalence of the Different Carpentier Classes of Mitral Regurgitation: A Stepping Stone for Future Therapeutic Research and Development. *J. Card Surg.* **2011**, *26*, 385–392. [CrossRef] [PubMed]
2. Grigioni, F.; Avierinos, J.-F.; Ling, L.H.; Scott, C.; Bailey, K.R.; Tajik, A.; Frye, R.L.; Enriquez-Sarano, M. Atrial fibrillation complicating the course of degenerative mitral regurgitation: Determinants and long-term outcome. *J. Am. Coll. Cardiol.* **2002**, *40*, 84–92. [CrossRef]
3. Essayagh, B.; Antoine, C.; Benfari, G.; Messika-Zeitoun, D.; Michelena, H.; Le Tourneau, T.; Mankad, S.; Tribouilloy, C.M.; Thapa, P.; Enriquez-Sarano, M. Prognostic Implications of Left Atrial Enlargement in Degenerative Mitral Regurgitation. *J. Am. Coll. Cardiol.* **2019**, *74*, 858–870. [CrossRef] [PubMed]
4. Eguchi, K.; Ohtaki, E.; Matsumura, T.; Tanaka, K.; Tohbaru, T.; Iguchi, N.; Misu, K.; Asano, R.; Nagayama, M.; Sumiyoshi, T.; et al. Pre-operative atrial fibrillation as the key determinant of outcome of mitral valve repair for degenerative mitral regurgitation. *Eur. Hear. J.* **2005**, *26*, 1866–1872. [CrossRef]
5. Klein, A.L.; Stewart, W.J.; Bartlett, J.; Cohen, G.I.; Kahan, F.; Pearce, G.; Husbands, K.; Bailey, A.S.; Salcedo, E.E.; Cosgrove, D.M. Effects of mitral regurgitation on pulmonary venous flow and left atrial pressure: An intraoperative transesophageal echocardiographic study. *J. Am. Coll. Cardiol.* **1992**, *20*, 1345–1352. [CrossRef] [PubMed]
6. Maruyama, T.; Kokawa, Y.; Nakamura, H.; Fukata, M.; Yasuda, S.; Odashiro, K.; Akashi, K. Pulmonary Venous Flow Pattern and Atrial Fibrillation: Fact and Controversy. In *Echocardiography—In Specific Disease*; Bajraktari, G., Ed.; InTech: Rijeka, Croatia, 2012; pp. 77–96.
7. Zoghbi, W.A.; Adams, D.; Bonow, R.O.; Enriquez-Sarano, M.; Foster, E.; Grayburn, P.A.; Hahn, R.T.; Han, Y.; Hung, J.; Lang, R.M.; et al. Recommendations for Noninvasive Evaluation of Native Valvular Regurgitation: A Report from the American Society of Echocardiography Developed in Collaboration with the Society for Cardiovascular Magnetic Resonance. *J Am Soc Echocardiogr.* **2017**, *30*, 303–371. [CrossRef]
8. Hindricks, G.; Potpara, T.; Dagres, N.; Arbelo, E.; Bax, J.J.; Blomström-Lundqvist, C.; Boriani, G.; Castella, M.; Dan, G.-A.; Dilaveris, P.; et al. ESC Scientific Document Group. 2020 ESC Guidelines for the Diagnosis and Management of Atrial Fibrillation Developed in Collaboration with the European Association for Cardio-Thoracic Surgery (EACTS): The Task Force for the Diagnosis and Management of Atrial Fibrillation of the European Society of Cardiology (ESC) Developed with the special Contribution of the European Heart Rhythm Association (EHRA) of the ESC. *Eur. Heart J.* **2021**, *42*, 373–498.
9. Hahn, R.T.; Abraham, T.; Adams, M.S.; Bruce, C.J.; Glas, K.E.; Lang, R.M.; Reeves, S.T.; Shanewise, J.S.; Siu, S.C.; Stewart, W.; et al. Guidelines for Performing a Comprehensive Transesophageal Echocardiographic Examination: Recommendations from the American Society of Echocardiography and the Society of Cardiovascular Anesthesiologists. *J. Am. Soc. Echocardiogr.* **2013**, *26*, 921–964. [CrossRef]
10. Tabata, T.; Thomas, J.D.; Klein, A.L. Pulmonary Venous Flow by Doppler Echocardiography: Revisited 12 Years Later. *J. Am. Coll. Cardiol.* **2003**, *41*, 1243–1250. [CrossRef]
11. Ren, W.D.; Visentin, P.; Nicolosi, G.L.; Canterin, F.A.; Dall'Aglio, V.; Lestuzzi, C.; Mimo, R.; Pavan, D.; Sparacino, L.; Cervesato, E.; et al. Effect of atrial fibrillation on pulmonary venous flow patterns: Transoesophageal pulsed Doppler echocardiographic study. *Eur. Hear. J.* **1993**, *14*, 1320–1327. [CrossRef]
12. Klein, A.L.; Tajik, A.J. Doppler Assessment of Pulmonary Venous Flow in Healthy Subjects and in Patients with Heart Disease. *J. Am. Soc. Echocardiogr.* **1991**, *4*, 379–392. [CrossRef]
13. Keren, G.; Bier, A.; Sherez, J.; Miura, D.; Keefe, D.; LeJemtel, T. Atrial contraction is an important determinant of pulmonary venous flow. *J. Am. Coll. Cardiol.* **1986**, *7*, 693–695. [CrossRef]
14. Klein, A.L.; Obarski, T.P.; Stewart, W.J.; Casale, P.N.; Pearce, G.L.; Husbands, K.; Cosgrove, D.M.; Salcedo, E.E. Transesophageal Doppler echocardiography of pulmonary venous flow: A new marker of mitral regurgitation severity. *J. Am. Coll. Cardiol.* **1991**, *18*, 518–526. [CrossRef] [PubMed]

15. Pu, M.; Griffin, B.P.; Vandervoort, P.M.; Stewart, W.J.; Fan, X.; Cosgrove, D.M.; Thomas, J.D. The Value of Assessing Pulmonary Venous Flow Velocity for Predicting Severity of Mitral Regurgitation: A Quantitative Assessment Integrating Left Ventricular Function. *J. Am. Soc. Echocardiogr.* **1999**, *12*, 736–743. [CrossRef]
16. Thiedemann, K.U.; Ferrans, V.J. Left atrial ultrastructure in mitral valvular disease. *Am. J. Pathol.* **1977**, *89*, 575–604. [CrossRef]
17. Shen, M.J.; Arora, R.; Jalife, J. Atrial Myopathy. *J. Am. Coll. Cardiol.* **2019**, *4*, 640–654. [CrossRef]
18. Purga, S.L.; Karas, M.G.; Horn, E.M.; Torosoff, M.T. Contribution of the left atrial remodeling to the elevated pulmonary capillary wedge pressure in patients with WHO Group II pulmonary hypertension. *J. Echocardiogr.* **2019**, *17*, 187–196. [CrossRef]
19. Güvenç, T.S.; Poyraz, E.; Güvenç, R.; Can, F. Contemporary usefulness of pulmonary venous flow parameters to estimate left ventricular end-diastolic pressure on transthoracic echocardiography. *Int. J. Cardiovasc. Imaging* **2020**, *36*, 1699–1709. [CrossRef]
20. Nagueh, S.F. Left Ventricular Diastolic Function: Understanding Pathophysiology, Diagnosis, and Prognosis with Echocardiography. *JACC Cardiovasc. Imaging* **2020**, *13 Pt 2*, 228–244. [CrossRef] [PubMed]
21. Writing Committee Members; Otto, C.M.; Nishimura, R.A.; Bonow, R.O.; Carabello, B.A.; Erwin, J.P.; Gentile, F.; Jneid, H.; Krieger, E.V.; Mack, M.; et al. 2020 ACC/AHA Guideline for the Management of Patients with Valvular Heart Disease: A Report of the American College of Cardiology/American Heart Association Joint Committee on Clinical Practice Guidelines. *J. Am. Coll. Cardiol.* **2021**, *77*, e25–e197.
22. Lazam, S.; Vanoverschelde, J.-L.; Tribouilloy, C.; Grigioni, F.; Suri, R.M.; Avierinos, J.-F.; de Meester, C.; Barbieri, A.; Rusinaru, D.; Russo, A.; et al. Twenty-Year Outcome After Mitral Repair Versus Replacement for Severe Degenerative Mitral Regurgitation. *Circulation* **2017**, *135*, 410–422. [CrossRef] [PubMed]

Journal of
Cardiovascular Development and Disease

MDPI

Article

Spatial and Temporal Non-Uniform Changes in Left Ventricular Myocardial Strain in Dogs with Duchenne Muscular Dystrophy

Bijan Ghaleh [1,2], Inès Barthélemy [3], Lucien Sambin [1], Alain Bizé [1], Daphné Corboz [1], Luc Hittinger [1,2], Stéphane Blot [3] and Jin Bo Su [1,*]

1 Inserm U955-IMRB, Team 3, UPEC, Ecole Nationale Vétérinaire d'Alfort, 94700 Maisons-Alfort, France; bijan.ghaleh@inserm.fr (B.G.); lucien.sambin@inserm.fr (L.S.); alain.bize@inserm.fr (A.B.); daphne.corboz@inserm.fr (D.C.); luc.hittinger@aphp.fr (L.H.)

2 Assistance Publique—Hôpitaux de Paris, Hôpital Henri Mondor, Service de Cardiologie, 94010 Créteil, France

3 Inserm U955-IMRB, Team10, UPEC, Ecole Nationale Vétérinaire d'Alfort, 94700 Maisons-Alfort, France; ines.barthelemy@vet-alfort.fr (I.B.); stephane.blot@inserm.fr (S.B.)

* Correspondence: jin-bo.su@inserm.fr

Abstract: Background: Understanding and effectively treating dystrophin-deficient cardiomyopathy is of high importance for Duchenne muscular dystrophy (DMD) patients due to their prolonged lifespan. We used two-dimensional speckle tracking echocardiography to analyze more deeply the non-uniformity of myocardial strain within the left ventricle during the progression of cardiomyopathy in golden retriever muscular dystrophy (GRMD) dogs. Methods: The circumferential strain (CS) and longitudinal strain (LS) of left ventricular (LV) endocardial, middle and epicardial layers were analyzed from three parasternal short-axis views and three apical views, respectively, in GRMD (n = 22) and healthy control dogs (n = 7) from 2 to 24 months of age. Results: In GRMD dogs, despite normal global systolic function (normal LV fractional shortening and ejection fraction), a reduction in systolic CS was detected in the three layers of the LV apex but not in the LV middle-chamber and base at 2 months of age. This spatial heterogeneity in CS progressed with age, whereas a decrease in systolic LS could be detected early at 2 months of age in the three layers of the LV wall from three apical views. Conclusions: Analyzing the evolution of myocardial CS and LS in GRMD dogs reveals spatial and temporal non-uniform alterations of LV myocardial strain, providing new insights into the progression of dystrophin-deficient cardiomyopathy in this relevant model of DMD.

Keywords: canine model of duchenne muscular dystrophy; dystrophin-deficient cardiomyopathy; heterogeneity; myocardial strain; speckle-tracking echocardiography

1. Introduction

Duchenne muscular dystrophy (DMD) is an X-linked hereditary disease affecting approximately 1 in 5000 male births worldwide and is caused by mutations in the gene that encodes the 427-kDa cytoskeletal protein dystrophin. Dystrophin forms a dystrophin protein complex with dystrophin-associated proteins including dystroglycans, sarcoglycans, integrins and caveolin in the sarcolemma, linking the internal cytoskeleton to the extracellular matrix in striated muscle and playing an important role in stabilizing the cell membrane and signal transduction during muscle contraction [1]. The vast majority of DMD patients lack the dystrophin protein, making the membrane susceptible to damage by mechanical stress which can lead to muscle degeneration. DMD is characterized by progressive muscle degeneration and weakness. Beginning as early as 2 to 3 years of age, the principal symptom of DMD is muscle weakness, affecting the proximal muscles first, then the distal limb muscles and usually the lower external muscles before the upper external muscles. Generally, DMD patients are wheelchair-bound by 12 years of age and die of respiratory failure in their late teens or early twenties. Although there is currently no effective treatment for this disease, patients with DMD live significantly longer thanks to improved respiratory ventilation and other supportive care. As a result, deaths from heart failure rather than respiratory failure have increased [2]. Therefore, understanding the development of dystrophin-deficient cardiomyopathy and effectively treating it has become very important for DMD patients.

Similar to DMD, golden retriever muscular dystrophy (GRMD) is also caused by the dystrophin gene mutation, a single nucleotide change that leads to exon skipping and an out-of-frame DMD transcript [3]. GRMD dogs develop symptoms and signs like DMD patients and are used to explore pathological changes and test novel therapeutic strategies for DMD [4–11].

Using image-processing algorithms for two-dimensional digital echocardiographic images, two-dimensional speckle tracking echocardiography (2D-STE) identifies small stable myocardial footprints called speckles generated by ultrasound-myocardial tissue interactions within a defined region of interest and tracks speckles frame-to-frame over the cardiac cycle. Distances between speckles or their spatiotemporal displacement provide information about global and segmental myocardial deformation. Despite some technical factors influencing strain value [12], 2D-STE has been developed into a reliable method to objectively quantify left ventricular (LV) regional and global myocardial function [12,13] since strain information is independent of the Doppler angle of incidence [13]. Studies have shown that 2D-STE can be used to reveal early pathological changes in the heart of DMD patients [14–16] and GRMD dogs and cardiac responses in GRMD therapeutic trials [8–10]. Interestingly, recent technological developments have enabled 2D-STE to analyze LV wall strain in more detail, allowing, for example, the analysis of endocardial, middle and epicardial strains in different regions of the LV wall. Therefore, the aim of this study was to evaluate the changes in myocardial circumferential strain (CS) and longitudinal strain (LS) of LV endocardial, middle and epicardial layers in GRMD dogs aged from 2 to 24 months. These GRMD dogs were compared to healthy control dogs to reveal alterations in LV myocardial strain during the pathological development of dystrophin-deficient cardiomyopathy. Our results showed that spatial and temporal non-uniform alterations of myocardial strain occur within the left ventricle during the progression of the disease. This finding may provide insight into the progression of cardiomyopathy due to dystrophin deficiency in this highly relevant canine model of DMD.

2. Materials and Methods

2.1. Animal Model

Twenty-two GRMD and seven healthy control dogs were provided by the Centre d'Elevage du Domaine des Souches (Mezilles, France) and were cared for by veterinarians throughout the study. GRMD was diagnosed by DNA analysis at 1 month of age. The experimental protocol was approved by the animal ethics committee (ComEth ANSES-ENVA-UPEC agreement #20/12/12–18) and the experimental procedures were performed in accordance with the European Union Directive 2010/63/EU.

2.2. Echocardiographic Image Acquisition and Analysis

Echocardiographic image acquisition and analysis were performed by the same investigator in GRMD dogs and their healthy littermates at 2, 6, 9, 12, 18 and 24 months of age. Using a Vivid 7 ultrasound (General Electric Medical System, Horten, Norway), echocardiographic images were acquired from conscious (i.e., without the use of sedatives or anesthetics) 2-month-old puppies in a standing position using a 7S cardiac sector array probe and from dogs of other ages in a standing position in a sling using a 5S or an M4S cardiac sector array probe after an adaptive period of 20–30 min. The standing position allows for the acquisition of images from all commonly used LV views. An ECG was recorded during the echocardiographic examination to calculate heart rate.

M-mode parasternal short-axis (PSAX) images at the mid-chamber (papillary muscles) level were recorded to measure LV end-diastolic (EDD) and end-systolic (ESD) diameters, end-diastolic and end-systolic posterior and interventricular septal wall dimensions and fractional shortening (FS).

High-frame-rate videos (ranging from 60 to 119 frames/s) were recorded in apical 2-chamber, 3-chamber and 4-chamber views. In some cases, the apical 5-chamber view was used when an adequate 3-chamber image could not be obtained. The PSAX-base view was acquired at the level of mitral valve leaflets. The PSAX-mid-chamber view was recorded at the level of papillary muscles. The PSAX-apex view was recorded when the LV cavity was as small as possible without visible papillary muscles. For each view, a cine loop of at least three consecutive cardiac cycles was stored digitally for offline analysis. To ensure the image quality for strain analysis, the images of young dogs were generally acquired with the highest frame rate possible.

Echocardiographic images were analyzed as recommended [17]. FS (%) was calculated as [(LV EDD − LV ESD)/LV EDD × 100%]. LV end-diastolic volume (EDV, mL), end-systolic volume (ESV, mL) and ejection fraction (EF, %) were calculated by the biplane Simpson's method using the apical 4-chamber and 2-chamber images.

Using dedicated software, 2D-STE was performed offline (EchoPac version 201, GE Healthcare, Horten, Norway). CS and LS were analyzed in endocardial (inner), middle and epicardial (outer) layers of GRMD and healthy control dogs of various ages using EchoPac version 201. The cardiac cycle length was measured from the beginning of systole. After delineating an area of interest within the LV wall and performing manual adjustments to include the entire LV wall, the software automatically divided the LV wall into 6 LV wall segments for each view. Each segment was divided into endocardial and epicardial parts and averaged to obtain endocardial, middle and epicardial strains. After viewing the validation results automatically generated by the software and adequately curve fitting the area of interest within the LV wall, the adequate tracking results were considered for analysis. It is often necessary to manually adjust the area of interest several times to obtain an adequate fitting. CS was analyzed in PSAX-apex, PSAX-mid-chamber and PSAX-base views. LS was analyzed in apical 3-chamber (or 5-chamber), 4-chamber and 2-chamber views.

2.3. Statistical Analysis

Continuous variables were expressed as mean ± SEM. Statistical analysis was performed with StatView (Version 5.0, Abacus Concepts Inc., Berkeley, CA, USA). The one-way ANOVA was used to test within-group differences over time (age). The ANOVA for repeated measurements over time was performed on echocardiographic data from 8 GRMD dogs and 4 healthy control dogs aged 2 to 24 months to test between-group differences. The two-tailed unpaired two-sample t-test was performed on data obtained in all dogs at each time point to determine the differences between GRMD and healthy control dogs. A difference was considered statistically significant at $p < 0.05$.

The assessment of inter-observer variability was not carried out in the study, because the acquisition and analysis of the echocardiographic images were carried out by a single investigator. To examine intra-observer variability, a set of images used for the calculation of EF, CS in the PSAX-apex view and LS in the 4-chamber view were taken from 6 randomly selected dogs used in the study and analyzed twice by the same sonographer in an interval of 24 h or more (3 heart beats were analyzed for each image). The interclass correlation coefficient (ICC) for these parameters was calculated using the Real Statistics Resource Pack. The coefficient of variation (CoV) for these parameters was calculated by the following equation: CoV (%) = standard deviation/mean × 100. The two measurements were used for the calculation of the ICC and the CoV for EF (0.908 and 3.1 ± 2.7%, respectively), endocardial CS (0.955 and −3.4 ± 2.9%), middle CS (0.941 and −3.8 ± 2.5%), epicardial CS (0.738 and −7.9 ± 5.7%), endocardial LS (0.958 and −3.1 ± 2.4%), middle LS (0.950 and −3.3 ± 2.7%) and epicardial LS (0.913 and −4.3 ± 4.2%).

3. Results

Of the 22 GRMD dogs included in the study, three were euthanized around the age of 6 months due to loss of ambulation; four between 9 and 12 months due to severely reduced mobility (n = 2), poor general conditions (n = 1) and severe bronchopneumonia (n = 1); three between 12 and 18 months of age due to reduced mobility (n = 2) and respiratory failure (n = 1); and two died of heart failure. No death occurred in healthy dogs throughout the study, and three of the seven healthy control dogs were rehomed after the 6-month examination.

GRMD dogs had significantly lower body weights than healthy control dogs at different ages (Table 1), notably reflecting a loss in muscle mass. In GRMD and healthy control dogs, the heart rate decreased with age, and the majority of GRMD dogs had slightly higher heart rates than healthy control dogs at the same age (Table 1).

Table 1. Body weight and LV dimensional and functional parameters measured by echocardiography in GRMD and healthy control dogs.

Parameter	Group Control GRMD	Age, Months						ANOVA p Value	
		2 n = 22 n = 7	6 n = 22 n = 7	9 n = 17 n = 4	12 n = 13 n = 4	18 n = 8 n = 4	24 n = 8 n = 4	Within-Group Effect	Between-Group Effect
body weight (kg)	Control	4.4 ± 0.4	20.1 ± 1.3	27.5 ± 2.2	29.5 ± 1.6	27.8 ± 1.6	26.2 ± 1.7	<0.0001	0.0003
	GRMD	3.1 ± 0.2 †	14.8 ± 0.7 †	18.3 ± 0.6 †	20.7 ± 0.9 †	20.5 ± 0.9 †	20.2 ± 0.9 †	<0.0001	
LV EDD (cm)	Control	2.3 ± 0.1	4.1 ± 0.2	4.4 ± 0.3	4.6 ± 0.3	4.4 ± 0.1	4.6 ± 0.3	<0.0001	0.0061
	GRMD	2.1 ± 0.1 *	3.5 ± 0.1 †	3.7 ± 0.1 *	4.2 ± 0.1	4.4 ± 0.1	4.5 ± 0.2	<0.0001	
LV ESD (cm)	Control	1.4 ± 0.1	2.5 ± 0.2	2.8 ± 0.2	3.0 ± 0.3	2.9 ± 0.2	2.9 ± 0.3	<0.0001	0.7718
	GRMD	1.3 ± 0.1	2.3 ± 0.1	2.5 ± 0.1	2.9 ± 0.1	3.1 ± 0.1	3.4 ± 0.2	<0.0001	
FS (%)	Control	37.4 ± 1.7	38.5 ± 0.9	35.3 ± 1.6	35.2 ± 1.6	35.2 ± 2.9	37.6 ± 2.5	0.5206	0.0015
	GRMD	38.3 ± 1.3	35.4 ± 1.1	32.8 ± 1.2	30.8 ± 1.1 *	29.6 ± 1.2 *	24.9 ± 1.6 †	<0.0001	
IVSWEDT (cm)	Control	0.49 ± 0.05	0.84 ± 0.06	1.00 ± 0.10	1.14 ± 0.10	1.12 ± 0.10	1.19 ± 0.11	<0.0001	0.0005
	GRMD	0.43 ± 0.01	0.70 ± 0.03 *	0.80 ± 0.03 †	0.71 ± 0.03 †	0.70 ± 0.04 †	0.73 ± 0.06 †	<0.0001	
IVSWTh (cm)	Control	0.29 ± 0.02	0.51 ± 0.04	0.64 ± 0.09	0.59 ± 0.08	0.52 ± 0.03	0.54 ± 0.01	<0.0001	0.0003
	GRMD	0.28 ± 0.02	0.45 ± 0.03	0.37 ± 0.03 †	0.42 ± 0.03 *	0.38 ± 0.04 *	0.28 ± 0.04 †	<0.0001	
%IVSWTh (%)	Control	62.5 ± 8.3	62.8 ± 6.3	65.2 ± 10.9	53.2 ± 10.1	48.1 ± 6.2	46.2 ± 4.4	0.3618	0.9705
	GRMD	67.1 ± 5.5	65.0 ± 4.0	46.4 ± 3.2 *	60.5 ± 4.9	54.7 ± 4.8	39.7 ± 6.4	0.0010	
PWEDT (cm)	Control	0.40 ± 0.02	0.75 ± 0.06	0.76 ± 0.03	0.93 ± 0.08	1.12 ± 0.10	1.08 ± 0.11	<0.0001	0.001
	GRMD	0.36 ± 0.03	0.59 ± 0.02	0.64 ± 0.03 *	0.73 ± 0.04 *	0.71 ± 0.06 *	0.73 ± 0.06 †	<0.0001	
PWTh (cm)	Control	0.30 ± 0.02	0.51 ± 0.04	0.57 ± 0.04	0.54 ± 0.04	0.60 ± 0.08	0.69 ± 0.06	<0.0001	0.0024
	GRMD	0.28 ± 0.01	0.36 ± 0.02 †	0.39 ± 0.03 *	0.36 ± 0.02 †	0.38 ± 0.05 *	0.28 ± 0.11 †	0.0028	
%PWTh (%)	Control	75.7 ± 8.9	71.0 ± 7.9	74.3 ± 4.9	58.7 ± 9.8	59.0 ± 7.6	65.1 ± 4.6	0.4770	0.0966
	GRMD	79.8 ± 4.8	61.7 ± 3.2	61.9 ± 6.0	51.3 ± 4.6	52.3 ± 5.4	40.3 ± 6.6 *	<0.0001	
Heart rate (beats/min)	Control	153.6 ± 5.5	98.4 ± 5.2	91.7 ± 2.4	81.7 ± 7.8	75.8 ± 5.1	83.1 ± 2.8	<0.0001	0.0751
	GRMD	161.0 ± 6.1	118.6 ± 3.5 †	108.2 ± 4.2	95.2 ± 3.6	102.1 ± 5.3 †	90.9 ± 6.6	<0.0001	
LV EDV (mL)	Control	10.8 ± 0.8	42.9 ± 5.3	63.4 ± 4.5	68.2 ± 5.8	76.2 ± 4.4	83.0 ± 7.8	<0.0001	0.0020
	GRMD	6.6 ± 0.4 †	30.8 ± 1.2 †	43.1 ± 2.5 †	49.5 ± 2.9 †	52.5 ± 3.3 †	61.5 ± 4.4 *	<0.0001	
LV ESV (mL)	Control	4.5 ± 0.4	15.9 ± 1.5	22.1 ± 1.7	27.2 ± 2.9	28.4 ± 2.8	34.2 ± 3.3	<0.0001	0.1450
	GRMD	2.7 ± 0.2 †	13.1 ± 0.5 *	20.1 ± 1.1	23.8 ± 2.0	26.5 ± 2.4	34.8 ± 3.0	<0.0001	
EF (%)	Control	58.8 ± 1.4	61.5 ± 3.0	64.3 ± 2.8	60.2 ± 1.8	63.1 ± 2.4	58.8 ± 0.5	0.4088	<0.0001
	GRMD	58.3 ± 1.2	57.3 ± 1.0	52.6 ± 1.3 †	52.5 ± 1.4 †	50.0 ± 2.0 †	43.8 ± 1.6 †	<0.0001	

Data were expressed as mean ± SEM. The one-way ANOVA was performed to test within-group differences. The ANOVA for repeated measurements over time was performed on echocardiographic data from 8 GRMD (golden retriever muscular dystrophy) and 4 healthy control dogs aged 2 to 24 months to test between-group differences. The two-tailed unpaired two-sample *t*-test was performed on data obtained in all dogs at each time point to determine the differences between GRMD and healthy control dogs. * $p < 0.05$ and † $p < 0.01$ versus healthy control dogs of the same age. EDD: end-diastolic diameter; EDV: end-diastolic volume; EF: ejection fraction; ESD: end-systolic diameter; ESV: end-systolic volume; FS: fractional shortening; IVSWEDT: interventricular septal wall end-diastolic thickness; IVSWTh: interventricular septal wall systolic thickening; % IVSWTh: percentage of interventricular septal wall systolic thickening; PWEDT: posterior wall end-diastolic thickness; LV: left ventricular; PWTh: posterior wall systolic thickening; % PWTh: percentage of posterior wall systolic thickening.

3.1. Changes in LV Dimensional and Functional Parameters Measured by Echocardiography in GRMD and Healthy Control Dogs at Different Ages

As shown in Table 1, the LV EDD of healthy control dogs increased with age until 9 months old. The LV EDD of GRMD dogs increased with age but was smaller than that of healthy control dogs until 9 months of age. Thereafter, LV EDD was similar in both groups. LV ESD increased with age in healthy control and GRMD dogs. As a result, these changes in LV EDD and ESD of GRMD dogs resulted in a significant reduction in FS at 12, 18 and 24 months ($p < 0.05$ or $p < 0.01$). The decrease in FS in some GRMD dogs reached a pathological value (i.e., less than 28%) at 18 and 24 months, whereas healthy control dogs had a stable FS throughout all ages examined. In healthy control dogs, interventricular septal wall end-diastolic thickness (IVSWEDT) and LV posterior wall end-diastolic thickness (PWEDT) increased with age and reached a stable thickness at 12 months. In contrast, IVSWEDT and PWEDT of GRMD dogs were smaller than those of healthy control dogs starting from 6 and 9 months of age, respectively. However, interventricular septal wall systolic thickening (% IVSWTh) was not significantly changed over time in healthy control dogs and decreased, without reaching significance, in GRMD dogs. Similarly, LV posterior wall systolic thickening (% PWTh) did not significantly change throughout the protocol in healthy control dogs, whereas it significantly decreased over time in GRMD dogs.

LV end-diastolic volume (LVEDV) increased with age in both healthy control and GRMD dogs, but GRMD dogs had smaller LVEDV at each age examined, which is certainly due to the marked smaller size and body weight of GRMD dogs. LV end-systolic volume (LVESV) increased with age in healthy control dogs whereas GRMD dogs had a smaller LVESV at 2 and 6 months of age than healthy control dogs but a similar LVESV from 9 months of age. Consequently, GRMD dogs had smaller EF and, contrasted with healthy control dogs, EF decreased progressively with age, starting at 9 months whereas healthy control dogs had stable EF at all ages examined (Table 1). The decrease in EF in some GRMD dogs reached a pathological value (i.e., less than 50%) at 18 and 24 months old.

These data obtained by conventional echocardiography indicated that significant alterations in LV global function (FS and EF) can be detected rather tardily (12–18 months of age) in GRMD dogs.

3.2. Changes in CS in the Three LV Wall Layers Analyzed by 2D-STE from the Three Short-Axis Views in GRMD and Healthy Control Dogs through Time

Figure 1 shows two typical examples of LV endocardial, middle and epicardial CS from a 2-month-old healthy control dog (panel A) and a 2-month-old GRMD dog (panel B) analyzed by 2D-STE from the PSAX-apex view. As shown in Table 2, in the LV apical region, the peak CS of endocardial, middle and epicardial layers remained rather stable with age in healthy control dogs. In contrast, GRMD dogs showed significant reduction in peak CS in the three examined layers of the LV apex (values being less negative) at 2 months, which were mainly caused by the significantly smaller peak CS of LV anterior and antero-lateral regions than those of healthy control dogs. It is worth noting that this smaller peak CS of epicardial and middle layers in the LV apical region of GRMD dogs could be seen at the different ages examined.

At the PSAX-mid-chamber level, GRMD had similar peak CS in the endocardial layer as healthy control dogs except at 2 and 24 months of age and had smaller peak CS in epicardial and middle layers at 18 and 24 months of age. In the endocardial layer, this parameter significantly decreased with age in both groups. However, in the middle and epicardial layer, peak CS significantly decreased with age in GRMD dogs, whereas no significant change was detected in healthy control dogs. At the base of the left ventricle, the peak CS of endocardial, middle and epicardial layers was basically similar for GRMD and healthy control dogs except for the epicardial layer at 9, 18 and 24 months and the middle and endocardial layers at 24 months, where GRMD dogs had smaller peak CS than healthy control dogs. In the epicardial layer, basal peak CS decreased significantly with age in GRMD dogs, whereas this parameter remained stable over time in healthy control dogs.

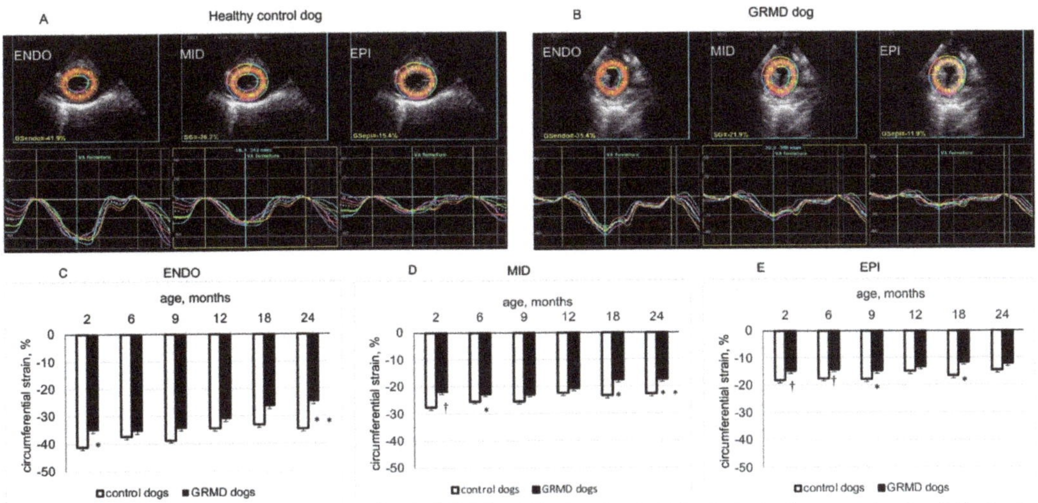

Figure 1. Circumferential strain (CS) of left ventricular (LV) endocardial (ENDO), middle (MID) and epicardial (EPI) layers analyzed from the parasternal short-axis-apex view. Panels (**A**,**B**) show the values and curves of 6 segments (showed by different colors) analyzed in each LV wall layer obtained in a 2-month-old healthy control dog and in an age-matched GRMD (golden retriever muscular dystrophy) dog. The curve in dotted line in each part of the LV wall is the average of the 6 curves. Panels (**C**–**E**) compare the peak systolic circumferential strain values of ENDO, MID and EPI layers of healthy control and GRMD dogs at different ages. Data were expressed as mean ± SEM. The one-way ANOVA was performed to test the within-group differences. The two-tailed unpaired two-sample *t*-test was performed on data obtained in all dogs at each time point to determine the difference between GRMD and healthy control dogs. n = 22, 22, 17, 13, 8 and 8 for GRMD dogs, and 7, 7, 4, 4, 4 and 4 for healthy control dogs at 2, 6, 9, 12, 18 and 24 months of age, respectively. * $p < 0.05$ and † $p < 0.01$ versus healthy control dogs of the same age.

These results indicated that GRMD dogs exhibited a non-uniform spatial alteration over time in CS, characterized by an early and persistent decrease in peak CS in the epicardial and middle layers of the LV apical region, mainly due to decreased peak CS in the apical anterior and antero-lateral regions. At the middle and basal levels of the left ventricle, decreased peak CS in GRMD dogs occurred later (at 18–24 months of age). In these regions of the left ventricle, the decrease in peak CS occurred earlier in epicardial and middle layers than in the endocardial layer.

3.3. Changes in LS in the Three LV Wall Layers Analyzed by 2D-STE from the Three Apical Views in GRMD and Healthy Control Dogs at Different Ages

Figure 2 shows two typical examples of LV endocardial, middle and epicardial LS from a 2-month-old healthy control dog (panel A) and a 2-month-old GRMD dog (panel B) analyzed by 2D-STE from the apical four-chamber view. As shown in Table 3, at the apical three-chamber view, GRMD dogs had significantly smaller peak LS than healthy control dogs at 2, 6, 9 and 12 months of age in the three layers of the LV wall. In the apical four-chamber view, peak LS of the three layers of LV wall were slightly but not significantly decreased with age in healthy control dogs. Contrastingly, GRMD dogs displayed a reduction with age and significantly smaller peak LS in the three layers of the

LV wall at 2, 6, 9 and 24 months of age (Figure 2 and Table 3). In the apical two-chamber view, GRMD had significantly smaller peak LS in the endocardial layer than healthy control dogs at 2, 6, 9 and 12 months and significantly smaller peak LS in epicardial and middle layer at 2, 6 and 12 months (Table 3).

Table 2. Circumferential strain in myocardial layers of the left ventricle analyzed by 2-dimensional speckle tracking echocardiography in healthy control and GRMD dogs at different ages.

Parameter	Group Control GRMD	Age, Months 2 n = 22 n = 7	6 n = 22 n = 7	9 n = 17 n = 4	12 n = 13 n = 4	18 n = 8 n = 4	24 n = 8 n = 4	ANOVA p Value Within−Group Effect	Between−Group Effect
Apical endocardial CS	Control GRMD	−41.2 ± 2.7 −35.1 ± 1.4 *	−37.4 ± 2.1 −35.5 ± 1.1	−38.8 ± 4.5 −34.4 ± 1.4	−34.5 ± 0.8 −31.1 ± 1.1	−33.2 ± 1.7 −26.5 ± 2.1	−34.7 ± 2.3 −24.8 ± 2.0 *	0.2656 <0.0001	0.0031
Apical middle layer CS	Control GRMD	−27.7 ± 1.2 −21.9 ± 0.6 †	−25.5 ± 1.2 −22.8 ± 0.5 *	−25.6 ± 2.2 −22.9 ± 0.9	−22.5 ± 0.7 −20.7 ± 0.6	−23.4 ± 0.8 −17.7 ± 1.3 †	−22.9 ± 1.1 −17.4 ± 1.3 †	0.0626 <0.0001	0.0004
Apical epicardial CS	Control GRMD	−18.2 ± 0.9 −14.8 ± 0.6 †	−17.6 ± 1.1 −14.3 ± 0.4 †	−18.0 ± 1.5 −14.8 ± 0.6 *	−15.0 ± 0.1 −13.3 ± 0.7	−16.5 ± 0.6 −11.7 ± 1.0 *	−14.7 ± 0.7 −12.2 ± 0.9	0.0881 0.0054	0.0025
Mid−chamber endocardial CS	Control GRMD	−37.3 ± 0.8 −33.2 ± 0.7 †	−31.9 ± 1.1 −33.0 ± 0.8	−30.9 ± 1.1 −31.9 ± 1.2	−32.2 ± 3.0 −30.7 ± 1.2	−29.8 ± 1.3 −25.9 ± 1.8	−31.9 ± 2.6 −22.9 ± 1.9 *	0.0068 <0.0001	0.1544
Mid−chamber middle layer CS	Control GRMD	−24.7 ± 0.8 −23.7 ± 0.5	−23.0 ± 0.9 −22.6 ± 0.5	−23.1 ± 0.8 −22.4 ± 0.9	−22.6 ± 1.2 −21.5 ± 0.7	−22.0 ± 0.8 −18.1 ± 0.7 †	−23.8 ± 1.3 −16.5 ± 0.8 †	0.2885 <0.0001	0.1028
Mid−chamber epicardial CS	Control GRMD	−15.7 ± 1.0 −16.5 ± 0.5	−16.7 ± 0.9 −15.1 ± 0.5	−17.3 ± 1.0 −15.8 ± 0.8	−15.5 ± 0.0 −14.6 ± 0.6	−16.4 ± 0.9 −12.4 ± 0.5 †	−18.2 ± 0.6 −11.7 ± 0.5 †	0.3164 <0.0001	0.1393
Basal endocardial CS	Control GRMD	−32.7 ± 1.5 −32.7 ± 0.9	−30.4 ± 1.0 −31.8 ± 1.1	−32.2 ± 1.5 −31.1 ± 1.5	−30.3 ± 2.5 −27.5 ± 1.4	−26.0 ± 1.7 −25.9 ± 1.5	−27.1 ± 1.6 −21.9 ± 1.3 *	0.0216 <0.0001	0.0406
Basal middle layer CS	control GRMD	−23.1 ± 1.0 −23.0 ± 0.6	−21.8 ± 0.5 −22.5 ± 0.7	−24.2 ± 1.2 −22.0 ± 1.0	−22.6 ± 1.1 −21.0 ± 1.0	−20.6 ± 1.0 −18.1 ± 1.2	−19.8 ± 1.3 −17.0 ± 1.4 *	0.0383 <0.0001	0.0069
Basal epicardial CS	Control GRMD	−16.7 ± 1.1 −16.2 ± 0.6	−15.6 ± 0.4 −16.0 ± 0.6	−18.4 ± 1.2 −15.2 ± 0.7 *	−16.7 ± 0.5 −16.5 ± 0.9	−17.0 ± 0.7 −13.1 ± 0.8 †	−14.6 ± 1.6 −13.6 ± 0.8 *	0.1231 0.0139	0.0023

Data were expressed as mean ± SEM. The one-way ANOVA was used to test within-group differences over time (age). The ANOVA for repeated measurements over time was carried out on echocardiographic data obtained from 8 GRMD (golden retriever muscular dystrophy) dogs and 4 healthy control dogs aged 2 to 24 months to test between-group differences. The two-tailed unpaired two-sample t-test was performed on data obtained in all dogs to determine the differences between GRMD and healthy control dogs at each time point. * $p < 0.05$ and † $p < 0.01$ versus healthy control dogs of the same age. CS: circumferential strain.

Table 3. Longitudinal strain in myocardial layers of the left ventricle analyzed by 2-dimensional speckle tracking echocardiography in healthy control and GRMD dogs at different ages.

Parameter	Group Control GRMD	Age, Months 2 n = 22 n = 7	6 n = 22 n = 7	9 n = 17 n = 4	12 n = 13 n = 4	18 n = 8 n = 4	24 n = 8 n = 4	ANOVA p Value Within−Group Effect	Between−Group Effect
3C endocardial LS	Control GRMD	−28.8 ± 1.9 −22.6 ± 0.6 †	−26.2 ± 1.7 −22.8 ± 0.8 *	−25.8 ± 0.9 −22.1 ± 1. 0 *	−26.1 ± 0.8 −21.9 ± 0.7 *	−23.5 ± 2.4 −22.1 ± 1.2	−21.7 ± 1.1 −19.5 ± 1.7	0.0702 0.3076	0.0010
3C middle layer LS	Control GRMD	−24.0 ± 1.8 −18.9 ± 0.5 †	−22.8 ± 1.5 −19.2 ± 0.6 *	−22.3 ± 0.8 −19.0 ± 0.7 *	−22.9 ± 1.0 −18.7 ± 0.8 *	−20.3 ± 2.2 −18.9 ± 0.9	−18.3 ± 0.6 −16.7 ± 1.6	0.1366 0.4422	0.0007
3C epicardial LS	Control GRMD	−19.9 ± 1.7 −15.9 ± 0.5 †	−19.9 ± 1.5 −16.3 ± 0.5 †	−19.3 ± 0.7 −16.5 ± 0.7	−20.1 ± 1.3 −16.2 ± 0.6 *	−17.6 ± 2.1 −16.2 ± 0.7	−15.5 ± 0.4 −14.4 ± 1.5	0.2452 0.5367	0.0010
4C endocardial LS	Control GRMD	−26.3 ± 1.3 −23.5 ± 0.6 *	−25.7 ± 1.2 −22.9 ± 0.5 *	−27.9 ± 2.1 −22.5 ± 1.0 *	−25.4 ± 1.5 −21.7 ± 0.9	−24.3 ± 0.6 −21.7 ± 1.3	−21.4 ± 0.4 −16.8 ± 0.7 †	0.0881 0.0002	0.0030
4C middle layer LS	Control GRMD	−22.8 ± 1.3 −20.0 ± 0.5 *	−22.3 ± 0.9 −19.6 ± 0.4 †	−23.7 ± 1.5 −19.1 ± 0.9 *	−21.6 ± 1.2 −18.5 ± 0.8	−20.3 ± 0.4 −18.7 ± 1.0	−18.7 ± 0.5 −14.4 ± 0.7 †	0.0863 0.0002	0.0034
4C epicardial LS	Control GRMD	−20.8 ± 1.4 −17.0 ± 0.5 *	−19.6 ± 0.8 −16.9 ± 0.4 †	−20.1 ± 1.0 −16.2 ± 0.8 *	−18.4 ± 1.0 −16.0 ± 0.7	−17.0 ± 0.5 −16.2 ± 0.8	−16.3 ± 0.6 −12.5 ± 0.7 †	0.1023 0.0006	0.0069
2C endocardial LS	Control GRMD	−26.0 ± 0.6 −23.2 ± 0.5 †	−25.9 ± 0.9 −22.6 ± 0.5 †	−25.2 ± 1.2 −21.8 ± 0.7 *	−25.6 ± 1.0 −20.0 ± 0.8 †	−22.6 ± 2.0 −19.7 ± 1.3	−22.1 ± 1.2 −19.4 ± 1.3	0.0277 0.0006	0.0054

Table 3. *Cont.*

Parameter	Group Control GRMD	Age, Months 2 n = 22 n = 7	6 n = 22 n = 7	9 n = 17 n = 4	12 n = 13 n = 4	18 n = 8 n = 4	24 n = 8 n = 4	ANOVA p Value Within −Group Effect	Between −Group Effect
2C middle layer LS	Control GRMD	−22.7 ± 0.6 −19.5 ± 0.4 †	−22.2 ± 0.9 −19.6 ± 0.4 †	−21.5 ± 1.2 −19.0 ± 0.7	−21.7 ± 0.7 −17.4 ± 0.7 †	−19.7 ± 1.4 −17.6 ± 1.2	−19.6 ± 0.9 −16.7 ± 1.1	0.0746 0.0088	0.0035
2C epicardial LS	Control GRMD	−20.1 ± 0.5 −16.4 ± 0.4 †	−19.1 ± 1.0 −17.2 ± 0.4 *	−18.4 ± 1.5 −16.8 ± 0.7	−18.3 ± 0.8 −15.3 ± 0.6 *	−17.2 ± 1.1 −15.8 ± 1.0	−17.5 ± 0.7 −14.4 ± 1.0	0.1672 0.0398	0.0032

Data were expressed as mean ± SEM. The one-way ANOVA determined within-group differences over time (age). The ANOVA for repeated measurements over time was carried out on echocardiographic data obtained from 8 GRMD (golden retriever muscular dystrophy) dogs and 4 healthy control dogs aged 2 to 24 months to test between-group differences. The two-tailed unpaired two-sample *t*-test was performed on data obtained in all dogs to determine the differences between GRMD and healthy control dogs at each time point. * $p < 0.05$ and † $p < 0.01$ versus healthy control dogs of the same age. LS: longitudinal strain; 2C, 3C and 4C: 2-chamber, 3-chamber and 4-chamber.

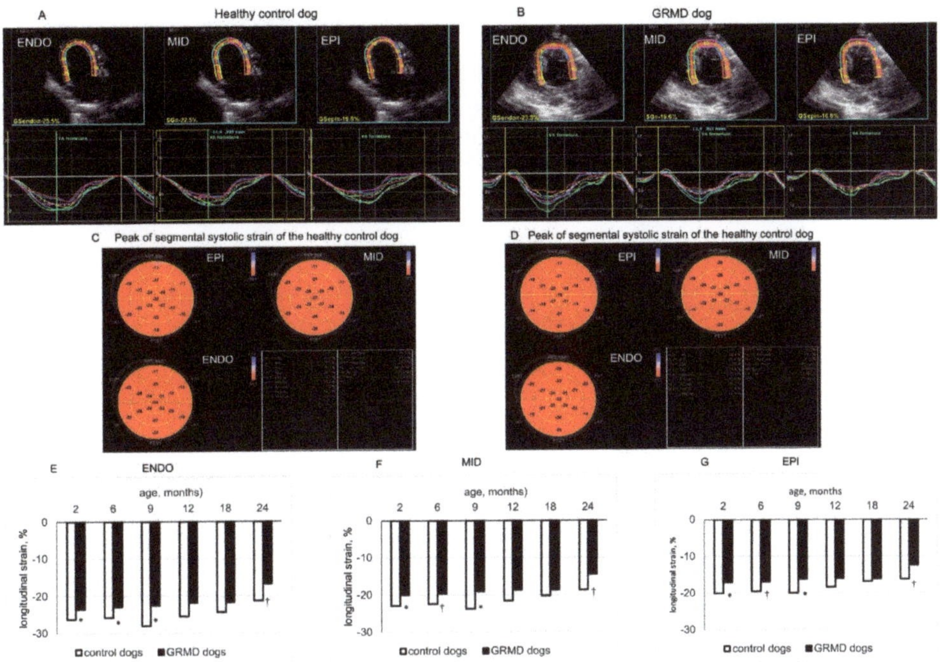

Figure 2. Longitudinal strain of left ventricular (LV) endocardial (ENDO), middle (MID) and epicardial (EPI) layers analyzed from the apical 4-chamber view. Panels (**A**,**B**) show the values and curves of 6 segments (showed by different colors) analyzed at each layer of the LV wall obtained in a 2-month-old healthy control dog and an age-matched GRMD (golden retriever muscular dystrophy) dog. The curve in dotted line in each part of the LV wall is the average of the 6 curves. Panels (**C**,**D**) are the bulls-eye presentations of segmental peak LS values obtained in each LV myocardial layer from 3 apical views of the above dogs. Panels (**E**–**G**) compare the longitudinal strain values of the ENDO, MID and EPI layers of healthy control and GRMD dogs at different ages. Data were expressed as mean ± SEM. The one-way ANOVA was performed to test within-group differences. The two-tailed unpaired two-sample t-test was performed on data obtained in all dogs at each time point to determine the differences between GRMD and healthy control dogs. n = 22, 22, 17, 13, 8 and 8 for GRMD dogs, and 7, 7, 4, 4, 4 and 4 for healthy control dogs at 2, 6, 9, 12, 18 and 24 months of age, respectively. * $p < 0.05$ and † $p < 0.01$ versus healthy control dogs of the same age.

Thus, from a young age, a significantly smaller peak LS could be detected in the three layers of the LV wall of GRMD dogs from three apical views. The difference in peak LS between GRMD and healthy control dogs became less evident at 18 and 24 months of age.

4. Discussion

In this longitudinal study, significant alteration in global LV systolic function (i.e., decreased FS and EF) was revealed late by conventional echocardiography in GRMD dogs, as previously reported [6,8]. The decline in LV systolic function with age reflects the natural progression of cardiomyopathy in GRMD dogs in the absence of specific treatment targeting cardiomyopathy.

Myocardial regional mechanics can be assessed by echocardiography in terms of four principal types of strain or deformation: circumferential, longitudinal, radial and rotational. A combined analysis of these strains can give a complete description of LV myocardial strain. At present, simultaneously analyzing myocardial strains of LV endocardial, middle and epicardial layers by echocardiography is technically available for CS and LS. This study analyzed myocardial strain in terms of the CS and LS of different LV wall layers of different regions, with the hope that assessing LV myocardial strain from two aspects gives a more detailed description of the changes in LV myocardial regional strain during the development of cardiomyopathy in GRMD dogs. In fact, more detailed analysis of LV myocardial CS and LS revealed different change trends in LV myocardial strain in both the circumferential and longitudinal directions, showing earlier alterations consistent with previous findings [6,8]. More importantly, these alterations in LV function were not uniform within the LV wall, showing differential progression of cardiomyopathy from the apex to the base and from the epicardium to the endocardium.

Clinical studies using cardiac magnetic resonance image [18], tissue Doppler imaging (TDI) [19] and 2D-STE [16] showed that DMD boys (less than 10 years old) had a decreased peak CS which worsened with age. Interestingly, a study in DMD boys (aged 14.8 ± 3.1 years old) showed that peak CS in the posterior wall analyzed by TDI exhibited smaller values, more frequently, in the outer layer than in the inner layer [20]. In the present study, an analysis of endocardial, middle and epicardial CS by 2D-STE from PSAX-apex, PSAX-mid-chamber and PSAX-base views demonstrated a non-uniform change in peak CS in GRMD dogs, which occurred early (2 months of age) and manifested as a significant and persistently smaller peak CS in the epicardial and middle layers of the LV apical anterior and antero-lateral wall (Figure 2 and Table 2). Meanwhile, at the mid-chamber and basal levels of the left ventricle, a smaller CS was detected relatively later in GRMD dogs (Table 2). These results suggest that analysis of CS in the LV apical region may be a useful tool to reveal early manifestations of cardiomyopathy in GRMD dogs, paralleling the pattern described in DMD patients. This non-uniform distribution of functional alteration between the apical and basal areas was complemented by differential timing of reduced contractile function from the epicardial to the endocardial layer.

Previous studies have shown that a reduction in global systolic LS can be detected in young DMD boys [14,16,19,21] and GRMD dogs [8,10]. Going further, this study analyzed LS more deeply in the three layers of the LV wall from three apical views and showed that systolic LS was lower in the three LV wall layers in GRMD dogs than in healthy control dogs from a young age, which is consistent with previous studies showing a worse global systolic LS in GRMD dogs [8,10]. These results suggest that analysis of LS remains a sensitive tool to detect early alterations in LV systolic function in GRMD dogs.

A preferential alteration in subendocardial contractile function has been demonstrated in many pathological conditions such as exercise under acute increase in afterload [22], LV hypertrophy [23], coronary heart disease [24], and heart failure [25]. Previous studies have shown an early alteration of subendocardial systolic velocity analyzed by TDI in GRMD dogs [4,8]. This non-uniform change in subendocardial-subepicardial function has been considered to contribute to the progression of the disease. Interestingly, the present study showed that the left ventricle of GRMD dogs exhibits spatial non-uniform alteration in myocardial strain that occurs particularly in the apical region for CS. Because this non-uniform alteration in myocardial strain occurs early, it is reasonable to speculate that it is an important factor contributing to the progression of LV global contractile dysfunction.

The study may have some limitations. (1). Due to the obvious physical differences between GRMD and healthy control dogs, it is impossible for the investigator to be blind to the study group, which may lead to study bias. (2). This study characterized the temporal changes of LV myocardial strain in GRMD dogs but did not provide cellular and molecular mechanisms to explain this early change in myocardial strain. Thus, further studies of cellular and molecular mechanisms are needed. (3). The LV myocardial wall is a three-dimensional object and has strain that can occur along three planes. During contraction, the heart is not only shortening along its long and short axis, but also rotating, tilting and displacing inside the chest. Thus, in addition to technical factors that may influence the analysis of strain [12], this may also affect linear strain analyzed by 2D-STE, which is based on a simplistic sense of lengthening, shortening, thickening or rotating. In addition, the small thickness of the myocardial wall of young dogs (to be further divided into different layers by the software) and the high heart rate may increase the difficulty for accurate analysis of myocardial strain and possibly affect the accuracy of results. Therefore, caution should be taken when interpreting these results. However, the results obtained in young and adult dogs regardless of their conditions (healthy or GRMD) provide consistent myocardial strain information which is consistent with classic notions about LV contractile function. For example, both CS and LS data showed that the myocardial strain of the subendocardial layer is stronger than that in the subepicardial layer, which is consistent with the classic concept that the subendocardial layer contracts more strongly than the subepicardial layer. Further development of three-dimensional STE may give a more physiological description of LV myocardial strain reflecting the complexity of the heart's three-dimensionality, and a recent study showed early impairment of LV 3-dimensional global LS in young patients with DMD [26].

5. Conclusions

In young dogs with DMD who have a normal global systolic function, a non-uniform reduction in systolic CS can be detected, especially in the LV apex, while decreased systolic LS can be detected in the three LV wall layers from three apical views. Our results suggest that analysis of myocardial strain by multi-layer 2D-STE may be a useful tool for monitoring the spatial evolution of alterations in LV systolic function and their progression with age in GRMD dogs. Given the similarity in pathogenesis, pathological changes, and clinical signs and symptoms between GRMD and DMD, our results suggest that assessing LV myocardial strain mechanics may be useful in detecting the early alteration of LV systolic function in early childhood of DMD patients and monitor its progression. The significance of these findings may warrant further investigation in DMD patients.

Author Contributions: Conceptualization, B.G., S.B. and J.B.S.; Methodology, J.B.S.; Validation, B.G. and J.B.S.; Formal Analysis, J.B.S.; Investigation, L.S., A.B. and J.B.S.; Resources, B.G., I.B. and S.B.; Data Curation, J.B.S.; Writing—Original Draft Preparation, J.B.S.; Writing—Review and Editing, B.G., I.B., A.B., D.C., L.H. and S.B., J.B.S.; Visualization, J.B.S.; Supervision, B.G.; Project Administration, B.G. and S.B.; Funding Acquisition, B.G., S.B. and J.B.S. All authors have read and agreed to the published version of the manuscript.

Funding: This research was supported by the Association Française Contre les Myopathies (Grant No. 18778) and EspeRare Foundation (Switzerland, Bale) who were not involved in the study design, data collection or analysis, nor manuscript preparation and submission.

Institutional Review Board Statement: The animal study protocol was approved by the Institutional Ethics Committee of ANSES-ENVA-UPEC (ComEth ANSES-ENVA-UPEC agreement #20/12/12–18).

Informed Consent Statement: Not applicable.

Data Availability Statement: All relevant data generated in this study are available in this article.

Acknowledgments: We thank the CEDS for providing GRMD and healthy dogs. We acknowledge Xavier Cauchois, Pablo Aguilar and the entire BNMS group in the ENVA for providing excellent cares to our canine patients. We thank Yi Su for her excellent technical support in the preparation of the figures.

Conflicts of Interest: The authors declare no conflict of interest.

Abbreviations

CS: circumferential strain; DMD: Duchenne muscular dystrophy; EDD: end-diastolic diameter; EDV: end-diastolic volume; EF: ejection fraction; ESD: end-systolic diameter; ESV: end-systolic volume; FS: fractional shortening; GRMD: golden retriever muscular dystrophy; LS: longitudinal strain; LV: left ventricular; IVSWEDT: interventricular septal wall end-diastolic thickness; IVSWTh: interventricular septal wall systolic thickening; % IVSWTh: percentage of interventricular septal wall systolic thickening: PSAX: parasternal short-axis; PWEDT: posterior wall end-diastolic thickness; PWTh: posterior wall systolic thickening; % PWTh: percentage of posterior wall systolic thickening; STE: speckle tracking echocardiography; TDI: tissue Doppler imaging; 2C, 3C and 4C: 2-chamber, 3-chamber and 4-chamber.

References

1. Allen, D.G.; Whitehead, N.P.; Froehner, S.C. Absence of Dystrophin Disrupts Skeletal Muscle Signaling: Roles of Ca^{2+}, Reactive Oxygen Species, and Nitric Oxide in the Development of Muscular Dystrophy. *Physiol. Rev.* **2016**, *96*, 253–305. [CrossRef] [PubMed]
2. Kamdar, F.; Garry, D.J. Dystrophin-Deficient Cardiomyopathy. *J. Am. Coll. Cardiol.* **2016**, *67*, 2533–2546. [CrossRef] [PubMed]
3. Kornegay, J.N. The Golden Retriever Model of Duchenne Muscular Dystrophy. *Skelet. Muscle* **2017**, *7*, 9. [CrossRef] [PubMed]
4. Chetboul, V. Tissue Doppler Imaging Detects Early Asymptomatic Myocardial Abnormalities in a Dog Model of Duchenne's Cardiomyopathy. *Eur. Heart J.* **2004**, *25*, 1934–1939. [CrossRef]
5. Townsend, D.; Turner, I.; Yasuda, S.; Martindale, J.; Davis, J.; Shillingford, M.; Kornegay, J.N.; Metzger, J.M. Chronic Administration of Membrane Sealant Prevents Severe Cardiac Injury and Ventricular Dilatation in Dystrophic Dogs. *J. Clin. Investig.* **2010**, *120*, 1140–1150. [CrossRef]
6. Su, J.B.; Cazorla, O.; Blot, S.; Blanchard-Gutton, N.; Mou, Y.A.; Barthélémy, I.; Sambin, L.; Sampedrano, C.C.; Gouni, V.; Unterfinger, Y.; et al. Bradykinin Restores Left Ventricular Function, Sarcomeric Protein Phosphorylation, and e/NNOS Levels in Dogs with Duchenne Muscular Dystrophy Cardiomyopathy. *Cardiovasc. Res.* **2012**, *95*, 86–96. [CrossRef]
7. Dabiré, H.; Barthélémy, I.; Blanchard-Gutton, N.; Sambin, L.; Sampedrano, C.C.; Gouni, V.; Unterfinger, Y.; Aguilar, P.; Thibaud, J.-L.; Ghaleh, B.; et al. Vascular Endothelial Dysfunction in Duchenne Muscular Dystrophy Is Restored by Bradykinin through Upregulation of ENOS and NNOS. *Basic Res. Cardiol.* **2012**, *107*, 240. [CrossRef]
8. Ghaleh, B.; Barthélemy, I.; Sambin, L.; Bizé, A.; Hittinger, L.; Blot, S.; Su, J.B. Alteration in Left Ventricular Contractile Function Develops in Puppies With Duchenne Muscular Dystrophy. *J. Am. Soc. Echocardiogr.* **2020**, *33*, 120–129.e1. [CrossRef] [PubMed]
9. Ghaleh, B.; Barthélemy, I.; Wojcik, J.; Sambin, L.; Bizé, A.; Hittinger, L.; Tran, T.D.; Thomé, F.P.; Blot, S.; Su, J.B. Protective Effects of Rimeporide on Left Ventricular Function in Golden Retriever Muscular Dystrophy Dogs. *Int. J. Cardiol.* **2020**, *312*, 89–95. [CrossRef]
10. Cazorla, O.; Barthélémy, I.; Su, J.B.; Meli, A.C.; Chetboul, V.; Scheuermann, V.; Gouni, V.; Anglerot, C.; Richard, S.; Blot, S.; et al. Stabilizing Ryanodine Receptors Improves Left Ventricular Function in Juvenile Dogs with Duchenne Muscular Dystrophy. *J. Am. Coll. Cardiol.* **2021**, *78*, 2439–2453. [CrossRef]
11. Martin, P.T.; Zygmunt, D.A.; Ashbrook, A.; Hamilton, S.; Packer, D.; Birch, S.M.; Bettis, A.K.; Balog-Alvarez, C.J.; Guo, L.-J.; Nghiem, P.P.; et al. Short-Term Treatment of Golden Retriever Muscular Dystrophy (GRMD) Dogs with RAAVrh74.MHCK7.GALGT2 Induces Muscle Glycosylation and Utrophin Expression but Has No Significant Effect on Muscle Strength. *PLoS ONE* **2021**, *16*, e0248721. [CrossRef]
12. Collier, P.; Phelan, D.; Klein, A. A Test in Context: Myocardial Strain Measured by Speckle-Tracking Echocardiography. *J. Am. Coll. Cardiol.* **2017**, *69*, 1043–1056. [CrossRef] [PubMed]
13. Gorcsan, J.; Tanaka, H. Echocardiographic Assessment of Myocardial Strain. *J. Am. Coll. Cardiol.* **2011**, *58*, 1401–1413. [CrossRef]
14. Cho, M.-J.; Lee, J.-W.; Lee, J.; Shin, Y.B. Evaluation of Early Left Ventricular Dysfunction in Patients with Duchenne Muscular Dystrophy Using Two-Dimensional Speckle Tracking Echocardiography and Tissue Doppler Imaging. *Pediatr. Cardiol.* **2018**, *39*, 1614–1619. [CrossRef]
15. Guo, L.-J.; Soslow, J.H.; Bettis, A.K.; Nghiem, P.P.; Cummings, K.J.; Lenox, M.W.; Miller, M.W.; Kornegay, J.N.; Spurney, C.F. Natural History of Cardiomyopathy in Adult Dogs With Golden Retriever Muscular Dystrophy. *J. Am. Heart Assoc.* **2019**, *8*, e012443. [CrossRef] [PubMed]

16. Amedro, P.; Vincenti, M.; De La Villeon, G.; Lavastre, K.; Barrea, C.; Guillaumont, S.; Bredy, C.; Gamon, L.; Meli, A.C.; Cazorla, O.; et al. Speckle-Tracking Echocardiography in Children with Duchenne Muscular Dystrophy: A Prospective Multicenter Controlled Cross-Sectional Study. *J. Am. Soc. Echocardiogr.* **2019**, *32*, 412–422. [CrossRef] [PubMed]
17. Lang, R.M.; Bierig, M.; Devereux, R.B.; Flachskampf, F.A.; Foster, E.; Pellikka, P.A.; Picard, M.H.; Roman, M.J.; Seward, J.; Shanewise, J.S.; et al. Recommendations for Chamber Quantification: A Report from the American Society of Echocardiography's Guidelines and Standards Committee and the Chamber Quantification Writing Group, Developed in Conjunction with the European Association of Echocardiography, a Branch of the European Society of Cardiology. *J. Am. Soc. Echocardiogr.* **2005**, *18*, 1440–1463. [CrossRef] [PubMed]
18. Hor, K.N.; Wansapura, J.; Markham, L.W.; Mazur, W.; Cripe, L.H.; Fleck, R.; Benson, D.W.; Gottliebson, W.M. Circumferential Strain Analysis Identifies Strata of Cardiomyopathy in Duchenne Muscular Dystrophy. *J. Am. Coll. Cardiol.* **2009**, *53*, 1204–1210. [CrossRef]
19. Ryan, T.D.; Taylor, M.D.; Mazur, W.; Cripe, L.H.; Pratt, J.; King, E.C.; Lao, K.; Grenier, M.A.; Jefferies, J.L.; Benson, D.W.; et al. Abnormal Circumferential Strain Is Present in Young Duchenne Muscular Dystrophy Patients. *Pediatr. Cardiol.* **2013**, *34*, 1159–1165. [CrossRef]
20. Mori, K.; Hayabuchi, Y.; Inoue, M.; Suzuki, M.; Sakata, M.; Nakagawa, R.; Kagami, S.; Tatara, K.; Hirayama, Y.; Abe, Y. Myocardial Strain Imaging for Early Detection of Cardiac Involvement in Patients with Duchenne's Progressive Muscular Dystrophy. *Echocardiography* **2007**, *24*, 598–608. [CrossRef]
21. Mertens, L.; Ganame, J.; Claus, P.; Goemans, N.; Thijs, D.; Eyskens, B.; Van Laere, D.; Bijnens, B.; D'hooge, J.; Sutherland, G.R.; et al. Early Regional Myocardial Dysfunction in Young Patients with Duchenne Muscular Dystrophy. *J. Am. Soc. Echocardiogr.* **2008**, *21*, 1049–1054. [CrossRef] [PubMed]
22. Su, J.B.; Hittinger, L.; Le Franc, P.; Crozatier, B. Limited Left Ventricular Inotropic Response to Exercise in Early Phase of Pressure Overload in Dogs. *Am. J. Physiol.* **1992**, *263*, H1011–H1016. [CrossRef] [PubMed]
23. Hittinger, L.; Ghaleh, B.; Chen, J.; Edwards, J.G.; Kudej, R.K.; Iwase, M.; Kim, S.-J.; Vatner, S.F.; Vatner, D.E. Reduced Subendocardial Ryanodine Receptors and Consequent Effects on Cardiac Function in Conscious Dogs with Left Ventricular Hypertrophy. *Circ. Res.* **1999**, *84*, 999–1006. [CrossRef]
24. Nagao, M.; Hatakenaka, M.; Matsuo, Y.; Kamitani, T.; Higuchi, K.; Shikata, F.; Nagashima, M.; Mochizuki, T.; Honda, H. Subendocardial Contractile Impairment in Chronic Ischemic Myocardium: Assessment by Strain Analysis of 3T Tagged CMR. *J. Cardiovasc. Magn. Reson.* **2012**, *14*, 14. [CrossRef] [PubMed]
25. Sinha, A.; Rahman, H.; Webb, A.; Shah, A.M.; Perera, D. Untangling the Pathophysiologic Link between Coronary Microvascular Dysfunction and Heart Failure with Preserved Ejection Fraction. *Eur. Heart J.* **2021**, *42*, 4431–4441. [CrossRef]
26. Yu, H.-K.; Xia, B.; Liu, X.; Han, C.; Chen, W.; Li, Z. Initial Application of Three-Dimensional Speckle-Tracking Echocardiography to Detect Subclinical Left Ventricular Dysfunction and Stratify Cardiomyopathy Associated with Duchenne Muscular Dystrophy in Children. *Int. J. Cardiovasc. Imaging* **2019**, *35*, 67–76. [CrossRef]

Journal of
Cardiovascular Development and Disease

MDPI

Article

Left Atrial Strain Imaging by Speckle Tracking Echocardiography: The Supportive Diagnostic Value in Cardiac Amyloidosis and Hypertrophic Cardiomyopathy

Ines Paola Monte [1,*,†], Denise Cristiana Faro [1,†], Giancarlo Trimarchi [2], Fabrizio de Gaetano [1], Mariapaola Campisi [3], Valentina Losi [1], Lucio Teresi [2], Gianluca Di Bella [2], Corrado Tamburino [1] and Cesare de Gregorio [2]

1 Department of Surgery and Medical-Surgical Specialties, University of Catania, Via Santa Sofia 78, 95123 Catania, Italy; denisefaro88@gmail.com (D.C.F.); fabridegafp7@gmail.com (F.d.G.); vale.losi@gmail.com (V.L.); tambucor@unict.it (C.T.)
2 Department of Clinical and Experimental Medicine, University Hospital of Messina, 98121 Messina, Italy; giancarlo.trimarchi18@gmail.com (G.T.); lucioteresi@gmail.com (L.T.); gianluca.dibella@unime.it (G.D.B.); cdegregorio@unime.it (C.d.G.)
3 Azienda Ospedaliera Provinciale di Catania, Santa Maria e Santa Venera Hospital, 95024 Acireale, Italy; campisi.mariapaola@gmail.com
* Correspondence: ines.monte@unict.it
† These authors contributed equally to this work.

Abstract: Background: Left atrial (LA) function is crucial for assessing left ventricular filling in various cardiovascular conditions. Cardiac Amyloidosis (CA) is characterized by atrial myopathy and LA function impairment, with diastolic dysfunction up to restrictive filling pattern, leading to progressive heart failure and arrhythmias. This study evaluates LA function and deformation using speckle tracking echocardiography (STE) in patients with CA compared to a cohort of patients with sarcomeric Hypertrophic Cardiomyopathy (HCM) and a control group. **Methods**: We conducted a retrospective, observational study (from January 2019 to December 2022) including a total of 100 patients: 33 with ATTR-CA, 34 with HCMs, and 33 controls. Clinical evaluation, electrocardiograms, and transthoracic echocardiography were performed. Echocardiogram images were analyzed in post-processing using EchoPac software for LA strain quantification, including LA-reservoir, LA-conduit, and LA-contraction strain. **Results**: The CA group exhibited significantly impaired LA function compared to HCMs and control groups, with LA-reservoir median values of −9%, LA-conduit −6.7%, and LA-contraction −3%; this impairment was consistent even in the CA subgroup with preserved ejection fraction. LA strain parameters correlated with LV mass index, LA volume index, E/e′, and LV-global longitudinal strain and were found to be associated with atrial fibrillation and exertional dyspnea. **Conclusions**: LA function assessed by STE is significantly impaired in CA patients compared to HCMs patients and healthy controls. These findings highlight the potential supportive role of STE in the early detection and management of the disease.

Keywords: Cardiac Amyloidosis; left-ventricle hypertrophy; diastolic dysfunction; heart failure; hypertrophic cardiomyopathy; speckle tracking echocardiography; atrial strain; amyloid atrial myopathy

1. Introduction

The assessment of left atrial (LA) morphology and function is paramount in gauging left ventricular filling amidst a variety of cardiovascular conditions, encompassing hypertension, heart failure, valvular heart disease, and cardiomyopathies.

The LA carries out three discrete functional phases, each accounting for approximately 50%, 30%, and 20% of left ventricle (LV) filling in healthy subjects, respectively.

The "reservoir" phase of the LA transpires during the isovolumetric contraction, ejection, and relaxation phase of the LV, with the mitral valve in a closed state. During this phase, the LA serves as a storage unit for potential energy.

The "conduit" phase occurs in the initial phase of ventricular diastole, beginning with the opening of the atrioventricular valves and continuing until the commencement of LA contraction. Throughout this phase, the LA functions as a pathway for blood from the pulmonary veins to the LV.

Lastly, during the "contraction" or "pump" phase, the contraction of the LA aids in augmenting left ventricular filling [1].

LA function is vital in averting heart failure as the LA initiates its inherent compensatory mechanisms in the event of left ventricular dysfunction. LA dilatation, as signified by a volume index (LAVi) exceeding 34 mL/m2, is a crucial indicator of LV filling and diastolic function [2].

Speckle tracking echocardiography (STE) can be used to investigate LA function, and LA strain, as quantified via the LA strain curve with two positive peaks corresponding to LA-reservoir and LA-pump function, serves as a sensitive indicator of LV filling pressure, superior to LA-volume and utilized for the early detection of preclinical LV dysfunction and remodeling [3,4]. Recent research suggests that atrial fibrosis precipitates impaired atrial contractility, preceding atrial remodeling, which forecasts cardiovascular morbidity and mortality [5].

LA dysfunction is influenced by LV remodeling and diastolic dysfunction amidst various cardiovascular disorders, including cardiomyopathies. A defining characteristic of restrictive cardiomyopathies is myocardial rigidity, denoted by diastolic dysfunction, hindering LV filling and conserving LV systolic function and LA enlargement/remodeling. Patients diagnosed with Sarcomeric Hypertrophic Cardiomyopathy (HCMs) are especially susceptible to adverse LA remodeling owing to heterogeneous myocardial hypertrophy, LV systolic and diastolic dysfunction, impaired LV global longitudinal strain (LV-GLS) and heightened mechanical dispersion [6], and progressive LA enlargement accompanied by morpho-functional impairment. This arises as a result of increased LV filling pressure, mitral insufficiency, outflow tract obstruction, and progressive LA fibrosis, culminating in what is referred to as "atrial myopathy". Certain studies have demonstrated that LA strain values in HCM are inferior to those in healthy subjects and are associated with adverse outcomes [7].

Cardiac Amyloidosis (CA) is induced by the intramyocardial deposition of abnormally folded amyloid fibrils, typically monoclonal immunoglobulin light chains in the context of systemic amyloidosis (AL) or transthyretin (ATTR), either in its hereditary (ATTRv) or acquired wild type (ATTRwt) form. This results in a steady increase in LV thickness, diastolic dysfunction, elevated filling pressures, and progressive LA dilatation and dysfunction [8–10]. Escalating LA-size has been correlated with adverse outcomes in patients with CA [11]. LA strain parameters, incorporating reservoir, conduit, and booster pump function, were compromised in individuals with CA and correlated well with the degree of LV dysfunction [12].

The aim of this study is to evaluate LA function and deformation using strain by STE in patients with CA compared to a cohort of patients with sarcomeric HCM and a control group and correlate the three LA strain parameters with echo (LV-mass, diastolic and systolic function, and LV-GLS) and clinical parameters. In addition to previous data from literature, we conducted this study to deepen the current knowledge by analyzing a subgroup of CA patients with preserved ejection fraction (pEF) to mitigate any potential influence on the echocardiographic and clinical parameters of diastolic dysfunction caused by reduced contractile function (systolic dysfunction), which is characteristic of advanced staged of Cardiac Amyloidosis. The goal was to make a comparison with HCMs, using a more similarly selected population in terms of EF.

2. Materials and Methods

2.1. Study Population

Our retrospective, observational study included patients aged over 18 years, who were referred to our Cardiology Units from January 2019 to December 2022. Patients were selected based on the following inclusion criteria and divided into two groups:

1. Patients affected by Transthyretin Cardiac Amyloidosis (ATTR), caused either by genetic mutation or wild type, diagnosed in accordance with the 2021 European Society of Cardiology (ESC) position statement [8]—using imaging criteria (transthoracic echocardiography [TTE] or cardiac magnetic resonance [CMR]) and total body 99mTc-PYP, DPD, or HMDP bone scintigraphy with SPECT (Perugini 2 or 3), after ruling out light chains amyloidosis (AL).
2. Patients diagnosed with Sarcomeric Hypertrophic Cardiomyopathies (HCMs), in line with the ESC 2014 guidelines [13], featuring TTE criteria: maximum wall thickness $\geq$15 mm (or $\geq$13 mm for family members), irrespective of the identification of the genetic mutation. Patients presenting with Obstructive HCM and LVOT gradient >30 mmHg were excluded from the analysis.

A control group (Co) of similar age range was introduced for comparison. The controls did not report any cardiac symptoms in their daily life, nor did they have pathological alterations found during physical examination, electrocardiogram (ECG), or basal echo or any organ damage. Some of them, consistent with the age range they belong to, were found during the visit to have office-measured borderline blood pressure values (normal-high) or to be within the range of grade 1 hypertension.

Upon enrolment, a thorough clinical evaluation was conducted, inclusive of a cardiomyopathy-oriented medical history and a comprehensive assessment of cardiovascular risk factors and major comorbidities. We executed ECG, 2D-color Doppler TTE, and dynamic-ECG (or ICD interrogation).

From the original database, we included all patients with optimal image quality (owing to an adequate acoustic window and/or patient's cooperation), suitable for speckle tracking analysis.

2.2. Echocardiography

Echocardiography was performed using an E95-GE machine equipped with a 1.5- and 3.6-MHz transducer, with a thorough assessment of parameters (chamber dimensions, systolic and diastolic function, and global longitudinal strain by STE) conforming to current recommendations [2,3,14]. Post-processing image analysis was performed using semi-automatic software (EchoPAC, ver. 2.02, GE, Chino, CA, USA) to achieve LV and LA strain quantification. GLS was analyzed from the apical views, at 60–70 fpm, from the average of 3 consecutive cardiac cycles.

2.3. LA Strain Assessment

The evaluation of LA strain was performed following the most recent EACVI consensus papers [3,15]. They advocate that it should be executed through dedicated image acquisition, from an LA-focused view (4 chambers or 2 chambers), with a narrow image sector, ensuring non-foreshortened images of the LA and acquiring 3–5 consecutive, regular beats. A high-quality ECG trace with a visible p wave is essential, and the acquisition of mitral and aortic valve Doppler waves can provide better retrospective definition of time intervals. Dedicated software should be utilized whenever possible. The region of interest (ROI) is defined by delineating the endocardial contour and encompassing the LA myocardium while avoiding the strong signal of the pericardium. Common tracking problems should be rectified by manual adjustment if required. LA strain is measured as GLS of the entire wall, and segmental strain is not considered. The zero reference is end-diastole, corresponding to mitral valve closure; following recommendations, we defined it by R wave at ECG (or simply the nadir of the atrial strain curve).

Phasic strain calculation involves calculating the deformation of atrial wall during three phases: reservoir strain (LASr), conduit strain (LAScd), and contraction strain (LASc). LASr, always positive, is calculated as the difference between the strain value at the curve peak and the end-diastolic value. LAScd, always negative, is calculated as the difference between the strain value at the onset of atrial contraction (*p*-wave) and the peak value (in atrial fibrillation (AF) patients, LAScd has the same value as LASr but with a negative sign) [15]. LASc is calculated from the difference between the strain value at end-diastole (R-wave) and the value at the onset of *p*-wave. It always exhibits a negative value and only occurs in sinus rhythm. See Figure 1 for details.

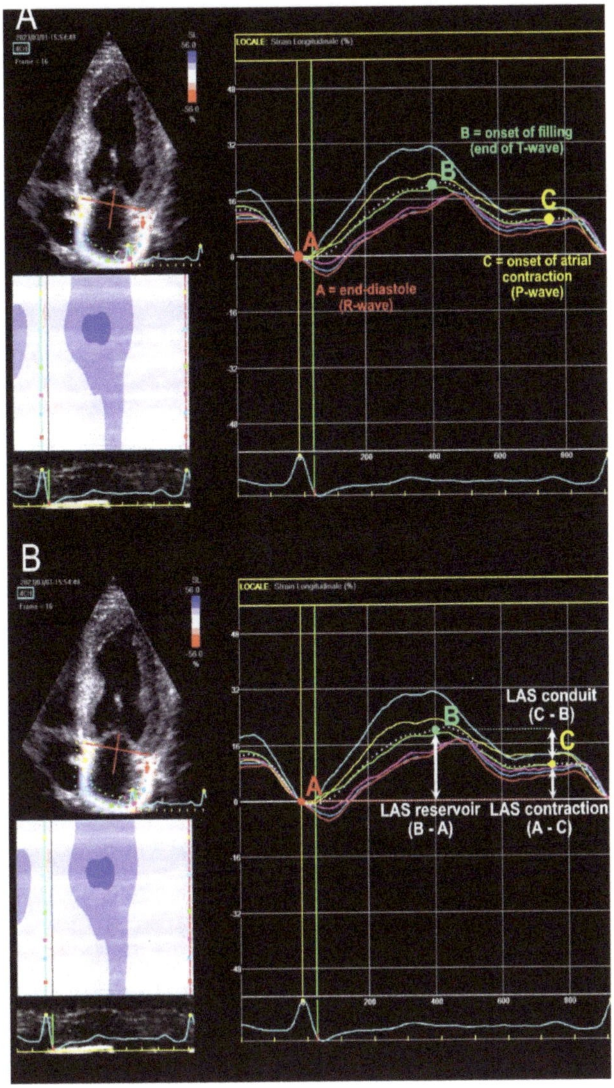

Figure 1. Left atrial strain (LAS) assessment. The white dotted line represents the average of the curves of the six atrial segments. (**A**): reference points for atrial function phases in relation to ECG waves and cardiac cycle. (**B**): here it is shown how to calculate the three LAS values from the reference points.

2.4. Clinical Outcomes Assessment

Arrhythmic episodes were reported during the patient's medical history interview: they were documented and recorded based on the medical reports provided by the patient. Arrhythmias were detected through Holter ECG monitoring or device interrogation in patients with an implanted cardioverter-defibrillator (ICD). We included episodes of ventricular fibrillation, sustained and non-sustained ventricular tachycardia, and AF.

Exertional dyspnea was assessed during patients' medical history interview: we inquired about the patient's current level of exercise tolerance (ordinary and extra-ordinary physical activity) and how it has changed over the past six months, asking specifically to quantify the impact of exertional dyspnea on their daily life based on effort intensity and whether there have been any alterations in the last six months compared to prior periods. Therefore, we expressed the reports according to the New York Heart Association (NYHA) classification.

2.5. Ethical Considerations

This study was conducted in accordance with the principles stated in the Declaration of Helsinki. Written informed consent was obtained from all participants at the time the tests were performed, according to the indications of the hospital.

2.6. Statistical Analysis

Data are expressed as median and inter-quartile range (IQR) for continue variables, in consideration of the relatively small sample size, regardless of distribution, and as number and percentage for categorical variables. Data were compared using the Mann–Whitney U test between two groups as appropriate, ANOVA or Kruskal–Wallis tests for comparison among more than two groups, and chi-square and Fisher's exact test for non-continuous variables: statistical significance was defined for $p < 0.05$, two-tailed test. We also applied the Pearson correlation and subsequently linear regression and binary logistic regression to examine the association between the echocardiographic parameters, and the association of selected clinical outcomes of interest with echocardiographic parameters. Analyses were performed using IBM SPSS Statistics ver.26 software.

3. Results

100 patients were included in this study, distributed as follows: 33 patients in the Cardiac Amyloidosis (CA) group, 34 patients in the Sarcomeric Hypertrophic Cardiomyopathy (HCM) group, and 33 patients in the control group (Co). In the CA group, the median age was 68 years, with 72.7% of the cohort being male. Most of the patients were categorized as NYHA class 2 (69.8%), while 21.2% were classified as NYHA class 1, and 9% were in NYHA class 3. Atrial fibrillation (AF) was reported for six patients (18.2%). Of these, four had permanent atrial fibrillation (which was also present during the examination, and therefore the atrial strain assessment was appropriately managed accordingly), while the other two reported episodes of paroxysmal atrial fibrillation in their medical history. Only one patient reported episodes of non-sustained ventricular tachycardia (NSVT).

For additional details regarding the general characteristics of the patients, please refer to Table 1.

Table 1. General characteristic of the three groups.

	CA N = 33	HCM N = 34	Co N = 33	*p* (All Groups)	CA vs. HCM	CA vs. Co	HCM vs. Co
Age (yo)	68 (62.5–77.5)	58.5 (38.7–63.2)	58 (53–65)	<0.001	<0.001	0.001	0.37
M	24 (72.7%)	23 (67.6%)	18 (54.5%)	0.31	0.79	0.20	0.32
F	9 (27.3%)	11 (32.4%)	15 (45.5%)	0.31	0.79	0.20	0.32
NYHA 1	7 (21.2%)	18 (52.9%)		<0.001	0.01	<0.001	<0.001
NYHA 2	23 (69.8%)	14 (41.2%)		<0.001	0.03	<0.001	<0.001
NYHA 3	3 (9%)	2 (5.9%)		0.28	0.38	0.06	0.49
NYHA 4	0	0		1	1	1	1
BSA	1.8 (1.7–1.9)	1.9 (1.6–2.0)	1.9 (1.7–2)	0.48	0.24	0.30	0.69
BP-sys, mmHg	125 (112.5–135)	130 (120–140)	135 (131–145)	0.001	0.11	<0.001	0.01
BP-dia, mmHg	80 (75–85)	80 (70–85)	85 (80.5–90)	0.03	0.13	0.07	0.004
HR, bpm	71 (65–78)	65 (60–74.7)	68 (60.5–75)	0.33	0.07	0.11	0.67
Fam. history SCD	2 (6.1%)	9 (26.5%)	0	0.001	0.04	0.49	0.002
Exertional dyspnoea	29 (87.9%)	14 (41.2%)	0	<0.001	<0.001	<0.001	<0.001
Syncope	1 (3%)	2 (5.9%)	0	0.65	1	1	0.49
AF	6 (18.2%)	3 (8.8%)	0	0.03	0.30	0.02	0.24
NSVT	1 (3%)	8 (23.5%)	0	0.001	0.031	1	0.005
ICD	1 (3%)	3 (8.8%)	0	0.31	0.61	1	0.23

Values are expressed as number and percentage for categorical ones, and as mean ± SD or median and interquartile range as appropriate. Abbreviations. AF = atrial fibrillation; BSA= body surface area; BP = blood pressure; HR = heart rate; ICD = implantable cardioverter defibrillator; NSVT = non sustained ventricular tachycardia; NYHA = New York Heart Association; SCD = sudden cardiac death.

From an echocardiographic point of view, they were all affected by left ventricular hypertrophy (median LVMi 150 g/sqm, IQR 123.5–188.5). The mean EF was 50%, and the median TAPSE was 18 mm [IQR 15–21]. These patients exhibited markers of altered diastolic function, with increased median LAVi (43.3 mL/sqm, IQR 37.4–53) and increased E/e′ ratio (median value 16.3). LV-GLS was markedly reduced (median −12%, IQR [−10, −14.2) with a typical apical sparing pattern. Atrial strain was compromised, with the following median values: LAS-reservoir 9%, LAS-conduit −6.7%, and LAS-contraction −3%.

When comparing the results with a group of patients with HCM, in CA patients we found a significantly lower LV-EF, significantly higher E/e′ ratio, and significantly lower LV-GLS ($p = 0.005$), with a different pattern of distribution of both hypertrophy (concentric vs. asymmetric) and strain alterations. Regarding atrial strain, we found significantly lower values for LAS-reservoir ($p = 0.009$), while LAS-conduit and LAS-contraction values were numerically lower but not significant ($p = 0.09$ and 0.14, respectively).

When comparing CA patients to the Co group, many of the examined parameters were significantly altered, both in terms of biventricular contractile function (significantly reduced LV-EF and tricuspid annular plane systolic excursion [TAPSE], both $p < 0.001$) and diastolic function (significantly increased LAVi and E/e′, $p < 0.001$), as well as LV-GLS (−12% vs. −19%, $p < 0.001$) (see Table 2 for further details).

All atrial strain parameters were significantly impaired in CA patients than in Co ($p < 0.001$ for all three comparisons) (See Table 2 and Figure 2).

Table 2. Echocardiographic parameters of all groups.

	CA N = 33	HCM N = 34	Co N = 33	p All Groups	CA vs. HCM	CA vs. Co	HCM vs. Co
EF, %	53 (40.5–58.5)	63.5 (58–69)	60 (56.5–63)	<0.001	<0.001	<0.001	0.08
LVMi (g/sqm)	150 (123.5–188.5)	130.2 (117.2–153)	79 (68–96.5)	<0.001	0.056	<0.001	<0.001
E/e′	16.3 (11.7–21.4)	10 (7.2–14.2)	6.5 (6–8.1)	<0.001	0.001	<0.001	<0.001
LAVi (mL/sqm)	43.3 (37.4–53)	40 (31.5–57.2)	25.6 (20.6–30.5)	<0.001	0.46	<0.001	<0.001
TAPSE mm	18 (15–21)	23 (20.5–25)	23 (20–26)	<0.001	<0.001	<0.001	0.92
LV-GLS, %	−12 (−10, −14.2)	−15 (−11.7, −18)	−19 (−18, −20.5)	<0.001	0.005	<0.001	<0.001
LAS-reservoir, %	9 (5.8–16.6)	14.5 (9.7–25)	32 (25–38)	<0.001	0.009	<0.001	<0.001
LAS-conduit, %	−6.7 (−4.2, −8.6)	−9 (−4.9, −15.3)	−15 (−12.1, −18.5)	<0.001	0.09	<0.001	0.005
LAS-contract., %	−3 (−0.9, −10.5)	−6 (−3, −9.7)	−14.3 (−10.5, −19.5)	<0.001	0.14	<0.001	<0.001

Values are expressed as mean ± SD or median and interquartile range [IQR] as appropriate. Abbreviations. EF = ejection fraction; LVMi = LV mass index; E/e′ = ratio between E wave of mitral flow and e′ at Tissue Doppler; LAVi = left atrial volume index; TAPSE: tricuspid annular plane systolic excursion; LV-GLS = left ventricle global longitudinal strain; LA: left atrium.

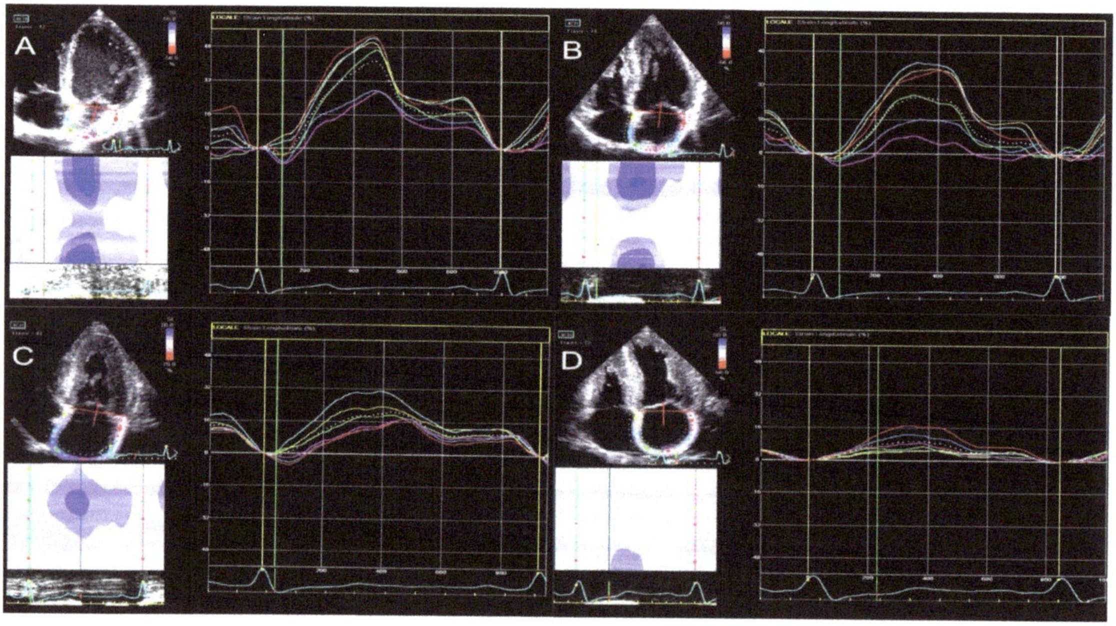

Figure 2. LA strain curves in comparison between subjects from the four groups. (**A**)—Co subject; (**B**)—HCM patient; (**C**)—CApEF patient; (**D**)—CArEF patient.

Applying Pearson's correlation, we found a significant correlation (r > 0.5) of LAS-reservoir with LVMi, LAVi, E/e′, GLS, (negative correlation), of LAS-conduit with age and GLS (positive), and of LAS-contraction with E/e′ and GLS (positive).

Applying binary logistic regression, AF was significantly associated with LAVi (OR 1.03 95% CI 1.005–1.069, $p = 0.025$), LA-reservoir (OR 0.77 95% CI 0.641–0.925, $p = 0.005$), LA-conduit (OR 1.274, 95% CI 1.034–1.570, $p = 0.023$), and LA-contraction (OR 1.14, 95% CI 1.003–1.304, $p = 0.046$).

NSVT were associated with LAVi (OR 1.045, 95% CI 1.010–1.080, $p = 0.010$), LAS-reservoir (OR 0.77, 95% CI 0.641–0.925, $p = 0.005$), LAS-contraction (OR 1.125, 95% CI 1.006–1.259, $p = 0.04$), and LV-GLS (OR 1.193, 95% CI 1.014–1.404, $p = 0.03$).

The presence of reported exertional dyspnea was found associated with LAVi, E/e′, LAS-reservoir, LAS-conduit, LAS-contraction, TAPSE, and EF (all p significant).

Applying linear regression, LAS-reservoir was found associated with LV-GLS (r 0.4–0.5).

Subanalysis of patients with CA was according to ejection fraction and comparison with other groups (HCM and control group).

Subsequently, we stratified the patients with Cardiac Amyloidosis based on their ejection fraction into two groups: preserved (CApEF, N = 20) if >50% or reduced (CArEF, N = 13) if <50%. We then analyzed the differential echocardiographic characteristics between these groups. The CApEF patients were significantly younger (median age 65.5 vs. 75, $p = 0.02$) and exhibited slightly higher systolic blood pressure values compared to the CArEF. The median ejection fraction (EF) was 55.5% in the CApEF group compared to 37% in the CArEF; left ventricular global longitudinal strain (LV-GLS) was significantly lower in patients with reduced EF ($p = 0.02$). Markers of diastolic function were more impaired in the CArEF group (both E/e′ ratio and LAVi), although the difference was not statistically significant. Atrial strain parameters were also numerically reduced in the CArEF compared to the CApEF group, but except for LAS-conduit, the difference did not reach statistical significance.

Therefore, to differentiate and exclude patients with reduced EF, who exhibited more altered parameters potentially linked to heart failure with systolic dysfunction and its hemodynamic consequences, we decided to compare the CApEF group with the HCM group. On comparing the CApEF group with the HCM group, we found a significant difference in EF ($p = 0.004$), E/e′ ratio, s′ wave, and TAPSE. The LAS-reservoir, LAS-conduit, and LAS-contraction values were numerically lower in the CApEF group compared to the HCM group (although without statistical significance) (Table 3 and Figure 3).

Table 3. Echocardiographic parameters in the two Cardiac Amyloidosis subgroups (with preserved EF and reduced EF) and comparison of CApEF group with HCM.

	CArEF N = 13	CApEF N = 20	HCM N = 34	CApEF vs. CArEF	CApEF vs. HCM
Age, yo	75 (66.5–82)	65.5 (57–72.5)	58.5 (38.7–63.2)	0.02	0.01
BP-sys, mmHg	115 (110–131.5)	130 (123.5–135)	130 (120–140)	0.03	0.77
BP-dia, mmHg	82 (77.5–85)	80 (75–88.7)	80 (70–85)	0.78	0.28
HR, bpm	69 (63–75)	76.5 (65–78.7)	65 (60–74.7)	0.23	0.06
NYHA 1, n (%)	2 (15)	5 (25)	18 (53)	0.67	0.05
NYHA 2	9 (60)	14 (70)	14 (41)	1	0.15
NYHA 3	2 (15)	1 (5)	2 (6)	0.54	1
AF, n (%)	3 (20)	3 (15)	3 (9)	0.65	0.66
EF, %	37 (34.5–41)	55.5 (54.2–60)	63.5 (58–69)	<0.001	0.004
LVMi, g/sqm	165.5 (129.7–206.7)	147.3 (119.8–176.8)	130.2 (117.2–153)	0.25	0.24
E/e′	16.3 (13.5–22.2)	15.9 (11.4–19.6)	10 (7.2–14.2)	0.43	0.001
S′, cm/s	4 (4–5.7)	5 (5,6)	7 (5–8)	0.06	0.002
LAVi, mL/sqm	47.4 (40.1–60.5)	41.9 (28.5–50.5)	40 (31.5–57.2)	0.08	0.85
TAPSE, mm	19 (11.5–24)	17.5 (15.7–19.2)	23 (20.5–25)	0.82	<0.001
LV-GLS, %	−10 (−7, −12)	−13 (−10, −15)	−15 (−11.7, −18)	0.02	0.07
LAS-reservoir, %	6.4 (3.9−13.5)	9.4 (7–18)	14.5 (9.7–25)	0.10	0.09
LAS-conduit, %	−5.2 (−3.3, −7.2)	−8 (−5, −9.7)	−9 (−4.9, −15.3)	0.04	0.35
LAS-contract. %	−3.5 (0.4, −10.2)	−3 (−1, −11)	−6 (−3, −9.7)	0.80	0.22

Values are expressed as mean ± SD or median and interquartile range (IQR) as appropriate. Abbreviations. AF = atrial fibrillation; CArEF = Cardiac Amyloidosis with reduced ejection fraction; CApEF = Cardiac Amyloidosis with preserved ejection fraction; BP-sys = blood pressure systolic; BP-dia = blood pressure diastolic; HR = heart rate; EF = ejection fraction; LVMi = LV mass index; E/e′ = ratio between E wave of mitral flow and e′ at Tissue Doppler; LAVi = left atrial volume index; NYHA = New-York Heart Association; TAPSE = tricuspid annular plane systolic excursion; LV-GLS= left ventricle global longitudinal strain; LA = left atrium.

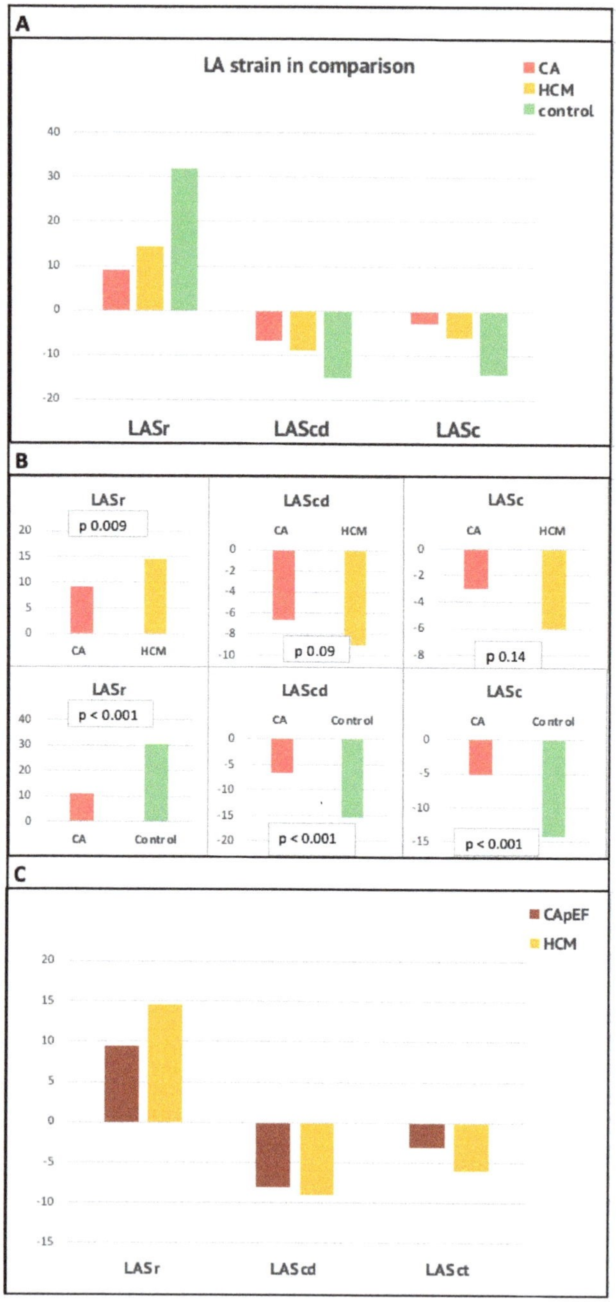

Figure 3. Comparison of LA strain values. (**A**)—Between the three study groups; (**B**)—between Cardiac Amyloidosis and HCM (upper panels) and between Cardiac Amyloidosis (CA) and controls (lower); (**C**)—between CApEF and HCM. Abbreviations. LASr = Left atrial strain reservoir; LAScd = Left atrial strain conduit; LASc = Left atrial strain contraction; CA = Cardiac Amyloidosis; HCM = hypertrophic cardiomyopathy; CApEF = Cardiac Amyloidosis with preserved ejection fraction.

4. Discussion

Our study assessed cardiac function and atrial strain in CA patients, comparing them to HCM patients and controls, offering valuable insights into atrial function in these populations.

CA, characterized by LV-hypertrophy, is difficult to distinguish from other LV hypertrophy-causing diseases, such as HCM and hypertensive cardiopathy. Previous studies demonstrated reductions in ventricular longitudinal strain parameters in CA patients and identified specific deformation parameters with discriminative capacity for differential diagnosis [16–19]. Our study supports these findings and expands on them by providing a detailed comparison between CA, HCM, and control subjects.

We found that CA patients had altered biventricular contractile and diastolic function, with reduced LV-GLS, increased LAVi, and elevated E/e′ ratio. Atrial strain was compromised, with lower values for LA-reservoir, LA-conduit, and LA-contraction. Sub-analysis of CA patients revealed differences in age, systolic-BP, exertion tolerance, and diastolic function markers between CApEF and CArEF groups.

Our study aimed firstly to compare HCMs patients to the whole CA patient population, at various stages of the disease. A subgroup of these CA patients had a reduced ejection fraction, indicative of a more advanced cardiac impairment with contractile dysfunction, typically seen in older patients. Our intent was to study the differing behaviors of atrial function in these two conditions, both characterized by myocardial hypertrophy and diastolic dysfunction, progressing to restrictive patterns in more advanced cases.

We subsequently isolated the subset of CApEF patients and compared them with HCMs patients, all of whom had preserved EF. This was conducted to compare two groups with similar ejection fraction, stripping away the possible repercussions on atrial dilation and dysfunction and symptoms due to compromised contractile function. The focus was to compare atrial function between these two groups, seeking differences with the aim of identifying early myocardial involvement and atrial myopathy in CA, while the ejection fraction is still preserved, to promote early initiation of therapy.

LA strain is an emerging marker of diastolic dysfunction. In Cardiac Amyloidosis, the left atrium is impaired like the left ventricle due to amyloid infiltration, leading to increased size, reduced ejection force, and strain. While LA dimension or volume can suggest chronic elevation of LA pressure, they are insufficient parameters to obtain detailed information about LA function [20].

Impaired atrial strain parameters in CA patients from our series are consistent with previous studies reporting reduced atrial function in CA, with peak LA strain correlated with LV-GLS and worse LA strain values in ATTRwt than AL [12]. A multicenter study found that LA reservoir and contraction correlated with LV-GLS and invasive LV-filling pressures, suggesting LA reservoir as an alternative marker of elevated filling pressure and LA compensation to maintain normal LV-filling pressure [21].

Aimo et al. explored multi-chamber speckle tracking imaging for assessing LA strain's diagnostic value in CA, demonstrating altered strain parameters, particularly in ATTR-CA, and good diagnostic accuracy in differentiating CA from other unexplained LV-hypertrophies [22]. They also found an association of severe impairment of peak atrial longitudinal strain (PALS) or LASc with a diagnosis of ATTR-CA.

Another study revealed increased LA volume and reduced LA strain in ATTR-CA patients, with stronger correlation of LA strain with LA volumes, E/e′, and LV-GLS for AL-CA than ATTR-CA, possibly due to a more acute disease course and less time for amyloid deposition in the LA-wall [23]. Our study supports these findings, with lower LA strain values in CA patients, but we did not include AL-CA patients for comparison.

Studies on HCM patients identified LA strain as a significant predictor of exercise tolerance, AF risk, appropriate ICD therapy, and HF incidence [24–27]. These findings emphasize the importance of evaluating LA strain in HCM patients to improve risk stratification, early intervention, and treatment outcomes.

Significant differences in LA strain parameters between CA and HCM patients and between CA patients and controls align with previous studies aiming to differentiate these conditions based on atrial function.

Rausch et al. examined LA strain for differentiating CA from hypertensive heart disease, finding good diagnostic accuracy and a similar reduction in LA strain values between ATTR and AL groups [28].

Our study also highlighted the diagnostic potential of left atrial strain in Cardiac Amyloidosis; however, we focused mostly on the comparison with HCM, while our control, healthy, or affected by mild hypertension groups did not have significant LV hypertrophy.

It has been reported an LA strain and four-chamber (4-CH) GLS significantly reduced in CA and HCM compared with control subjects, with CA patients showing the lowest values, and LV-EF significantly reduced in CA patients in association with major adverse cardiac events (MACE), suggesting that the severity of LV systolic dysfunction could influence cardiac events and a prognostic influence of LA on MACE and AF incidence [10,29,30].

Lucas et al. demonstrated a significant difference in PALS and contraction-phase strain between the two groups CA and HCM patients [31]. LA dysfunction in CA has been shown to be likely caused by amyloid deposition in the LA wall, as confirmed by atrial wall LGE in CMR study [10,31].

Another study revealed reduced atrial deformation during atrial systole in hypertrophic ATTR-CA patients independent of LA size, unlike HCM, with LA strain rate being the only independent predictor of atrial arrhythmias [32].

4.1. LA Strain: Prognostic Value

Our study's findings on LA strain parameters' association with echocardiographic and clinical markers in CA patients align with previous research, which reported a prognostic value for LA strain and a relationship between LA strain and arrhythmia susceptibility, such as AF and NSVT.

Huntjens et al. found that peak LA strain had the strongest association with survival, and LA strain combined with LV-GLS and RV-free wall strain had the highest prognostic value in a longitudinal study of CA patients [33].

Oike et al. found reduced LA strain values in patients with cardiovascular death during follow-up and noted that LASr was independently associated with cardiovascular death and HF-related hospitalization in patients with ATTRwt [34].

In CA, LASr and LASc are often compromised, regardless of LA size [12], suggesting both raised LV-filling pressures and direct atrial amyloid infiltration contribute to dysfunction. Consequently, atrial and left appendage thrombi may develop, increasing embolic stroke risk and mortality [35,36]. The right ventricle is also commonly impacted, leading to decreased TAPSE, tissue Doppler systolic velocity, and longitudinal strain [37].

Bandera et al. found that LA infiltration was associated with greater disease severity, worse prognosis, impaired three-phasic atrial function, and "atrial electromechanical dissociation". This phenomenon, with an absence of atrial contraction in 22.1% despite sinus rhythm, had risks and prognosis like patients with AF, worse than those with sinusal rythm and effective mechanical contraction [38]. This highlights atrial strain's utility in detecting atrial myopathy and preventing thromboembolic complications, independently and before AF development.

4.2. Insights about Cut-Off Values from Literature

In the study of LA strain, various cut-off points are emerging as potential indicators of LA dysfunction. Rausch et al. proposed an LAS-reservoir cut-off value of 20%, suggesting it could aid in distinguishing Cardiac Amyloidosis from hypertensive heart disease, especially in clinically uncertain cases with increased LV wall thickness where an LAS-reservoir <20% increases the likelihood of Cardiac Amyloidosis as a differential diagnosis [28]. De Gregorio et al. offered specific cut-offs for LA reservoir and pump function ($\leq$20,05% and ≤ -1.4%, respectively) to differentiate hypertrophic phenotypes [10].

Aimo et al. suggest the first quartiles of PALS or PACS (<6.65% or <3.62%) as potential diagnostic cut-offs, particularly beneficial for patients with unexplained hypertrophy, considering the independent diagnostic value of the combination of both parameters and their ability to reclassify patient risk of ATTR-CA [22].

Regarding survival prognosis, Kado et al. pointed to a cut-off of 8.05 (peak strain) [30], while Oike indicated an optimal LAS reservoir cut-off of 6.69% for predicting cardiovascular death [34].

Cut-off values for LAS reservoir were proposed in relation to LV diastolic function, that was therefore categorized into four categories: LAS reservoir ≥35% (grade 0), ≥24% to <35% (grade 1), ≥19% to <24% (grade 2), and <19% (grade 3), with grade 2+ associated with incident heart failure in the elderly, independent of LAVI [4,39]. Inoue and Nagueh's works emphasized an 18% cut-off for LAS reservoir to differentiate between normal and elevated LV filling pressure (when defining PCWP > 12 mmHg as elevated, and 16% when using PCWP ≥ 15 mmHg). However, they cautioned that this parameter is most accurate in estimating high filling pressure in patients with depressed EF (<50%), and less in patients with preserved EF [21,40].

At the current stage, there's no single universal cut-off applicable to all scenarios. While useful, these cut-offs are not without limitations. The fluctuating accuracy of LAS reservoir in estimating LV filling pressures, especially in relation to ejection fraction, underscores the need for it not to be a standalone diagnostic tool. Future research should strive to refine these cut-offs, exploring their applicability across patient populations and conditions.

4.3. Strengths and Clinical—Practical Implications

Our study's notable strength is the in-depth analysis of atrial strain parameters across different CA patient subgroups based on LV-EF (preserved vs. reduced), which provides valuable insights into LV-EF's potential influence on atrial dysfunction in CA patients, an aspect previously under-investigated. Our findings have significant clinical implications. LA strain may help clinicians differentiate CA from other conditions like HCM and hypertension; moreover, understanding LA strain parameters in CA can improve patients' risk stratification and management and enable more personalized therapeutic approaches, such as initiating anticoagulation therapy or closer monitoring for AF development. Our study highlights the need for further research to investigate atrial strain's prognostic implications in CA patients. Longitudinal follow-up data can provide insights into atrial strain's role in predicting outcomes like HF, stroke, and mortality. Future research could explore treatment strategies' impact on LA strain parameters and their potential role in monitoring treatment response. Additionally, investigating associations between LA strain parameters and echocardiographic markers, arrhythmias, and symptoms in CA patients could enhance our understanding of CA pathophysiology, contributing to novel therapeutic approaches targeting atrial dysfunction and potentially improving patient outcomes and quality of life.

4.4. Study Limitations and Future Perspectives

Our study has limitations, including a relatively small sample size, limiting generalizability, and a lack of longitudinal follow-up analysis to assess atrial strain parameters' prognostic value in CA patients. Future studies with larger cohorts and longitudinal follow-up data are needed to confirm these findings and address these limitations, investigate atrial strain's prognostic implications, and explore treatment strategies' impact on atrial strain parameters, focusing on understanding pathophysiological mechanisms, refining diagnostic criteria, and optimizing patient management strategies.

5. Conclusions

In conclusion, our study contributes valuable insights into atrial function in CA patients, showing significantly LA strain parameters in ATTR-CA patients compared to HCMs and control groups (this impairment remains consistent even in the subgroup with preserved EF). These findings highlight the potential role of LA strain in differentiating between CA and other conditions, identifying patients at higher risk of arrhythmias and evaluating cardiac involvement severity and response to therapy.

Author Contributions: I.P.M. and C.d.G. contributed to the conception and design of the work and coordination. D.C.F. and I.P.M. performed data acquisition analysis and interpretation, drafted the manuscript, and revised it critically for important intellectual content; G.T., F.d.G., M.C., V.L. and L.T., gave their contribution for data collection; G.D.B. and C.T. overviewed the study. All authors have read and agreed to the published version of the manuscript.

Funding: This research received no external funding.

Institutional Review Board Statement: The study was conducted in accordance with the Declaration of Helsinki. Ethical review and approval were waived due to the observational retrospective nature of the study.

Informed Consent Statement: Informed consent was obtained from all subjects involved in the study at the time of first visit.

Data Availability Statement: The data presented in this study are available on request from the corresponding author. The data underlying this article will be shared on reasonable request to the corresponding author.

Conflicts of Interest: The authors declare no conflict of interest.

References

1. Prioli, A.; Marino, P.; Lanzoni, L.; Zardini, P. Increasing degrees of left ventricular filling impairment modulate left atrial function in humans. *Am. J. Cardiol.* **1998**, *82*, 756–761. [CrossRef]
2. Nagueh, S.F.; Smiseth, O.A.; Appleton, C.P.; Byrd, B.F.; Dokainish, H.; Edvardsen, T.; Flachskampf, F.A.; Gillebert, T.C.; Klein, A.L.; Lancellotti, P.; et al. Recommendations for the Evaluation of Left Ventricular Diastolic Function by Echocardiography: An Update from the American Society of Echocardiography and the European Association of Cardiovascular Imaging. *J. Am. Soc. Echocardiogr.* **2016**, *29*, 277–314. [CrossRef]
3. Badano, L.P.; Kolias, T.J.; Muraru, D.; Abraham, T.P.; Aurigemma, G.; Edvardsen, T.; D'Hooge, J.; Donal, E.; Fraser, A.G.; Marwick, T.; et al. Standardization of left atrial, right ventricular, and right atrial deformation imaging using two-dimensional speckle tracking echocardiography: A consensus document of the EACVI/ASE/Industry Task Force to standardize deformation imaging. *Eur. Heart J. Cardiovasc. Imaging* **2018**, *19*, 591–600. [CrossRef]
4. Singh, A.; Addetia, K.; Maffessanti, F.; Mor-Avi, V.; Lang, R.M. LA Strain for Categorization of LV Diastolic Dysfunction. *JACC Cardiovasc. Imaging* **2017**, *10*, 735–743. [CrossRef]
5. Bisbal, F.; Baranchuk, A.; Braunwald, E.; Bayés de Luna, A.; Bayés-Genís, A. Atrial Failure as a Clinical Entity: JACC Review Topic of the Week. *J. Am. Coll. Cardiol.* **2020**, *75*, 222–232. [CrossRef]
6. Faro, D.C.; Losi, V.; Rodolico, M.S.; Licciardi, S.; Monte, I.P. Speckle tracking echocardiography-derived parameters as new prognostic markers in hypertrophic cardiomyopathies. *Eur. Heart J. Open* **2023**, *3*, oead014. [CrossRef]
7. Fujimoto, K.; Inoue, K.; Saito, M.; Higashi, H.; Kono, T.; Uetani, T.; Aono, J.; Nagai, T.; Nishimura, K.; Suzuki, J.; et al. Incremental value of left atrial active function measured by speckle tracking echocardiography in patients with hypertrophic cardiomyopathy. *Echocardiography* **2018**, *35*, 1138–1148. [CrossRef]
8. Garcia-Pavia, P.; Rapezzi, C.; Adler, Y.; Arad, M.; Basso, C.; Brucato, A.; Burazor, I.; Caforio, A.L.P.; Damy, T.; Eriksson, U.; et al. Diagnosis and treatment of cardiac amyloidosis: A position statement of the ESC Working Group on Myocardial and Pericardial Diseases. *Eur. Heart J.* **2021**, *42*, 1554–1568. [CrossRef]
9. Versteylen, M.O.; Brons, M.; Teske, A.J.; Oerlemans, M. Restrictive Atrial Dysfunction in Cardiac Amyloidosis: Differences between Immunoglobulin Light Chain and Transthyretin Cardiac Amyloidosis Patients. *Biomedicines* **2022**, *10*, 1768. [CrossRef]
10. De Gregorio, C.; Dattilo, G.; Casale, M.; Terrizzi, A.; Donato, R.; Di Bella, G. Left Atrial Morphology, Size and Function in Patients With Transthyretin Cardiac Amyloidosis and Primary Hypertrophic Cardiomyopathy–Comparative Strain Imaging Study. *Circ. J.* **2016**, *80*, 1830–1837. [CrossRef]
11. Mohty, D.; Pibarot, P.; Dumesnil, J.G.; Darodes, N.; Lavergne, D.; Echahidi, N.; Virot, P.; Bordessoule, D.; Jaccard, A. Left atrial size is an independent predictor of overall survival in patients with primary systemic amyloidosis. *Arch. Cardiovasc. Dis.* **2011**, *104*, 611–618. [CrossRef] [PubMed]
12. Nochioka, K.; Quarta, C.C.; Claggett, B.; Roca, G.Q.; Rapezzi, C.; Falk, R.H.; Solomon, S.D. Left atrial structure and function in cardiac amyloidosis. *Eur. Heart J. Cardiovasc. Imaging* **2017**, *18*, 1128–1137. [CrossRef] [PubMed]
13. Elliott, P.M.; Anastasakis, A.; Borger, M.A.; Borggrefe, M.; Cecchi, F.; Charron, P.; Hagege, A.A.; Lafont, A.; Limongelli, G.; Mahrholdt, H.; et al. 2014 ESC Guidelines on diagnosis and management of hypertrophic cardiomyopathy: The Task Force for the Diagnosis and Management of Hypertrophic Cardiomyopathy of the European Society of Cardiology (ESC). *Eur. Heart J.* **2014**, *35*, 2733–2779. [PubMed]

14. Galderisi, M.; Cosyns, B.; Edvardsen, T.; Cardim, N.; Delgado, V.; Di Salvo, G.; Donal, E.; Sade, L.E.; Ernande, L.; Garbi, M.; et al. Standardization of adult transthoracic echocardiography reporting in agreement with recent chamber quantification, diastolic function, and heart valve disease recommendations: An expert consensus document of the European Association of Cardiovascular Imaging. *Eur. Heart J. Cardiovasc. Imaging* **2017**, *18*, 1301–1310. [PubMed]
15. Voigt, J.U.; Mălăescu, G.G.; Haugaa, K.; Badano, L. How to do LA strain. *Eur. Heart J. Cardiovasc. Imaging* **2020**, *21*, 715–717. [CrossRef] [PubMed]
16. Koyama, J.; Ray-Sequin, P.A.; Falk, R.H. Longitudinal myocardial function assessed by tissue velocity, strain, and strain rate tissue Doppler echocardiography in patients with AL (primary) cardiac amyloidosis. *Circulation* **2003**, *107*, 2446–2452. [CrossRef]
17. Pagourelias, E.D.; Duchenne, J.; Mirea, O.; Vovas, G.; Van Cleemput, J.; Delforge, M.; Kuznetsova, T.; Bogaert, J.; Voigt, J.-U. The Relation of Ejection Fraction and Global Longitudinal Strain in Amyloidosis: Implications for Differential Diagnosis. *JACC Cardiovasc. Imaging* **2016**, *9*, 1358–1359. [CrossRef]
18. Ternacle, J.; Bodez, D.; Guellich, A.; Audureau, E.; Rappeneau, S.; Lim, P.; Radu, C.; Guendouz, S.; Couetil, J.-P.; Benhaiem, N.; et al. Causes and Consequences of Longitudinal LV Dysfunction Assessed by 2D Strain Echocardiography in Cardiac Amyloidosis. *JACC Cardiovasc. Imaging* **2016**, *9*, 126–138. [CrossRef]
19. Pagourelias, E.D.; Mirea, O.; Duchenne, J.; Van Cleemput, J.; Delforge, M.; Bogaert, J.; Kuznetsova, T.; Voigt, J.U. Echo Parameters for Differential Diagnosis in Cardiac Amyloidosis: A Head-to-Head Comparison of Deformation and Nondeformation Parameters. *Circ. Cardiovasc. Imaging* **2017**, *10*, e005588. [CrossRef]
20. Inoue, K.; Kawakami, H.; Akazawa, Y.; Higashi, H.; Higaki, T.; Yamaguchi, O. Echocardiographic Assessment of Atrial Function: From Basic Mechanics to Specific Cardiac Diseases. *J. Cardiovasc. Dev. Dis.* **2022**, *9*, 68. [CrossRef]
21. Inoue, K.; Khan, F.H.; Remme, E.W.; Ohte, N.; García-Izquierdo, E.; Chetrit, M.; Moñivas-Palomero, V.; Mingo-Santos, S.; Andersen, Ø.S.; Gude, E.; et al. Determinants of left atrial reservoir and pump strain and use of atrial strain for evaluation of left ventricular filling pressure. *Eur. Heart J. Cardiovasc. Imaging* **2021**, *23*, 61–70. [CrossRef]
22. Aimo, A.; Fabiani, I.; Giannoni, A.; Mandoli, G.E.; Pastore, M.C.; Vergaro, G.; Spini, V.; Chubuchny, V.; Pasanisi, E.M.; Petersen, C.; et al. Multi-chamber speckle tracking imaging and diagnostic value of left atrial strain in cardiac amyloidosis. *Eur. Heart J. Cardiovasc. Imaging* **2022**, *24*, 130–141. [CrossRef]
23. Aimo, A.; Fabiani, I.; Spini, V.; Chubuchny, V.; Pasanisi, E.M.; Petersen, C.; Poggianti, E.; Taddei, C.; Cameli, M.; E Mandoli, G.; et al. Left atrial strain in cardiac amyloidosis. *Eur. Heart J.* **2021**, *42*, ehab724-1794. [CrossRef]
24. Tayal, B.; Malahfji, M.; Buergler, J.M.; Shah, D.J.; Nagueh, S.F. Hemodynamic determinants of left atrial strain in patients with hypertrophic cardiomyopathy: A combined echocardiography and CMR study. *PLoS ONE* **2021**, *16*, e0245934. [CrossRef]
25. Candan, Ö.; Geçmen, Ç.; Kahyaoğlu, M.; Çelik, M.; Şimşek, Z.; Dindaş, F.; Doğduş, M.; Zehir, R.; Kırma, C. Left Atrial Dysfunction as Marker of Arrhythmic Events in Patients with Hypertrophic Cardiomyopathy. *Anatol. J. Cardiol.* **2022**, *26*, 771–777. [CrossRef]
26. Teixeira, K.L.M.; Correia, E.B.; Tressino, C.G.; Peçanha, M.M.; Melchior, W.A.; Barretto, R.B.D.M.; de Medeiros, B.G.; Le Bihan, D. Echocardiographic assessment of atrial function in patients with hypertrophic cardiomyopathy with and without paroxysmal atrial fibrillation. *Rev. Port. Cardiol.* **2022**, *41*, 771–779. [CrossRef]
27. Lee, H.J.; Kim, H.K.; Rhee, T.M.; Choi, Y.-J.; Hwang, I.-C.; Yoon, Y.E.; Park, J.-B.; Lee, S.-P.; Kim, Y.-J.; Cho, G.-Y. Left Atrial Reservoir Strain-Based Left Ventricular Diastolic Function Grading and Incident Heart Failure in Hypertrophic Cardiomyopathy. *Circ. Cardiovasc. Imaging* **2022**, *15*, e013556. [CrossRef]
28. Rausch, K.; Scalia, G.M.; Sato, K.; Edwards, N.; Lam, A.K.-Y.; Platts, D.G.; Chan, J. Left atrial strain imaging differentiates cardiac amyloidosis and hypertensive heart disease. *Int. J. Cardiovasc. Imaging* **2021**, *37*, 81–90. [CrossRef]
29. Iio, C.; Inoue, K.; Nishimura, K.; Fujii, A.; Nagai, T.; Suzuki, J.; Okura, T.; Higaki, J.; Ogimoto, A. Characteristics of Left Atrial Deformation Parameters and Their Prognostic Impact in Patients with Pathological Left Ventricular Hypertrophy: Analysis by Speckle Tracking Echocardiography. *Echocardiography* **2015**, *32*, 1821–1830. [CrossRef]
30. Kado, Y.; Obokata, M.; Nagata, Y.; Ishizu, T.; Addetia, K.; Aonuma, K.; Kurabayashi, M.; Lang, R.M.; Takeuchi, M.; Otsuji, Y. Cumulative Burden of Myocardial Dysfunction in Cardiac Amyloidosis Assessed Using Four-Chamber Cardiac Strain. *J. Am. Soc. Echocardiogr.* **2016**, *29*, 1092–1099.e2. [CrossRef]
31. Lucas, C.; Martel, H.; Ruimy, A.; Fabre, C.; Gardenat, A.; Rique, A.; Michel, N.; Dernys, A.; Jacquier, A.; Habib, G. Multimodal imaging assessment of left atrial strain in cardiac amyloidosis and hypertrophic cardiomyopathies. *Eur. Heart J. Cardiovasc. Imaging* **2022**, *23*, jeab289-045. [CrossRef]
32. Henein, M.Y.; Suhr, O.B.; Arvidsson, S.; Pilebro, B.; Westermark, P.; Hörnsten, R.; Lindqvist, P. Reduced left atrial myocardial deformation irrespective of cavity size: A potential cause for atrial arrhythmia in hereditary transthyretin amyloidosis. *Amyloid* **2018**, *25*, 46–53. [CrossRef] [PubMed]
33. Huntjens, P.R.; Zhang, K.W.; Soyama, Y.; Karmpalioti, M.; Lenihan, D.J.; Gorcsan, J., 3rd. Prognostic Utility of Echocardiographic Atrial and Ventricular Strain Imaging in Patients With Cardiac Amyloidosis. *JACC Cardiovasc. Imaging* **2021**, *14*, 1508–1519. [CrossRef] [PubMed]
34. Oike, F.; Usuku, H.; Yamamoto, E.; Yamada, T.; Egashira, K.; Morioka, M.; Nishi, M.; Komorita, T.; Hirakawa, K.; Tabata, N.; et al. Prognostic value of left atrial strain in patients with wild-type transthyretin amyloid cardiomyopathy. *ESC Heart Fail.* **2021**, *8*, 5316–5326. [CrossRef] [PubMed]

35. Martinez-Naharro, A.; Gonzalez-Lopez, E.; Corovic, A.; Mirelis, J.G.; Baksi, A.J.; Moon, J.C.; Garcia-Pavia, P.; Gillmore, J.D Hawkins, P.N.; Fontana, M. High Prevalence of Intracardiac Thrombi in Cardiac Amyloidosis. *J. Am. Coll. Cardiol.* **2019**, *73* 1733–1734. [CrossRef]
36. Akintoye, E.; Majid, M.; Klein, A.; Hanna, M. Prognostic Utility of Left Atrial Strain to Predict Thrombotic Events and Mortality in Amyloid Cardiomyopathy. *J. Am. Coll. Cardiol. Imaging*, 2023; in press. [CrossRef]
37. Dorbala, S.; Ando, Y.; Bokhari, S.; Dispenzieri, A.; Falk, R.H.; Ferrari, V.A.; Fontana, M.; Gheysens, O.; Gillmore, J.D.; Glaudemans A.W.J.M.; et al. ASNC/AHA/ASE/EANM/HFSA/ISA/ SCMR/SNMMI Expert Consensus Recommendations for Multimodality Imaging in Cardiac Amyloidosis: Part 1 of 2—Evidence Base and Standardized Methods of Imaging. *Circ. Cardiovasc. Imaging* **2021**, *14*, e000029.
38. Bandera, F.; Martone, R.; Chacko, L.; Ganesananthan, S.; Gilbertson, J.A.; Ponticos, M.; Lane, T.; Martinez-Naharro, A.; Whelan C.; Quarta, C.; et al. Clinical Importance of Left Atrial Infiltration in Cardiac Transthyretin Amyloidosis. *JACC Cardiovasc. Imaging* **2022**, *15*, 17–29. [CrossRef]
39. Potter, E.L.; Ramkumar, S.; Kawakami, H.; Yang, H.; Wright, L.; Negishi, T.; Marwick, T.H. Association of Asymptomatic Diastolic Dysfunction Assessed by Left Atrial Strain With Incident Heart Failure. *JACC Cardiovasc. Imaging.* **2020**, *13*, 2316–2326. [CrossRef]
40. Nagueh, S.F.; Khan, S.U. Left Atrial Strain for Assessment of Left Ventricular Diastolic Function: Focus on Populations With Normal LVEF. *JACC Cardiovasc. Imaging* **2023**, *16*, 691–707. [CrossRef]

MDPI AG
Grosspeteranlage 5
4052 Basel
Switzerland
Tel.: +41 61 683 77 34

Journal of Cardiovascular Development and Disease Editorial Office
E-mail: jcdd@mdpi.com
www.mdpi.com/journal/jcdd

www.ingramcontent.com/pod-product-compliance
Lightning Source LLC
Chambersburg PA
CBHW062054220926
51850CB00010B/2763
* 9 7 8 3 7 2 5 8 7 0 5 4 7 *